Craniofacial Distraction

Editor

ROBERTO L. FLORES

CLINICS IN PLASTIC SURGERY

www.plasticsurgery.theclinics.com

July 2021 • Volume 48 • Number 3

ELSEVIER

1600 John F. Kennedy Boulevard • Suite 1800 • Philadelphia, Pennsylvania, 19103-2899

http://www.theclinics.com

CLINICS IN PLASTIC SURGERY Volume 48, Number 3
July 2021 ISSN 0094-1298, ISBN-13: 978-0-323-79468-8

Editor: Stacy Eastman
Developmental Editor: Jessica Nicole B. Cañaberal

Clinics in Plastic Surgery (ISSN 0094-1298) is published quarterly by Elsevier Inc., 360 Park Avenue South, New York, NY 10010-1710. Months of issue are January, April, July, and October. Business and Editorial Offices: 1600 John F. Kennedy Blvd., Suite 1800, Philadelphia, PA 19103-2899. Periodicals postage paid at New York, NY and additional mailing offices. Subscription prices are $543.00 per year for US individuals, $1210.00 per year for US institutions, $100.00 per year for US students and residents, $607.00 per year for Canadian individuals, $1252.00 per year for Canadian institutions, $675.00 per year for international individuals, $1252.00 per year for international institutions, $100.00 per year for Canadian and $305.00 per year for international students/residents. To receive student/resident rate, orders must be accompanied by name of affiliated institution, date of term, and the *signature* of program/residency coordinator on institution letterhead. Orders will be billed at individual rate until proof of status is received. Foreign air speed delivery is included in all *Clinics* subscription prices. All prices are subject to change without notice. **POSTMASTER:** Send address changes to *Clinics in Plastic Surgery*, Elsevier Health Sciences Division, Subscription Customer Service, 3251 Riverport Lane, Maryland Heights, MO 63043. **Customer Service: 1-800-654-2452 (US and Canada). From outside of the United States and Canada, call 314-447-8871. Fax: 314-447-8029. E-mail: JournalsCustomerService-usa@elsevier.com (for print support); JournalsOnline-Support-usa@elsevier.com (for online support).**

Reprints. For copies of 100 or more of articles in this publication, please contact the Commercial Reprints Department, Elsevier Inc., 360 Park Avenue South, New York, New York 10010-1710. Tel.: +1-212-633-3874; Fax: +1-212-633-3820; E-mail: reprints@elsevier.com.

Clinics in Plastic Surgery is covered in *Current Contents, EMBASE/Excerpta Medica, Science Citation Index, MEDLINE/PubMed (Index Medicus), ASCA,* and *ISI/BIOMED.*

Contributors

EDITOR

ROBERTO L. FLORES, MD
Joseph G. McCarthy Associate Professor of
Reconstructive Plastic Surgery, Director, Cleft
Lip and Palate, Director, Craniofacial Surgery
Fellowship, Hansjörg Wyss Department of
Plastic Surgery, Cleft and Craniofacial Surgery,
NYU Langone Health, New York, New York,
USA

AUTHORS

ERIC ARNAUD, MD
Unité fonctionnelle de chirurgie craniofaciale,
Service de Neurochirurgie Pédiatrique, Hôpital
Necker – Enfants Malades, Assistance
Publique – Hôpitaux de Paris, Centre de
Référence Maladies Rares CRANIOST, Filière
Maladies Rares TeteCou, Université Paris
Descartes, ERN Cranio, Paris, France; Clinique
Marcel Sembat, Ramsay Générale de Santé,
Boulogne, France

SHAYNA AVINOAM, DDS, MS
Craniofacial Orthodontic Fellow, Hansjörg
Wyss Department of Plastics Surgery, NYU
Langone Health, New York, New York, USA

SCOTT P. BARTLETT, MD
Mary Downs Endowed Chair in Pediatric
Craniofacial Treatment and Research,
Perelman School of Medicine, University of
Pennsylvania, Professor of Surgery, Division of
Plastic and Reconstructive Surgery, The
Children's Hospital of Philadelphia,
Philadelphia, Pennsylvania, USA

CURTIS BUDDEN, MD, MEd, FRCSC
Assistant Professor, Department of Surgery,
Faculty of Medicine and Dentistry, University of
Alberta, Edmonton, Alberta, Canada

RICHARD G. BURTON, DDS, MS, FACS
Clinical Professor and Vice Chair, Oral and
Maxillofacial Surgery, Hospital Dentistry
Institute, University of Iowa Hospitals and
Clinics, Iowa City, Iowa, USA

MARCUS V. COLLARES MD, PhD
Rio Grande do Sul Federal University Medical
School, Hospital de Clinicas de Porto Alegre,
Rio Grande do Sul Federal University, Porto
Alegre, Brazil

**EVELLYN M. DEMITCHELL-RODRIGUEZ,
BS**
Research Fellow, Hansjörg Wyss Department
of Plastic Surgery, NYU Langone Health, New
York, New York, USA

RAFAEL DENADAI, MD
Institute of Plastic and Craniofacial Surgery,
SOBRAPAR Hospital, Campinas, São Paulo,
Brazil

**DAVID J. DUNAWAY, MBChB, FDSRCS,
FRCS(plast)**
Professor of Craniofacial Surgery, Consultant
Craniofacial and Plastic Surgeon, Great
Ormond Street Hospital for Children, London,
United Kingdom

ELÇIN ESENLIK, DDS, PhD
Professor, Chair of the Orthodontics
Department, Faculty of Dentistry, Department
of Orthodontics, Akdeniz University, Konyaaltı,
Antalya, Turkey

AARON D. FIGUEROA, DDS, FACS
Clinical Assistant Professor, Oral and
Maxillofacial Surgery, Hospital Dentistry
Institute, University of Iowa Hospitals and
Clinics, Iowa City, Iowa, USA

ALVARO A. FIGUEROA, DDS, MS
Adjunct Associate Professor, Rush
Craniofacial Center, Division of Plastic Surgery,
Department of Surgery, Rush University
Medical Center, Chicago, Illinois, USA; Private
Practice of Orthodontics, Naperville and
Winnetka, Illinois, USA

ROBERTO L. FLORES, MD
Joseph G. McCarthy Associate Professor of
Reconstructive Plastic Surgery, Director, Cleft
Lip and Palate, Director, Craniofacial Surgery
Fellowship, Hansjörg Wyss Department of
Plastic Surgery, Cleft and Craniofacial Surgery,
NYU Langone Health, New York, New York,
USA

ENRICO GHIZONI, MD, PhD
Institute of Plastic and Craniofacial Surgery,
SOBRAPAR Hospital, Campinas, Department
of Neurology, University of Campinas
(UNICAMP), São Paulo, Brazil

WALEED GIBREEL, MBBS
Division of Plastic and Maxillofacial Surgery,
Children's Hospital Los Angeles, Los Angeles,
California, USA

SAMER ELIE HABER, MD
Unité fonctionnelle de chirurgie craniofaciale,
Service de Neurochirurgie Pédiatrique, Hôpital
Necker – Enfants Malades, Assistance
Publique – Hôpitaux de Paris, Centre de
Référence Maladies Rares CRANIOST, Filière
Maladies Rares TeteCou, Université Paris
Descartes, ERN Cranio, Paris, France

JEFFREY A. HAMMOUDEH, MD, DDS
Division of Plastic and Maxillofacial Surgery,
Division of Dentistry and Orthodontics,
Children's Hospital Los Angeles, Division of
Plastic and Reconstructive Surgery, Keck

School of Medicine of USC, Division of Oral
and Maxillofacial Surgery, University of
Southern California, Los Angeles, California,
USA

RICHARD A. HOPPER, MD, MS
Professor, The Craniofacial Center, Seattle
Children's Hospital, Division of Plastic Surgery,
Department of Surgery, University of
Washington, Seattle, Washington, USA

LAURA S. HUMPHRIES, MD
Assistant Professor, Division of Plastic and
Reconstructive Surgery, University of
Mississippi Medical Center, Children's of
Mississippi Hospital, Jackson, Mississippi,
USA

**GREG JAMES, PhD, FRCS (Eng), FRCS
(NeuroSurg)**
Consultant Paediatric Neurosurgeon, Great
Ormond Street Hospital for Children, London,
United Kingdom

SYRIL JAMES, MD
Unité fonctionnelle de chirurgie craniofaciale,
Service de Neurochirurgie Pédiatrique, Hôpital
Necker – Enfants Malades, Assistance
Publique – Hôpitaux de Paris, Centre de
Référence Maladies Rares CRANIOST, Filière
Maladies Rares TeteCou, Université Paris
Descartes, ERN Cranio, Paris, France; Clinique
Marcel Sembat, Ramsay Générale de Santé,
Boulogne, France

**NOOR UL OWASE JEELANI, MBA, MPhil
(Medical Law), FRCS (NeuroSurg)**
Consultant Paediatric Neurosurgeon, Great
Ormond Street Hospital for Children, London,
United Kingdom

HITESH KAPADIA, PhD
Assistant Professor, The Craniofacial Center,
Seattle Children's Hospital, Division of Plastic
Surgery, Department of Surgery, Department
of Orthodontics, School of Dentistry, University
of Washington, Seattle, Washington, USA

ROMAN HOSSEIN KHONSARI, MD, PhD
Unité fonctionnelle de chirurgie craniofaciale,
Service de Neurochirurgie Pédiatrique, Hôpital
Necker – Enfants Malades, Assistance
Publique – Hôpitaux de Paris, Centre de
Référence Maladies Rares CRANIOST, Filière

Maladies Rares TeteCou, Université Paris Descartes, ERN Cranio, Paris, France; Service de chirurgie maxillofaciale et chirurgie plastique, Hôpital Necker – Enfants Malades, Assistance Publique – Hôpitaux de Paris, Centre de Référence Maladies Rares CRANIOST, Filière Maladies Rares TeteCou, Université de Paris, Université Paris Descartes, Paris, France

JOSEPH LOPEZ, MD, MBA
Section of Plastic Surgery, Department of Surgery, Yale School of Medicine, New Haven, Connecticut, USA

EZGI MERCAN, PhD
Scientist, The Craniofacial Center, Seattle Children's Hospital, Seattle, Washington, USA

PAUL A. MITTERMILLER, MD
Hansjörg Wyss Department of Plastic Surgery, NYU Langone Health, New York, New York, USA

KERRY A. MORRISON MD
Hansjörg Wyss Department of Plastic Surgery, NYU Langone Health, New York, New York, USA

JULING ONG, FRCS(plast)
Craniofacial and Plastic Surgeon, Great Ormond Street Hospital for Children, London, United Kingdom

GIOVANNA PATERNOSTER, MD
Unité fonctionnelle de chirurgie craniofaciale, Service de Neurochirurgie Pédiatrique, Hôpital Necker – Enfants Malades, Assistance Publique – Hôpitaux de Paris, Centre de Référence Maladies Rares CRANIOST, Filière Maladies Rares TeteCou, Université Paris Descartes, ERN Cranio, Paris, France

CONNOR J. PECK, BS
Section of Plastic Surgery, Department of Surgery, Yale School of Medicine, New Haven, Connecticut, USA

CASSIO EDUARDO RAPOSO-AMARAL, MD, PhD
Institute of Plastic and Craniofacial Surgery, SOBRAPAR Hospital, Campinas, Department of Neurology, University of Campinas (UNICAMP), São Paulo, Brazil

CESAR AUGUSTO RAPOSO-AMARAL, MD
Institute of Plastic and Craniofacial Surgery, SOBRAPAR Hospital, Campinas, São Paulo, Brazil

SAMEER SHAKIR, MD
Chief Resident, Division of Plastic Surgery, Perelman School of Medicine, University of Pennsylvania, Philadelphia, Pennsylvania, USA

PRADIP R. SHETYE, DDS, BDS, MDS
Associate Professor of Plastic Surgery (Orthodontics), Director of Craniofacial Orthodontics, Director of Craniofacial Orthodontic Fellowship Program, Hansjörg Wyss Department of Plastics Surgery, NYU Langone Health, New York, New York, USA

JOHN T. SMETONA, MD
Section of Plastic Surgery, Department of Surgery, Yale School of Medicine, New Haven, Connecticut, USA

DAVID A. STAFFENBERG, MD, DSc (Hon)
Vice Chair of Pediatric Plastic Surgery, Hansjörg Wyss Department of Plastic Surgery, NYU Langone Health, New York, New York, USA

DEREK M. STEINBACHER, MD, DMD, FACS
Chief of Oral and Maxillofacial Surgery, Professor of Plastic Surgery, Yale School of Medicine, New Haven, Connecticut, USA

JORDAN W. SWANSON, MD, MSc
Assistant Professor of Surgery, Division of Plastic and Reconstructive Surgery, The Children's Hospital of Philadelphia, Philadelphia, Pennsylvania, USA

JESSE A. TAYLOR, MD
Professor of Surgery, Peter Randall Endowed Chair and Chief, Division of Plastic and Reconstructive Surgery, The Children's Hospital of Philadelphia, Pennsylvania, USA

CHRISTINA TRAGOS, MD
Director, Rush Craniofacial Center, Division of Plastic Surgery, Department of Surgery, Rush University Medical Center, Chicago, Illinois, USA

MARK M. URATA, MD, DDS
Division of Plastic and Maxillofacial Surgery,
Division of Dentistry and Orthodontics,
Children's Hospital Los Angeles, Division of
Plastic and Reconstructive Surgery, Keck
School of Medicine of USC, Division of Oral
and Maxillofacial Surgery, University of
Southern California, Los Angeles, California,
USA

PEDRO HENRIQUE VIEIRA, MD
Institute of Plastic and Craniofacial Surgery,
SOBRAPAR Hospital, Campinas, São Paulo,
Brazil

HOWARD D. WANG, MD
Fellow, The Craniofacial Center, Seattle
Children's Hospital, Division of Plastic Surgery,

Department of Surgery, University of
Washington, Seattle, Washington, USA

JORDAN R. WLODARCZYK, MD, MS
Division of Plastic and Maxillofacial Surgery,
Children's Hospital Los Angeles, Division of
Plastic and Reconstructive Surgery, Keck
School of Medicine of USC, Los Angeles,
California, USA

ERIK M. WOLFSWINKEL, MD
Division of Plastic and Maxillofacial Surgery,
Children's Hospital Los Angeles, Los Angeles,
California, USA

STEPHEN YEN, DMD, PhD
Division of Plastic and Maxillofacial Surgery,
Division of Dentistry and Orthodontics,
Children's Hospital Los Angeles, Los Angeles,
California, USA

Contents

Pierre Robin sequence is defined by the clinical triad: mandibular hypoplasia, glossoptosis, and airway obstruction. Mandibular distraction osteogenesis (MDO) is a standard treatment of Robin sequence associated with severe airway obstruction and is the only intervention that directly corrects the underlying anatomic pathologic condition. Compared with tongue-lip adhesion, MDO has demonstrated more success in treating airway obstruction in infants with Pierre Robin sequence, including patients with syndromic diagnoses and concomitant anomalies. This article provides a current, comprehensive review of neonatal mandibular distraction and offers treatment guidelines based on a combined surgical experience of more than 400 patients.

Phenotypic severity dictates the timing and type of surgical intervention required. Mandibular distraction in children without respiratory and feeding difficulties remains controversial with regard to long-term mandibular growth outcomes and reducing surgical burden. Early mandibular distraction does not obviate secondary orthognathic surgery at skeletal maturity; it provides improved functional, aesthetic, and psychosocial outcomes, at least in the short term. Costochondral rib grafting for Pruzansky type IIB and III mandibles can produce reliable results, especially when combined with subsequent mandibular distraction. Secondary 2-jaw orthognathic surgery plus genioplasty at skeletal maturity benefits from improved bone volume from prior mandibular distraction.

Distraction osteogenesis is a viable treatment option for patients with a cleft associated with severe maxillary retrusion. A rigid external distraction device and a hybrid internal maxillary distractor have been used to advance the maxilla allowing for predictable and stable results. These techniques can be applied by itself or as an adjunct to traditional orthognathic procedures. The technical aspects are presented. These procedures tend to be simpler and demonstrate great stability compared to traditional surgical methods. The reasons for stability are discussed.

Maxillary hypoplasia is a commonly seen dentofacial anomaly in patients with cleft lip and palate after surgical repair of the cleft anomaly. To facilitate large horizontal movements of the maxilla, distraction osteogenesis is used to slowly stretch the soft tissue envelope with the skeletal advancement preventing tissue recoil and skeletal relapse. Internal distraction devices have the advantage of reducing the amount of physical and psychological stress placed on patients, families, and caregivers. The technique has been successful in producing stable results for large advancements of the facial skeleton when compared with conventional Le Fort I advancement and fixation of the maxilla.

Alveolar distraction osteogenesis (ADO) has been used for the reconstruction of atrophic alveolus for decades. The advantage of this technique is that it augments the bone and soft tissues together, creating a better alveolar platform for subsequent surgeries and dental rehabilitation. It is especially useful in patients with large and/or complex alveolar clefts for which approximating the alveolar segments reduces the size of the bony cleft and associated fistula. Displacement of the transported segment is the most frequently encountered complication of ADO but can be managed by constructing case-specific distractors.

Treacher Collins syndrome (TCS) is a genetic disorder that presents with a variety of craniofacial deformities. One classic feature of TCS is a steep, counterclockwise rotation of the occlusal plane, and microretrognathia with bony deficiencies in both the body and ramus of the mandible. This morphology commonly necessitates reconstruction by the craniofacial surgeon. This article discusses strategies and considerations for surgically correcting the mandibular deformity associated with TCS using mandibular distraction osteogenesis and other related techniques. The proper implementation of these techniques can yield excellent results that greatly improve quality of life in this challenging patient population.

Anatomic studies have identified that patients with Treacher Collins syndrome and some cases of bilateral craniofacial microsomia are characterized by multilevel airway obstruction as a result of hypoplasia and clockwise rotation of the maxillomandibular complex. Patients often remain tracheostomy-dependent despite multiple airway surgeries. Counterclockwise craniofacial distraction osteogenesis aims to correct the facial skeletal deformity and expand the upper airway volume by rotating the subcranial complex en bloc around the nasofrontal junction. Early results have demonstrated significant increases in the nasopharyngeal and oropharyngeal airway volumes with successful decannulation in a majority of patients who have undergone this operation.

Posterior cranial vault distraction osteogenesis is a powerful, reliable, low-morbidity method to achieve intracranial expansion. It is particularly useful in treating turribrachycephaly seen in syndromic craniosynostosis, allowing for gradual expansion of the bone while stretching the soft tissues over several weeks allowing greater volumetric expansion than conventional techniques. Posterior cranial vault distraction osteogenesis constitutes a more gradual remodeling modality, with infrequent complications. As a first step in intracranial expansion, it preserves the frontal cranium for future frontofacial procedures. A drawback is the need for a second surgery to remove the device, and this must be taken into account during counseling.

deformity and play a role in the management of ocular exposure, intracranial hypertension, and upper airway obstruction. Facial bipartition distraction corrects the intrinsic facial deformities of Apert syndrome. Both procedures are associated with relatively high complication rates principally related to ascending infection and persistent cerebrospinal fluid leaks. Modern perioperative management has resulted in a significant decline in complications. External distractors allow fine tuning of distraction vectors and improve outcome but are less well tolerated than internal distractors.

Cassio Eduardo Raposo-Amaral, Pedro Henrique Vieira, Rafael Denadai, Enrico Ghizoni, and Cesar Augusto Raposo-Amaral

Monobloc and facial bipartition combined with distraction osteogenesis (MFBDO) has gained popularity over the past several years as a treatment of syndromic craniosynostosis, in part because this surgical technique effectively removes many stigmatic clinical features associated with the syndromic face. The objective of this study is to detail the surgical planning used to achieve medialization of the orbits and describe the authors' experience using MFBDO to destigmatize the syndromic face. By using MFBDO, hypertelorism, vertical orbital dystopia, and downslanting of the palpebral fissure were surgically corrected in all patients, thereby destigmatizing the syndromic face.

Shayna Avinoam and Pradip R. Shetye

A combined surgical and orthodontic approach to midface and mandibular distraction optimizes stability and outcomes. Orthodontic considerations include proper planning of the distraction vector, appropriate device use, and thorough follow-up through the consolidation and postoperative period. The dental occlusion must be managed throughout treatment in order to achieve ideal results.

CLINICS IN PLASTIC SURGERY

ISSUE OF RELATED INTEREST

Facial Plastic Surgery Clinics
https://www.facialplastic.theclinics.com/
Otolaryngologic Clinics
https://www.oto.theclinics.com/

THE CLINICS ARE AVAILABLE ONLINE!
Access your subscription at:
www.theclinics.com

CLINICS IN PLASTIC SURGERY

FORTHCOMING ISSUES

October 2021
Melanoma
Brian R. Gastman and Michael W. Neumeister, Editors

January 2022
Rhinoplasty
Alan Matarasso and Sam P. Most, Editors

April 2022
Plastic Surgery for Men
Douglas S. Steinbrech, Editor

RECENT ISSUES

April 2021
Contemporary Approach to Lower Extremity Reconstruction
Lee L.Q. Pu, Editor

January 2021
Breast Augmentation
Bradley P. Bengtson, Editor

October 2020
Microsurgery: Global Perspectives, An Update
Jin Bo Tang and Michel Saint-Cyr, Editors

ISSUE OF RELATED INTEREST

Facial Plastic Surgery Clinics
https://www.facialplastic.theclinics.com/
Otolaryngic Clinics
https://www.oto.theclinics.com/

Preface
Craniofacial Distraction–The Thirty-Year Journey

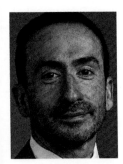

Roberto L. Flores, MD
Editor

Thirty years ago, a study published in *Plastic and Reconstructive Surgery* by McCarthy and colleagues[1] reported on a technique of bone lengthening, applied to the mandible in a child with craniofacial microsomia. At that time, distraction osteogenesis was a well-characterized orthopedic surgery technique in which an external fixation frame was attached to the lower extremity to gradually lengthen bone over time. The technique was developed and popularized by the Russian orthopedic surgeon, Gavrill Ilizarov, who, practicing in Siberia, was an unknown to the rest of the world. Dr Ilizarov achieved national recognition after successfully treating Valeriy Brumel, the Soviet 1964 Olympic High Jump champion, for a chronic nonunion of the lower extremity. International fame followed after the successful treatment of Carlo Mauri, an Italian explorer and photojournalist who harbored a poorly healed tibial fracture 10 years after a skiing accident.

Ironically, Dr Ilizarov, himself, was an inpatient at New York University (NYU) while Dr Joseph McCarthy was developing the technique of craniofacial distraction in dogs, prior to human application. Excitedly, Dr McCarthy visited Dr Ilizarov and presented his idea of applying the principles of distraction osteogenesis to the mandible. As would be recorded in NYU lore, Dr Ilizarov dismissed Dr McCarthy's idea, claiming that it would never work.

Now, 30 years later, distraction osteogenesis is a standard part of the craniofacial surgeon's repertoire: craniofacial exposure, craniofacial osteotomies, harvesting bone, grafting bone, splitting bone, remodeling bone, *distracting bone*. Craniofacial fellowship training programs accredited by the Accreditation Council for Graduate Medical Education specifically mandate that competency in craniofacial distraction procedures is confirmed though milestones reporting.

The collection of articles in this issue of *Clinics in Plastic Surgery* represents the state-of-the-art in distraction osteogenesis of the craniofacial skeleton, authored by the international leaders of the field. Each article focuses on a specific treatment intervention as well as a condition. As craniofacial distraction has evolved, we came to appreciate that the same intervention can be guided by different technical nuances and principles of care depending on the patient's underlying diagnosis. Mandibular distraction is as good example: application in a neonate with Pierre Robin sequence, a child with craniofacial microsomia, or a patient with Treacher Collins syndrome requires distinct planning and surgical endpoints and, therefore, each deserves a stand-alone discussion.

Despite the breadth of craniofacial distraction osteogenesis techniques described in this issue, there are important, recurring themes that the reader will notice. These include the following:

1. Close partnership with a craniofacial orthodontist when transporting adult teeth and leveraging orthodontic techniques to refine and inform the surgical plan
2. Incorporation of increasingly complex distraction movements: curvilinear mandibular

Clin Plastic Surg 48 (2021) xiii–xiv
https://doi.org/10.1016/j.cps.2021.03.006
0094-1298/21/© 2021 Published by Elsevier Inc.

distraction, composite counterclockwise rotation of the midface, rounding the curve of the maxillary arch

3. Importance of function (normative intracranial pressure, protection of the globes, functional occlusion, patent airway) to guide surgical indications and optimize clinical outcomes

4. Long-term view of surgical indications: when is the best time to distract, when is it better to wait

5. How distraction fits into the overall care plan of comprehensive craniofacial rehabilitation

I would like to dedicate this Craniofacial Distraction issue of *Clinics in Plastic Surgery* to my mentor, Dr Joseph G. McCarthy, and the faculty, past and present, of the Hansjörg Wyss Department of Plastic Surgery at NYU Langone Health, who have given me training, opportunity, partnership, and friendship in this inspiring world of academic plastic surgery. My hope is that, over the next 30 years, craniofacial distraction continues to evolve through the innovative work of the next generation of craniofacial surgeons or is relegated to the Smithsonian, by the next breakthrough in craniofacial bone replacement.

Roberto L. Flores, MD
Hansjörg Wyss Department of
Plastic Surgery
NYU Langone Health
222 East 41st Street
22nd Floor, Room 22-017
New York, NY 10017, USA

E-mail address:
roberto.flores@nyulangone.org

REFERENCES

1. McCarthy JG, Schreiber J, Karp N, et al. Lengthening the Human Mandible by Gradual Distraction. Plastic and Reconstructive Surgery 1992;89(1):1–8.

Robin Sequence
Neonatal Mandibular Distraction

Kerry A. Morrison, MD[a], Marcus V. Collares, MD, PhD[b], Roberto L. Flores, MD[c],*

KEYWORDS

- Mandibular distraction osteogenesis • Pierre Robin sequence • Neonate • Polysomnography
- Sleep study • Mandibular morphology • Micrognathia • Glossoptosis

KEY POINTS

- In properly selected patients, neonatal mandibular distraction osteogenesis can resolve tongue-based airway obstruction and obviate tracheostomy in Pierre Robin sequence patients with severe airway obstruction.
- Understanding mandibular morphology in Robin sequence is crucial to plan and to properly place osteotomies and vectors.
- The complication rate associated with neonatal mandibular distraction is low in both occurrence and level of acuity.
- Specific indications for neonatal mandibular distraction have not been codified, but it is a critical next step toward the standardization of care.

INTRODUCTION

Pierre Robin sequence is defined by the clinical triad: mandibular hypoplasia, glossoptosis, and airway obstruction. In his 1923 publication, Robin first described the eponymous constellation of respiratory distress associated with glossoptosis in the presence of mandibular micrognathia.[1,2] Cleft palate is not a criterion for the diagnosis of Robin sequence despite the fact that up to 90% of affected patients have a concomitant U-shaped or V-shaped cleft of the posterior palate.[2–5] With Robin sequence, nosologic confusion is evidenced by the wide variability in defining the clinical entity, which is highlighted in a survey of American Cleft Palate-Craniofacial Association providers.[6] Inaccurate use of the correct Robin sequence definition hinders communication between specialists and thwarts the development of standardized care protocols.

A multidisciplinary approach to Robin sequence evaluation and treatment is critical and includes neonatologists, geneticists, pulmonologists, developmental pediatricians, otolaryngologists, plastic surgeons, pediatric gastroenterologists, nurse feeding specialists, and speech-language pathologists.[7] Although there are multiple conservative interventions available for infants expressing mild to moderate airway obstruction, this article addresses the implementation of mandibular distraction in severely affected infants and neonates. Direct laryngoscopy/bronchoscopy, and polysomnography (PSG) should be performed, whenever possible, for patients under consideration for surgical intervention.

[a] Hansjörg Wyss Department of Plastic Surgery, NYU Langone Medical Center, 222 East 41st Street, New York, NY, 10017, USA; [b] Rio Grande do Sul Federal University Medical School, Hospital de Clinicas de Porto Alegre, Rio Grande do Sul Federal University, Rua Hilário Ribeiro 202, cj 406, Porto Alegre, Brazil; [c] Hansjörg Wyss Department of Plastic Surgery, Cleft and Craniofacial Surgery, NYU Langone Health, 222 East 41st Street, 22nd floor, New York, NY, 10017, USA
* Corresponding author.
E-mail address: Roberto.Flores@nyulangone.org

Clin Plastic Surg 48 (2021) 363–373
https://doi.org/10.1016/j.cps.2021.03.005
0094-1298/21/© 2021 Elsevier Inc. All rights reserved.

Although drug-induced sleep endoscopy (DISE) from nasal aperture to bronchus is the yardstick to assess glossoptosis and other associated airway anomalies, the degree of glossoptosis may not correlate with the severity of respiratory dysfunction.[8–10]

PSG remains the gold standard to quantify the severity of airway obstruction and to identify the presence of central sleep apnea.[11] However, PSG interpretation is not standardized for neonates.[12,13] A severe obstructive index in neonates has been reported from greater than 6 to greater than 24, thereby representing a wide range of interpretation in the literature.[14–16] Most craniofacial surgeons select an apnea-hypopnea index (AHI) of 11 to 29 as their minimum for surgical intervention.[17] Thus, PSG indications for neonatal mandibular distraction osteogenesis (MDO) for Robin sequence are currently based largely on clinical judgment.[18] Establishment of reference values for neonates will provide a helpful construct to further standardize polysomnographic findings in the complex Robin sequence population. The senior authors' protocol of care includes PSG on all neonates under consideration for MDO unless the patient is intubated or PSG is not tolerated/possible. A maxillofacial computed tomography (CT) scan is obtained to evaluate the quality of the bone stock as well as mandibular and temporomandibular joint (TMJ) morphology.[19] Concomitantly, under the same anesthetic before MDO, a pediatric otolaryngologist performs a DISE.[19] Neonates with Robin sequence may also have secondary airway abnormalities that compound respiratory distress, such as laryngomalacia, bronchial stenosis, bronchomalacia, or tracheomalacia,[20,21] which may influence the decision to proceed with MDO.

Previously, laryngomalacia was deemed a contraindication to successful distraction in Robin sequence patients.[22–25] However, Tholpady and colleagues[26] demonstrated that properly selected patients with Robin sequence and laryngomalacia can successfully undergo MDO and avoid tracheostomy. It is important to note that close collaboration with an experienced pediatric otolaryngologist is critical to proper patient indications, and certain patients will require supraglottoplasty before, concurrent with, or after MDO.

SURGICAL MANAGEMENT

Robin sequence patients with severe airway obstruction, who fail nonsurgical management, are considered for surgical intervention, including tracheostomy, tongue-lip adhesion (TLA), MDO, or subperiosteal release of the floor of mouth.[27]

Tracheostomy is a direct, effective method to establish the airway, which relies on subsequent mandibular growth to facilitate decannulation.[28] As tracheostomy is associated with multiple morbidities, including laryngeal stenosis, tracheomalacia, chronic pneumonia, and extensive nursing care, it is usually reserved for patients in which no other intervention is deemed to be a viable option.[29–35] More recently, tracheostomy has been shown to be associated with increased financial costs compared with MDO.[36–39] Despite these limitations, tracheostomy is still a life-saving intervention, especially for medically complex patients with multiple sites of airway obstruction.[21,22,40]

TLA is a staged surgical technique that translates the base of the tongue anteriorly until airway obstruction is definitively alleviated by lower jaw growth. Although there is supportive evidence that TLA can relieve airway obstruction caused by Robin sequence,[41] most comprehensive analyses demonstrate that clinical outcomes are inferior to mandibular distraction.[29,42–45] The success of TLA is predicated upon compensatory "catch-up" growth of the mandible to relieve airway obstruction, which remains a debated concept.[29,46–50]

Clinically introduced and popularized by McCarthy and colleagues,[51] MDO is a safe and effective intervention for relieving airway obstruction in infants with severe Robin sequence.[22,29,40,49,52–59] Its use, even in neonates weighing less than 4 kg with severe airway obstruction, slowly became more popular after the first publications of Collares and colleagues (2000), Denny and colleagues (2002), and Monasterio and colleagues (2002).[60–63] The benefit of neonatal distraction lies in direct anterior translation of the mandible and tongue base, thus increasing airway patency as glossoptosis is decreased.[64] Current indications for MDO include PSG demonstrating no or limited central sleep apnea and either an AHI greater than 20 (New York University [NYU])/greater than 6 (Hospital de Clinicas de Porto Alegre [HCPA]), or Sao_2 less than 90% more than 1% of sleep time (HCPA), or significant carbon dioxide retention,[60] and absence of severe neurologic or cardiac pathologic condition or secondary airway pathologic condition, which could preclude successful restoration of the airway. Because MDO can be effective for correction of tongue-based airway obstruction and tracheostomy avoidance, it has become the first-line surgical option for Robin sequence patients at many institutions.[22,28,29,52,55,58]

MDO has been found to be a superior intervention to relieve tongue-based airway obstruction compared with TLA by multiple studies. In nonsyndromic patients, MDO results in shorter time to extubation, a higher postoperative oxygen saturation level, a greater decrease in AHI, and a lower incidence of tracheostomy when compared with TLA.[43] In a subsequent comparative study that included both Robin sequence syndromic diagnoses and significant medical comorbidities, superior airway outcomes were demonstrated using MDO compared with TLA despite a 5-fold increase in syndromic diagnosis and large increase in central nervous system anomalies in the MDO cohort.[29] These data points have been corroborated by other institutional studies and meta-analyses.[40,44,45,65]

SURGICAL CONSIDERATIONS IN MANDIBULAR DISTRACTION

As most Robin sequence cases have primary hypoplasia of the mandibular body, a horizontal vector is commonly used. In contrast, several other institutions do use a vertical vector for the mandibular distraction.[22,49] Duarte and Collares,[66] comparing pre-MDO and post-MDO, showed horizontal vectors resulted in an increase of 11% for ramus, and 36% in body length, whereas the vertical vectors showed an elongation of 34% in ramus and 27.5% in body length. Vertical vectors were used in 30% of their series with no TMJ damage. They stated vertical vectors should be carefully considered when the ramus is impaired. Ultimately, substantial airway enlargement occurs after mandibular distraction, and no difference in final airway volumes has been demonstrated between the use of horizontal or vertical vectors.[67] However, prudent judgment should be exercised when committing to the vertical vector in the Robin sequence patient population, as it risks iatrogenic damage to the TMJ.[24] This iatrogenic injury can result either directly by placement of the device and screws too close to the condyle or indirectly by forcing the vector of distraction into the glenoid fossa. TMJ ankylosis in the infant is a morbid complication reported in a small percentage of cases and can be a challenging sequela to treat.[22,68] However, iatrogenic TMJ ankylosis can be avoided by using a horizontal vector.[19,24,29,54]

Considerations for Osteotomy Technique

Among craniofacial surgeons performing MDO, 39% of surgeons perform an inverted L ramus osteotomy, 37% perform a mandibular angle osteotomy, 17% perform a mandibular body osteotomy, and the remainder perform a horizontal ramus osteotomy.[17] Although the inverted L-osteotomy requires the most dissection and the other osteotomies are simpler to perform, the inverted L-osteotomy and the horizontal ramus osteotomy design provide the best opportunity to preserve developing tooth buds and lower-lip sensibility. Although piezoelectric saws can theoretically accomplish this as well, clinical outcomes in the neonatal population are pending.

Surgical Techniques

MDO can be performed with external or internal devices. The choice between techniques is dependent on the volume of mandibular bone as well as the desired vector of distraction,[69] and the surgeon/institutional surgical preference is based on experience.[70] Despite the differences in the techniques, there are certain shared surgical principles.

Surgical exposure

Mandibular distraction is performed through an extraoral approach for direct exposure to the mandible without the risk of oral contamination. A transoral approach is certainly a viable option; however, precision in vector and screw placement can be compromised by this approach. A Risdon incision is placed 1 cm inferior to the mandibular border. Sharp dissection is performed to and through the platysma, and a small superior and inferior platysma flap is mobilized to facilitate layered closure at the end of the procedure. Wide subperiosteal exposure of the ramus, angle, distal body, and sigmoid notch is obtained. The condyle is not dissected.

Corticotomy/osteotomy

A subtotal osteotomy (corticotomy) is performed before placement of the device. This subtotal osteotomy will preserve native mandibular form and position, facilitating accurate device positioning. After the device is secured, the osteotomy is completed. The bony edges are then broadly separated, and any remaining bony bridges are separated. This separation will avoid "premature consolidation" of the bony edges, which is more likely an incomplete osteotomy.

Internal Devices: Mandibular Distraction Osteogenesis: New York University Technique

Internal devices are more easily tolerated by infants, but require repeat surgery for removal.[64] Most craniofacial surgeons use internal devices (79.9%),[17] and there are a variety of osteotomy techniques, distraction devices, and surgical approaches. The senior author's (R.L.F.) preferred technique is described in detail with an accompanying surgical video in the reference by Diep and colleagues.[19] This reference delineates and the surgical video demonstrates the preferred patient markings, extraoral approach, inverted L-osteotomy, and semiburied distraction device used by the senior author (R.L.F.).[19]

Osteotomy

A coronoidectomy is performed with a sagittal saw or 2-mm Kerrison punch. A near-complete vertical ramus osteotomy is then performed from the sigmoid notch to the antegonial notch. A full corticotomy is made over the buccal face of the mandible and along the superior and inferior aspects of the lingual surface of the mandible, leaving a small lingual bony bridge along the horizontal axis of the jaw. The purpose of the near-complete osteotomy is to maintain alignment of the mandible during placement of the distractor devices. Importantly, the vertical ramus osteotomy avoids injury to the inferior alveolar nerve and the developing tooth buds. Alternatively, one can consider using an ultrasonic bone cutter to make the described inverted L-osteotomy or a mandibular body osteotomy.[19,24,29]

Hardware application

A 20-mm semiburied, uniplane distraction device (Micro Zurich mandibular distractor; KLS Martin, Jacksonville, FL, USA) with a ratchet is primarily used. In cases of extreme micrognathia, longer devices are occasionally used. The ratchet system on the device is protective, as it prevents backing of the activation by parental error or inadvertent manipulation by the infant. The device is affixed to the lower border of the mandible, and the activation arm exits percutaneously behind the earlobe. To affix the footplates to the mandible, high-profile screws are used, as they are easy to apply and more easily removed compared with 1-mm screws. When using a ratchet system distractor, high-profile screws can impinge on the ratchet during full activation; thus, the placement and type of screws should be carefully considered by the craniofacial surgeon.[19,24,29]

Once the device is secured to the mandible, the distractor is activated for several millimeters, and there should be no resistance on the device once activated. The osteotomy on the lingual surface may be completed by activation of the device alone. Completion of the mandibular osteotomy should be confirmed by palpation using an osteotome or a suction cannula, as direct vision will not suffice for confirming that the osteotomy is complete. Once a full osteotomy is confirmed, the bony edges are opposed, and the initial Risdon incision is closed meticulously in layers.[19,24,29]

Distraction and postoperative management

After a latency period of 5 days, activation is commenced at a rate of 1 mm per day to the maximal permissible length of the distraction device, or until the deemed appropriate maxillomandibular distraction is achieved. In the interim, serial cephalograms are obtained to closely monitor the distraction progress, to confirm symmetric bilateral advancement, and to identify any device failures. Last, the devices are removed in a second operation after 6 weeks of consolidation.[19,24,29]

Following completion of mandibular distraction, the patient should be followed by a plastic surgeon and a pediatric otolaryngologist or pulmonologist to monitor mandibular development and the recurrence of obstructive breathing patterns. In addition, a follow-up PSG is obtained within 3 months of distractor removal.[19,24]

External Devices: Mandibular Distraction Osteogenesis: Porto Alegre Technique

External devices are easy to adjust and remove, facilitate shorter surgeries, and have the capability of remodeling and adjusting the vector mid-distraction. The preferred surgical technique by the senior author is demonstrated. They also have the versatility to be reused as devices, and the overall treatment costs tend to be lower, which is of particular interest in developing countries. External devices are well tolerated by neonates (**Fig. 1**).

The main disadvantage of external devices is poor scarring, although it is mostly inconspicuous in neonates.[71] In reviewing clinical outcomes of MDO, it is key to interpret findings judiciously, as analyses of internal device outcomes may not be extrapolated to external devices.[52]

Osteotomy

A near-complete osteotomy is then performed with a thin reciprocating saw. A full corticotomy is made over the retromolar area and the posterior/inferior border of the mandible, leaving a lingual bony bridge to keep the segments aligned for pin placement along the chosen vector. An inverted L on the ramus/angle is preferred over a vertical/oblique osteotomy, on the distal body/angle, to protect the inferior alveolar nerve and the developing tooth buds (**Fig. 2**). In 30% of the authors' cases, they use a horizontal osteotomy on the ramus, for vertical vectors, which also keeps the nerve and tooth buds safe (**Fig. 3**). The horizontal/oblique vectors range from 10° to −20°, and vertical vectors have an inclination of 80° to 120° both related to the mandibular plane.

Hardware application

A neonate external, unidirectional, 2-rotational boxes, and 4-pin distraction device (Neonate External Mandibular Distractor; Engimplan, Rio Claro, SP, Brazil) is used. After the first part of the planned osteotomy is performed, the 4 pins are placed through 4 1-mm 11-blade incisions,

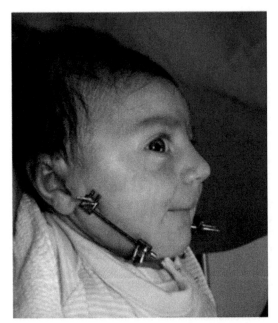

Fig. 1. Robin sequence patient after complete distraction demonstrating that external devices are well tolerated by neonates. (Clinical photograph is courtesy of Marcus V. Collares, MD PhD.)

following the chosen vector. The pins are introduced using a manual wire driver or a very low rotation drill and should surpass the lingual cortical by 2 mm to secure traction. When the distraction device is placed and secured into the pins, 5-mm activation is performed to gently complete the osteotomy, and if it is not achieved, a delicate chisel can be used carefully. Then, the device is activated to reach a 10-mm gap between the bony edges, and to confirm appropriate use. The inferior alveolar nerve can often be visualized. It

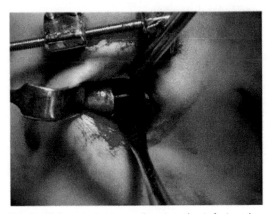

Fig. 2. Oblique osteotomy showing the inferior alveolar nerve intact. (Clinical photograph is courtesy of Marcus V. Collares, MD PhD.)

is important to notice that the boxes of the device are rotational, so one can be inserted upside down. Therefore, optionally, 2 pins can be in a line parallel to the others, keeping the vector preserved, and this facilitates pin placement in very small jaws. Finally, the bony edges are brought together, and the incision is closed in layers.

Distraction and postoperative management

On postoperative day 1, the activation period starts, at a rate of 0.5 mm twice a day. Parents perform all activation. The activation phase is kept until the mandibular gingiva is 2 to 3 mm forward in relationship to maxillary gingiva. Ideally, DISE should be performed at this point to confirm glossoptosis correction; if not feasible, it will be performed at the time of device removal. Complete external device activation is not typically necessary. In the last 12 years, no X rays or CT scans were routinely taken while the device was in place, unless a complication was suspected. The consolidation period is 30 days. The external device is then removed, under sedation in a 5-minute outpatient procedure.[62] A PSG is obtained 3 to 6 months following distraction. Patients are monitored by the Robin sequence team regarding all aspects of the anomaly on a regular basis until adolescence.

Predictors of Failure in Mandibular Distraction

Although MDO is an effective option for patients with Robin sequence associated with severe airway obstruction, critical appraisal of the literature reveals that the definition of success varies widely across studies.[23,42,43,49,52,58,59,61,71] "Success" has been defined as avoidance of tracheostomy or mortality, resolution of apnea as measured by PSG improvement or physical examination, and changes in airway obstruction patterns.[23,42,43,49,52,58,59,61,71,72]

The myriad of definitions for success creates variability in determining the characteristics predictive of MDO failure.[28,52,72] Also attributable is the low incidence of Robin sequence, inconsistent evaluation and diagnosis of comorbidities, and inclusion/exclusion criteria of clinically significant anomalies in statistical analyses between institutions.[28,52,72] For example, according to Runyan and colleagues,[28] failure of MDO to avoid tracheostomy can be predicted by syndromic status, neurologic impairment, and low birth weight. Whereas Hammoudeh and colleagues[72] demonstrated central nervous system abnormalities, laryngomalacia and preoperative intubation had a significant impact on MDO failure rate. Moreover, Murage and colleagues[52] found that failure of MDO was significantly associated with an intact palate,

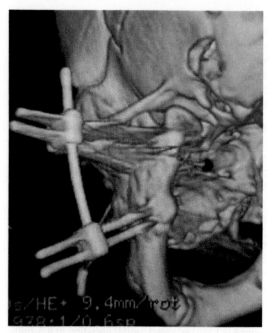

Fig. 3. Three-dimensional CT demonstrating appropriate bone formation and remodeling in a vertical vector distraction. (Imaging is courtesy of Marcus V. Collares, MD PhD.)

gastroesophageal reflux disease, and need for Nissen fundoplication.

To further address the need for standardized assessment of surgical outcomes in the Robin sequence population, Flores and colleagues[42] constructed a preoperative tool to predict failures of MDO. Flores and colleagues[42] identified the following patient variables associated with failure as defined by postprocedure tracheostomy, persistent elevation in AHI, or death by apnea: Gastroesophageal Reflux (GER), age greater than 30 days at the time of surgery, neurologic anomaly, airway anomalies other than laryngomalacia, intact palate, and preoperative intubation. Notably, Robin sequence patients less than 30 days of age at the time of MDO were more likely to be successful than children older than 2 months.[42] This finding is in accordance with previous research seen in the GILLS score for TLA.[73] Murage and colleagues[52] make the astute point that the associated failures of MDO in patients with an intact palate could be ascribed to a degree of micrognathia insufficient to create a palatal cleft, but comparable with an additional respiratory abnormality to lead to failed improvement with jaw lengthening.

Complications of Mandibular Distraction Osteogenesis

In reviewing MDO complications, Davidson and colleagues[69] previously described the complication profile using a classification system of perioperative incident stratification events, delineated as major, moderate, and minor.[24,54] Overall, the average complication rate of mandibular distraction in the Robin sequence patient population is 34% with most complications classified as minor or moderate (**Table 1**).[24,54,69]

With respect to timing, early complications following MDO can include surgical site infection, device failure, hematoma, neuropraxia, fibrous nonunion, facial fracture, hypertrophic scarring, inappropriate vector of distraction, and relapse of tongue-based airway obstruction.[43,54,60,69,71,74,75] Long-term complications from MDO can include TMJ ankylosis, trismus, facial nerve injury, inferior alveolar nerve injury, tooth bud injury, asymmetry, and disturbance to facial growth.[43,54,60,69,71,74,75]

Table 1
Incidence of complications associated with neonatal mandibular distraction

Complication rate of mandibular distraction in the Robin sequence patient populations is 34%		
Minor Complications (15%)	Moderate Complications (15%)	Major Complications (9%)
Event that does not lead to adverse outcomes and can be resolved with or without noninvasive therapy	Event that could result in an adverse outcome but can be resolved with invasive therapy	Event that results in an adverse outcome and did not or could not be resolved with invasive therapy
Surgical site infection treated with antibiotics	Surgical site infection requiring surgery	Dental injury
Facial neuropraxia	Device fracture	Residual anterior open bite
Self-extubation	Widened neck scars	TMJ ankyloses
Hypertrophic scarring	Device exposure	Death
Device loosening	Incomplete osteotomy Bilateral odontomas	

With respect to dental complications, Steinberg and colleagues[74] reported injury to the first permanent mandibular molar in 50% of cases, which was restorable in more than 75% of cases when recognized. Injury to the marginal mandibular nerve and resultant lower-lip depressor weakness is more common than previously reported at 15% on the operated side.[74] Interestingly, permanent inferior alveolar nerve injury was comparatively infrequent (2.5%), despite it frequently being cited as a common risk of MDO.[74] Finally, in a systematic review of the published literature over 4 decades, fewer complications overall were seen in internal MDO compared with external MDO.[71] Ultimately, the complication rate associated with MDO in the Robin sequence population is low in both occurrence and level of acuity.

LONG-TERM OUTCOMES OF MANDIBULAR DISTRACTION OSTEOGENESIS

A dearth of primary literature exists on long-term outcomes of MDO, given it is a newer treatment modality than tracheostomy and TLA. A robust meta-analysis review of MDO surgical outcomes in the Robin sequence literature from 1960 to 2017 demonstrates 95% avoidance of tracheostomy, 80% decannulation, 87% full oral feeds at follow-up, and a 4% to 6% rate of reoperation.[40] MDO patients were found to have 6.1 times increased odds of successful resolution of obstructive apnea compared with TLA patients, after controlling for age at operation, gender, body mass index at postoperative polysomnogram, and presence of a syndromic diagnosis.[40] In addition, MDO patients were found to have 1.3 times increased odds of successful resolution of

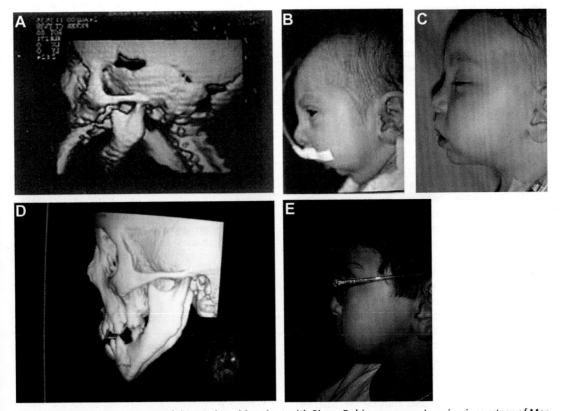

Fig. 4. (*A*) Preoperative CT scan of this 12-day-old patient with Pierre Robin sequence. Imaging is courtesy of Marcus V. Collares, MD, PhD. (*B*) Preoperative photograph of this 12-day-old patient with Pierre Robin sequence. Clinical photograph is courtesy of Marcus V. Collares, MD, PhD. (*C*) Postoperative photograph of this same patient now 12 months old with Pierre Robin sequence after MDO with external distractor at the time of palatoplasty. Clinical photograph is courtesy of Marcus V. Collares, MD, PhD. (*D*) Postoperative imaging of this same patient now 12 years old with Pierre Robin sequence after MDO with external distractor for longitudinal follow-up. Imaging is courtesy of Marcus V. Collares, MD, PhD. (*E*) Postoperative photograph of this 12-year-old patient with Pierre Robin sequence after MDO with external distractor for longitudinal follow-up. (Clinical photograph is courtesy of Marcus V. Collares, MD, PhD.)

obstructive apnea compared with TLA patients, after controlling for preoperative AHI score.[40]

To date, only 1 level II evidence and 3 level III evidence comparison studies exist demonstrating the efficacy of MDO over TLA with a mean follow-up of 1.75 years using both internal nonresorbable and external devices.[43,76–78] Long-term results of MDO with internal resorbable distraction systems in Robin patients demonstrate significantly shorter mandibular lengths following MDO compared with no distraction after a mean follow-up time of 6.8 years.[79]

Despite the mounting evidence for the efficacy of MDO, operative indications for neonates with Robin sequence remain controversial. Specifically, concerns for higher surgical complexity when simpler procedures are proven to be effective, nerve injury, tooth injury, and detrimental effect on future mandibular growth in patients are all reported.[22,46,58,73,80] Nevertheless, prospective analyses demonstrate that Robin sequence patients can successfully be selected for an appropriate treatment modality to obviate tracheostomy[77] (**Fig. 4**). Neonatal MDO should only be performed by experienced, high-volume distraction centers with expert pediatric anesthesiologists and neonatal intensive care units to ensure patient safety.[60]

FUTURE DIRECTIONS

Surgical treatment in this challenging patient population has been previously hindered by noncomparative analyses of techniques and low-level evidence recommendations that are largely based on expert opinion. Although there has been a steady improvement in the scientific quality of clinical outcomes reports over the last 10 years, further research is required. Currently, there is a paucity of high-level evidence regarding diagnosis, treatment, and long-term outcomes of infants with Robin sequence. Given the relative low incidence of Robin sequence in conjunction with the multiple factors involved in the clinical decision to use MDO for treatment, and the ethical challenges of randomization, there are currently no level 1 evidence outcomes studies, nor are these studies likely to happen. Thus, future directions in the field of neonatal MDO for Robin sequence should include coordinated multicenter studies, preferably prospective trials, investigating standardized diagnostic and management algorithms for these infants. Additional studies are needed on the long-term effects of MDO on clinical outcomes and growth of the mandible. Based on the outcomes of these proposed studies, definitive indications for distraction can be codified as, at present, nonexistent.

Most importantly, universal language should be used when discussing a patient with Robin sequence (defined by micrognathia, glossoptosis, and airway obstruction); surgeons treating infants with Pierre Robin sequence should use a well-documented, protocol-driven care plan, which includes preoperative and postoperative PSG to quantify the preoperative severity and postoperative resolution of disease, and there should be an expectation for further evolution in care as many unanswered questions remain.

CLINICS CARE POINTS

- Consensus on the definition of Robin sequence is paramount to facilitate future prospective and comparative research studies examining treatment protocols and clinical outcomes in this challenging, heterogenous patient population.
- A validated evaluation protocol is needed to standardize patient care. Specifically, objective studies to evaluate the severity of airway obstruction, namely polysomnography, must be universally incorporated into such protocol.
- Mandibular distraction is proven to be a safe and effective intervention for neonates with Robin sequence with severe airway obstruction. Furthermore, the complication profile associated with mandibular distraction remains low.
- Future directions in the field of neonatal mandibular distraction for Robin sequence include prospective and coordinated multicenter studies to investigate standardized diagnostic and management algorithms for these infants.

DISCLOSURE

The authors have nothing to disclose.

REFERENCES

1. Robin P. La glossoptosis son diagnostic, ses consequences, son traitment. Paris: Bulletin de l'Academie National de Medecine; 1923.
2. Hsieh ST, Woo AS. Pierre Robin sequence. Clin Plast Surg 2019;46(2):249–59.
3. Vatlach S, Maas, Poets CF. Birth prevalence and initial treatment of Robin sequence in Germany: a prospective epidemiologic study. Orphanet J Rare Dis 2014;9:9.

4. Printzlau A, Anderson M. Pierre Robin sequence in Denmark: a retrospective population-based epidemiologic study. Cleft Palate Craniofac J 2004;41: 47–52.

5. Caouette-Laberge L, Bayet B, Larocque Y. The Pierre Robin sequence review of 125 cases and evolution of treatment modalities. Plast Reconstr Surg 1994;93(5):934–42.

6. Breugem CC, Courtemanche DJ. Robin sequence: clearing nosologic confusion. Cleft Palate Craniofac J 2010;47(2):197–200.

7. Bookman LB, Melton KR, Pan BS, et al. Neonates with tongue-based airway obstruction: a systematic review. Otolaryngol Head Neck Surg 2012;146:8–18.

8. de Sousa TV, Marques IL, Carneiro AF, et al. Nasopharyngoscopy in Robin sequence: clinical and predictive value. Cleft Palate Craniofac J 2003;40(6): 618–23.

9. Manica D, Schweiger C, Sekine L, et al. Diagnostic accuracy of current glossoptosis classification systems: a nested cohort cross-sectional study. Laryngoscope 2018;128(2):502–8.

10. Manica D, Schweiger C, Sekine L, et al. Severity of clinical manifestations and laryngeal exposure difficulty predicted by glossoptosis endoscopic grades in Robin sequence patients. Int J Pediatr Otorhinolaryngol 2016;90:270–5.

11. Lee JJ, Thottam PJ, Ford MD, et al. Characteristics of sleep apnea in infants with Pierre-Robin sequence: is there improvement with advancing age? Int J Pediatr Otorhinolaryngol 2015;79:2059–67.

12. DeHaan KL, Seton C, Fitzgerald DA, et al. Polysomnography for the diagnosis of sleep disordered breathing in children under 2 years of age. Pediatr Pulmonol 2015;50:1346–53.

13. Katz ES, Mitchell RB, D'Ambrosio CM. Obstructive sleep apnea in infants. Am J Respir Crit Care Med 2012;185:805–16.

14. van Lieshout MJ, Joosten KF, Hoeve HL, et al. Unravelling Robin sequence: considerations of diagnosis and treatment. Laryngoscope 2014;124: E203–9.

15. Daniel M, Bailey S, Walker K, et al. Airway, feeding, and growth in infants with Robin sequence, and sleep apnea. Int J Pediatr Otorhinolaryngol 2013; 77:499–503.

16. Cladis F, Kumar A, Grunwaldt L, et al. Pierre Robin sequence: perioperative review. Anesth Analg 2014;119:400–12.

17. Fan KL, Mandelbaum M, Buro J, et al. Current trends in surgical airway management of neonates with Robin sequence. Plast Reconstr Surg Glob Open 2018;6(11):e1973.

18. Bekisz JM, Wang MM, Rickert SM, et al. Sleep-disordered breathing and airway assessment using polysomnography in pediatric patients with craniofacial disorders. J Craniofac Surg 2020;31(3):720–6.

19. Diep GK, Eisemann BS, Flores RL. Neonatal mandibular distraction osteogenesis in infants with Pierre Robin sequence. J Craniofac Surg 2020; 31(4):1137–41.

20. Knapp K, Powitzky R, Digoy P. Subglottic stenosis: another challenge for intubation and potential mechanism of airway obstruction in Pierre Robin sequence. Int J Pediatr Otorhinolaryngol 2011;75:1075–7.

21. Cruz MJ, Kerschner JE, Beste DJ, et al. Pierre Robin sequences: secondary respiratory difficulties and intrinsic feeding abnormalities. Laryngoscope 1999;109:1632–6.

22. Andrews BT, Fan KL, Roostaeian J, et al. Incidence of concomitant airway anomalies when using the University of California, Los Angeles, protocol for neonatal mandibular distraction. Plast Reconstr Surg 2013;131:1116–23.

23. Denny AD, Talisman R, Hanson PR, et al. Mandibular distraction osteogenesis in very young patients to correct airway obstruction. Plast Reconstr Surg 2001;108:302–11.

24. Flores RL. Neonatal mandibular distraction osteogenesis. Thieme Medical Publishers. Semin Plast Surg 2014;28:199–206.

25. Morovic CG, Monasterio L. Distraction osteogenesis for obstructive apneas in patients with congenital craniofacial malformations. Plast Reconstr Surg 2000;105(7):2324–30.

26. Tholpady SS, Costa MA, Hadad I, et al. Mandibular distraction for Robin sequence associated with laryngomalacia. J Craniofac Surg 2015;26:826–30.

27. Caouette-Laberge L, Borsuk DE, Bortoluzzi PA. Subperiosteal release of the floor of the mouth to correct airway obstruction in Pierre Robin sequence: review of 31 cases. Cleft Palate Craniofac J 2012;49(1):14–20.

28. Runyan CM, Uribe-Rivera A, Tork S, et al. Management of airway obstruction in infants with Pierre Robin sequence. Plast Reconstr Surg Glob Open 2018;6(5):e1688.

29. Greathouse ST, Costa M, Ferrera A, et al. The surgical treatment of Robin sequence. Ann Plast Surg 2016;77(4):413–9.

30. Zeitouni A, Manoukian J. Tracheostomy in the first year of life. J Otolaryngol 1993;22:431–4.

31. Tomaski SM, Zalzal GH, Saal HM. Airway obstruction in the Pierre Robin sequence. Laryngoscope 1995; 105(2):111–4.

32. Arola MK. Tracheostomy and its complications. A retrospective study of 794 tracheostomized patients. Ann Chir Gynaecol 1981;70:96–106.

33. Guilleminault C, Simmons FB, Motta J, et al. Obstructive sleep apnea syndrome and tracheostomy. Long-term follow up experience. Arch Intern Med 1981;141:985–8.

34. Sasaki CT, Horiuchi M, Koss N. Tracheostomy-related subglottic stenosis: bacteriologic pathogenesis. Laryngoscope 1979;89:857–65.

35. Singer LT, Kercsmar C, Legris G, et al. Developmental sequelae of long-term infant tracheostomy. Dev Med Child Neurol 1989;31:224–30.

36. Runyan CM, Uribe-Rivera A, Karlea A, et al. Cost analysis of mandibular distraction versus tracheostomy in neonates with Pierre Robin sequence. Otolaryngol Head Neck Surg 2014;151(5):811–8.

37. Paes EC, Fouche JJ, Muradin MS, et al. Tracheostomy versus mandibular distraction osteogenesis in infants with Robin sequence: a comparative cost analysis. Br J Oral Maxillofac Surg 2014;52(3):223–9.

38. Hong P, Bezuhly M, Mark Taylor S, et al. Tracheostomy versus mandibular distraction osteogenesis in Canadian children with Pierre Robin sequence: a comparative cost analysis. J Otolaryngol Head Neck Surg 2012;41(3):207–14.

39. Lee M, Ho ES, Forrest CR. Pierre Robin sequence: cost analysis and qualitative assessment of 89 patients at the hospital for sick children. Plast Surg (Oakv) 2019;27(1):14–21.

40. Zhang RS, Hoppe IC, Taylor JA, et al. Surgical management and outcomes of Pierre Robin sequence: a comparison of mandibular distraction osteogenesis and tongue-lip adhesion. Plast Reconstr Surg 2018;142(2):480–509.

41. Viezel-Mathieu A, Safran T, Gilardino MS. A systematic review of the effectiveness of tongue lip adhesion in improving airway obstruction in children with Pierre Robin sequence. J Craniofac Surg 2016;27(6):1453–6.

42. Flores RL, Greathouse ST, Costa M, et al. Defining failure and its predictors in mandibular distraction for Robin sequence. J Craniomaxillofac Surg 2015;43:1614–9.

43. Flores RL, Tholpady SS, Sati S, et al. The surgical correction of Pierre Robin sequence: mandibular distraction osteogenesis versus tongue-lip adhesion. Plast Reconstr Surg 2014;133:1433–9.

44. Resnick CM, Calabrese CE, Sahdev R, et al. Is tongue-lip adhesion or mandibular distraction more effective in relieving obstructive apnea in infants with Robin sequence? J Oral Maxillofac Surg 2019;77(3):591–600.

45. Almajed A, Viezel-Mathieu A, Gilardino MS, et al. Outcome following surgical interventions for micrognathia in infants with Pierre Robin sequence: a systematic review of the literature. Cleft Palate Craniofac J 2017;54(1):32–42.

46. Kirschner RE, Low DW, Randall P, et al. Surgical airway management in Pierre Robin sequence: is there a role for tongue-lip adhesion? Cleft Palate Craniofac J 2003;40(1):13–8.

47. Denny AD, Amm CA, Schaefer RB. Outcomes of tongue-lip adhesion for neonatal respiratory distress caused by Pierre Robin sequence. J Craniofac Surg 2004;15:819–23.

48. Schaefer RB, Stadler JA 3rd, Gosain AK. To distract or not to distract: an algorithm for airway management in isolated Pierre Robin sequence. Plast Reconstr Surg 2004;113:1113–25.

49. Denny AD. Distraction osteogenesis in Pierre Robin neonates with airway obstruction. Clin Plast Surg 2004;31:221–9.

50. Hoffman W. Outcome of tongue-lip plication in patients with severe Pierre Robin sequence. J Craniofac Surg 2003;14:602–8.

51. McCarthy JG, Schreiber K, Karp N, et al. Lengthening the human mandible by gradual distraction. Plast Reconstr Surg 1992;89:1–8 [discussion 9].

52. Murage KP, Tholpady SS, Friel M, et al. Outcomes analysis of mandibular distraction osteogenesis for the treatment of Pierre Robin sequence. Plast Reconstr Surg 2013 Aug;132(2):419–21.

53. Monasterio FO, Molina F, Berlanga F, et al. Swallowing disorders in Pierre Robin sequence: its correction by distraction. J Craniofac Surg 2004;15:934–41.

54. Murage KP, Costa MA, Friel MT, et al. Complications associated with neonatal mandibular distraction osteogenesis in the treatment of Robin sequence. J Craniofac Surg 2014;25:383–7.

55. Hammoudeh J, Bindingnavele VK, Davis B, et al. Neonatal and infant mandibular distraction as an alternative to tracheostomy in severe obstructive sleep apnea. Cleft Palate Craniofac J 2012;49:32–8.

56. Scott AR, Tibesar RJ, Lander TA, et al. Mandibular distraction osteogenesis in infants younger than 3 months. Arch Facial Plast Surg 2011;13:173–9.

57. Genecov DG, Barcelo CR, Steinberg D, et al. Clinical experience with the application of distraction osteogenesis for airway obstruction. J Craniofac Surg 2009;20(Suppl 2):1817–21.

58. Burstein FD, Williams JK. Mandibular distraction osteogenesis in Pierre Robin sequence: application of a new internal single-stage resorbable device. Plast Reconstr Surg 2005;115:61–7 [discussion 68].

59. Tahiri Y, Viezel-Mathieu A, Aldekhayel S, et al. The effectiveness of mandibular distraction in improving airway obstruction in the pediatric population. Plast Reconstr Surg 2014;133:352e–9e.

60. Tahiri Y, Greathouse ST, Tholpady SS, et al. Mandibular distraction osteogenesis in low-weight neonates with Robin sequence: is it safe? Plast Reconstr Surg 2015;136(5):1037–44.

61. Denny A, Kalantarian B. Mandibular distraction in neonates: a strategy to avoid tracheostomy. Plast Reconstr Surg 2002;109:896–904 [discussion 905-6].

62. Collares MVM, Pinto RADP, Berlim GL, et al. Use of osteogenic mandibular distraction in neonates with severe airway obstruction. Braz J Craniomaxillofac Surg 2000;3(2):7–12.

63. Monasterio FO, Drucker M, Molina F, et al. Distraction osteogenesis in Pierre Robin sequence and

related respiratory problems in children. J Craniofac Surg 2002;13(1):79–83 [discussion 84].

64. Evans KN, Sie KC, Hopper RA, et al. Robin sequence: from diagnosis to development of an effective management plan. Pediatrics 2011; 127(5):936–48.

65. Hong P, McNeil M, Kearns DB, et al. Mandibular distraction osteogenesis in children with Pierre Robin sequence: impact on health-related quality of life. Int J Pediatr Otorhinolaryngol 2012;76(8): 1159–63.

66. Duarte DW, Collares MVM. Mandibular distraction osteogenesis and mandibular morphology in Pierre Robin sequence patients. Universidade Federal do Rio Grande do Sul; 2020. Available at: http://hdl.handle.net/10183/212723.

67. Zellner EG, Mhlaba JM, Reid RR, et al. Does mandibular distraction vector influence airway volumes and outcome? J Oral Maxillofac Surg 2017; 75(1):167–77.

68. Ramly EP, Yu JW, Eisemann BS, et al. Temporomandibular joint ankylosis in pediatric patients with craniofacial differences: causes, recurrence, and clinical outcomes. J Craniofac Surg 2020;31(5): 1343–7.

69. Davidson EH, Brown D, Sheyte PR, et al. The evolution of mandibular distraction: device selection. Plast Reconstr Surg 2010;126:2061–70.

70. Li WY, Poon A, Courtemanche D, et al. Airway management in Pierre Robin sequence: the Vancouver classification. Plast Surg (Oakv) 2017;25:14–20.

71. Paes E, Mink van der Molen AB, Muradin MM, et al. A systematic review on the outcome of mandibular distraction osteogenesis in infants suffering Robin sequence. Clin Oral Investig 2013;178:1807–20.

72. Hammoudeh JA, Fahradyan A, Brady C, et al. Predictors of failure in infant mandibular distraction osteogenesis. J Oral Maxillofac Surg 2018;76(9): 1955–65.

73. Rogers GF, Murphy AS, LaBrie RA, et al. The GILLS score: part 1. Patient selection for tongue-lip adhesion in Robin sequence. Plast Reconstr Surg 2011; 128:243–51.

74. Steinberg JP, Brady CM, Waters BR, et al. Mid-term dental and nerve-related complications of infant distraction for Robin sequence. Plast Reconstr Surg 2016;138(1):82e–90e.

75. Master DL, Hanson PR, Gosain AK. Complications of mandibular distraction osteogenesis. J Craniofac Surg 2010;21:1565–70.

76. Susarla SM, Mundinger GS, Chang CC, et al. Gastrostomy placement rates in infants with Pierre Robin sequence: a comparison of tongue-lip adhesion and mandibular distraction osteogenesis. JAMA Facial Plast Surg 2016;18(2):95–100.

77. Khansa I, Hall C, Madhoun LL, et al. Airway and feeding outcomes of mandibular distraction, tongue-lip adhesion, and conservative management in Pierre Robin sequence: a prospective study. Plast Reconstr Surg 2017;139(4):975e–83e.

78. Papoff P, Guelfi G, Cicchetti R, et al. Outcomes after tongue-lip adhesion or mandibular distraction osteogenesis in infants with Pierre Robin sequence and severe airway obstruction. Int J Oral Maxillofac Surg 2013;42(11):1418–23.

79. Paes EC, Bittermann GK, Bittermann D, et al. Long-term results of mandibular distraction osteogenesis with a resorbable device in infants with Robin sequence: effects on developing molars and mandibular growth. Plast Reconstr Surg 2016; 137(2):375e–83e.

80. Evans AK, Rahbar R, Rogers GF, et al. Robin sequence: a retrospective review of 115 patients. Int J Pediatr Otorhinolaryngol 2006;70(6):973–80.

Modern Mandibular Distraction Applications in Hemifacial Microsomia

Sameer Shakir, MD[a], Scott P. Bartlett, MD[b],*

KEYWORDS

- Hemifacial microsomia • Craniofacial microsomia • Goldenhar syndrome
- Mandibular distraction osteogenesis • Costochondral rib grafting • Orthognathic surgery

KEY POINTS

- Phenotypic severity dictates the timing and type of surgical intervention required.
- Mandibular distraction in children without respiratory and feeding difficulties remains controversial with regard to long-term mandibular growth outcomes and reducing surgical burden.
- Early mandibular distraction does not obviate secondary orthognathic surgery at skeletal maturity; it provides improved functional, aesthetic, and psychosocial outcomes, at least in the short term.
- Costochondral rib grafting for Pruzansky type IIB and III mandibles can produce reliable results, especially when combined with subsequent mandibular distraction.
- Secondary 2-jaw orthognathic surgery plus genioplasty at skeletal maturity benefits from improved bone volume from prior mandibular distraction.

SURGICAL HISTORY

The historical management of bony and soft tissue hemifacial microsomia (HFM) largely paralleled advances in reconstructive surgery: bone grafts, osteotomies, dermis-fat grafts, locoregional flaps, microvascular free flaps, and autologous fat grafting. Maxillomandibular osteotomies and autologous bone grafts remained the gold standard for mandibular reconstruction during the 1980s.[1,2] However, the introduction of distraction osteogenesis represented a paradigm shift in the treatment of mandibular hypoplasia. Initially described by Ilizarov and colleagues[3] for the endochondral bones of the extremities and applied to the craniofacial skeleton by Snyder and colleagues,[4] mandibular distraction osteogenesis (MDO) was popularized in 1992 by McCarthy and colleagues[5] at New York University. Using an external fixator–like device secured to the mandible with transcutaneous pins and a Risdon approach, McCarthy and colleagues[5] showed mandibular bony lengthening of 18 to 24 mm in a series of 4 patients, obviating autologous bone grafts, blood transfusion, and/or maxillomandibular fixation. MDO provided several advantages compared with existing modalities, including a simpler technique, decreased morbidity (eg, infection blood loss, operative time), and ability to lengthen the mandible at a younger age. Compared with bone grafting, successful MDO vertically lengthens the mandible, improves the quality of bone stock, improves soft tissue asymmetry, allows improved vector control of bony regenerate, and may be associated with less relapse.[6–15]

TREATMENT ALGORITHM

The reconstructive requirements of patients with HFM relate to anatomic and functional deficiencies

[a] Division of Plastic Surgery, Perelman Center for Advanced Medicine, 3400 Civic Center Blvd, South Pavilion, 14th Fl, Philadelphia, PA 19104, USA; [b] Division of Plastic Surgery, Department of Surgery, Children's Hospital of Philadelphia, 3401 Civic Center Boulevard, Philadelphia, PA 19014, USA
* Corresponding author.
E-mail address: bartletts@email.chop.edu

Clin Plastic Surg 48 (2021) 375–389
https://doi.org/10.1016/j.cps.2021.02.001
0094-1298/21/© 2021 Elsevier Inc. All rights reserved.

in the setting of patient age. The observed composite soft tissue and bony deformities may lead to impaired respiratory, otologic, masticatory, speech, and psychosocial well-being, necessitating early multidisciplinary treatment beyond simple "bone carpentry." This article focuses on the skeletal deformity of the jaws. However, augmentation of the soft tissue deficiency warrants a brief discussion. At the time of operative skeletal intervention (eg, mandibular distraction, rib grafting, and orthognathic surgery), the authors perform fat grafting ad seriatim, which significantly improves the soft tissues over time and frequently obviates more complex augmentation procedures such as free tissue transfers. The treatment of mandibular hypoplasia, specifically, depends on age and severity. Age can be divided into 3 periods: (1) neonatal, (2) school age, and (3) skeletal maturity. Severity is determined by a dichotomized Pruzansky classification: (1) type I/IIA (mild/moderate) versus (2) type IIB/III (severe).

During the neonatal period, which is defined as the first 28 days after birth, respiratory and feeding concerns dictate early interventions. Obstructive sleep apnea and other respiratory deficiencies secondary to severe mandibular hypoplasia, micrognathia, and glossoptosis may require tracheostomy, although neonatal MDO may obviate this morbid procedure if respiratory insufficiency is limited to a single-level obstruction.[16–18]

The timing of surgical treatment remains controversial for patients without severe mandibular hypoplasia and consequent respiratory insufficiency beyond the neonatal period. Is early surgical intervention deleterious in the context of craniofacial growth and overall appearance? Does early intervention in the form of MDO, which is associated with decreased operative time and invasiveness compared with major osteotomies, prevent further deformity or impair otherwise normal growth?[19–22] Poswillo[23] and Obwegeser[24] argued against osteotomies before skeletal maturity because they thought early intervention interfered with the underlying functional matrix and consequently deterred craniofacial growth. Instead, Obwegeser[23] advocated rib graft reconstruction of the temporomandibular joint (TMJ) and zygomatic arch and definitive orthognathic correction consisting of Le Fort 1 and bilateral sagittal split osteotomy[22] (BSSO) with genioplasty during adulthood.[24] Proponents of early intervention include Dingman and Grabb,[25] who reconstructed the hypoplastic ramus using metatarsal bone graft. Converse and colleagues[26] similarly advocated staged, early treatment during mixed dentition in order to avoid difficulties with soft

tissue hypoplasia in adulthood and to achieve greater benefit from surgical-orthodontic therapy during periods of growth. Munro and colleagues,[27] Murray and colleagues,[28] and Lauritzen and colleagues[29] similarly recommended childhood osteotomies and costochondral rib grafting with subsequent growth of the rib-mandible constructs. In general, surgical intervention for mild mandibular hypoplasia (ie, Pruzansky type I) can be successfully managed with orthodontics during childhood. Alternatively, more severe Pruzansky type I and IIA phenotypes are associated with occlusal cants and facial asymmetries that have the potential of worsening during the period of mixed dentition and may benefit from early surgical intervention. McCarthy and coworkers' experience with early MDO during childhood for patients with mild to moderate unilateral HFM (ie, Pruzansky type I and IIA) showed efficacy in achieving satisfactory outcomes through adhering to proper vector selection, overcorrection, and close orthodontic managment.[30] The vector of distraction depends on mandibular morphology, with overall goals to lengthen the deficient ramus, upright the condyle, and create a gonial angle; type IIA mandibles characterized by deficient ramal height benefit from a vertical vector of distraction, whereas type IIB mandibles characterized by vertical and horizontal ramal and body deficiencies benefit from a more oblique vector of distraction.[13,31–35] The authors have adopted a similar philosophy consisting of early MDO for patients with mild to moderate mandibular hypoplasia and facial asymmetry without respiratory insufficiency, which are discussed later in detail.[36]

For patients with severe mandibular hypoplasia (type IIB/III) during childhood, the authors recommend costochondral rib reconstruction with or without subsequent mandibular distraction of the construct.[37] In addition, we recommend conventional maxillomandibular orthognathic surgery in skeletally mature patients with HFM regardless of prior surgical interventions.

NEONATAL MANDIBULAR DISTRACTION

In cases of mild to moderate respiratory insufficiency associated with HFM mandibular hypoplasia, conservative measures that are similarly used for the treatment of Robin sequence, such as prone positioning, supplemental oxygen, nasopharyngeal airways, and continuous positive airway pressure, may provide adequate symptomatic relief.[18,38,39] In more severe cases of unilateral or bilateral hypoplasia requiring intubation, MDO may prevent progression to tracheostomy. Although neonatal distraction is discussed in detail elsewhere in this issue, this article briefly comments on relevant principles.

Our preferred technique for MDO independent of age involves an osteotomy (vertical or oblique >horizontal vector) of 1 or both sides of the deficient mandible with the application of an internal, semiburied distractor through a Risdon approach. Advantages of internal devices include decreased visibility, cutaneous scarring, and likelihood of trauma and infection.[40] Advantages of external devices include increased ability to mold the regenerate and alter the distraction vector after osteotomy, and precise placement of distracting pins without wide periosteum undermining in the setting of a severely hypoplastic mandible.[41] We typically favor a vector oblique to the maxillary occlusal plane in order to obtain expansion in both the vertical and sagittal dimensions, although the exact vector orientation depends on the underlying mandibular morphology. The semiburied distractor, which is secured with bicortical screws, typically exits the skin near the retroauricular region. A piezoelectric saw is used to perform a near-complete osteotomy distal to the developing tooth roots. While considering the inferior alveolar nerve, a full corticotomy over the buccal surface of the mandible and superior and inferior surfaces of the lingual mandible completes the osteotomy. The distractor device is then activated for several millimeters to ensure advancement without interference. An osteotome may be used to carefully separate adjoining bony edges while preserving the nerve. Once confirming a complete osteotomy, the engaged bony edges are opposed and the incision closed in layers with resorbable suture.

After a latency period of approximately 1 to 2 days in neonates, distraction during the activation phase proceeds at a rate of 1 mm/d (potentially 2 mm/d) to avoid premature consolidation and to reduce the length of endotracheal intubation. Clinical end points for the activation phase in patients with unilateral HFM include (1) overcorrection of the occlusal plane, (2) inferior displacement of the ipsilateral oral commissure, and (3) and movement of the chin point beyond the midline. In neonates with bilateral HFM, activation continues until the mandibular anterior teeth are anterior to the maxillary anterior teeth (ie, class III malocclusion–like appearance). An additional criterion for cessation of distraction in respiratory-compromised neonates includes evidence of improved retroglossal airspace on lateral radiograph or endoscopy. Adherence to these principles has led to successful extubation and improved maxillomandibular relation in 92% to 100% of patients (**Fig. 1**).[18]

MILD OR MODERATE MANDIBULAR HYPOPLASIA

Perhaps the most controversial decision in the surgical management HFM relates to patients with mild or moderate mandibular hypoplasia without functional compromise. Early on, MDO improves facial appearance by lengthening the mandible and expanding the overlying soft tissues; however, the correction may be prone to relapse and require future interventions.[9,30,36,42] Whether the distracted mandible fails to grow or the deformity relapses, the outcome nevertheless results in the need for orthognathic correction at skeletal maturity. Moreover, the potential benefit must be considered in the context of potential complications, including tooth bud injury, facial nerve injury, premature bony consolidation, and hardware failure.[43,44]

Our preferred technique for early unilateral MDO largely mirrors the technique described for neonatal MDO, but with a few caveats. Our experience with early MDO highlights the importance of comprehensive orthodontic care and orthodontic splint therapy to negate the effects of masseter muscle contraction on the regenerate, control maxillary dentoalveolar elongation, and subsequent preservation of mandibular regenerate length and volume. Predistraction orthodontic management may involve removal of dental compensations, expansion of the maxillary arch width, maintenance of the mandibular lingual arch, and forced eruption of molar tooth buds away from planned mandibular osteotomies. For patients undergoing early MDO, the procedure inherently generates a posterior open bite on the affected side. Intraoperatively, we secure orthodontic bone anchors on the hypoplastic mandible. Intermaxillary guiding elastics can be used during the active phase of distraction to mold the generate and adjust the distraction vector to achieve a planned occlusion. During the activation and consolidation phases, the use of elastics further guides vertical growth of the maxilla. Following removal of the distractor, the patient is fitted with a custom splint to maintain the surgically created open bite. Gradual burring down of the splint allows for selective eruption and growth of the maxillary dentition and alveolar bone closing the open bite and maintaining the mandibular correction. Our anecdotal experience suggests overcorrection can further level the maxillary dental arch and provide an improved functional and aesthetic outcome. These properly positioned orthodontic devices and splints not only preserve regenerate volume but may also promote regenerate and maxillary growth. Judicious care coordination

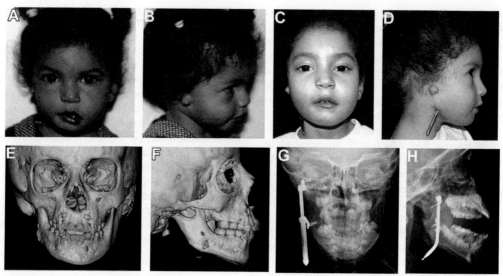

Fig. 1. Vertical mandibular distraction of Pruzansky type IIA mandible. (*A, B*) Patient with Pruzansky type IIA mandible in setting of Goldenhar syndrome affecting the right face. (*C, D*) During activation of initial vertical MDO at age 4 years. (*E, F*) Three-dimensional (3D) computed tomography reconstruction after primary MDO with evidence of undercorrection (ie, right-sided upward occlusal cant of 10°). (*G, H*) Radiographic imaging during activation phase of secondary MDO at age 9 years with goal of overcorrection. (*I, J*) At age 16 years showing persistent right-sided upward occlusal cant. (*K–M*) Preoperative virtual surgical planning (VSP) imaging of planned orthognathic correction at age 20 years consistent with class II malocclusion and microgenia. (*N–P*) Planned VSP imaging showing bony movements involving Le Fort 1 advancement, BSSO of the mandible, and sliding osseous genioplasty. (*Q–T*) Long-term follow-up at age 21 years showing excellent occlusal relationships and aesthetic reconstruction. Note that the patient underwent multiple rounds of concurrent fat grafting to augment the overlying deficient soft tissue.

with the orthodontist should not be underemphasized.

In order to lengthen the deficient mandibular ramus, we prefer a more vertical or oblique vector of distraction. When using a more vertical vector (ie, horizontal osteotomy in line with maxillary occlusal plane), the proximal segment distraction force generates counterclockwise rotation about the condyle and TMJ impaction, leading to generalized joint dysmorphology, including flattening, hypertrophy, ankylosis, and/or dislocation.[45–49] Some investigators even promote coronoidectomy at the time of MDO to prevent these untoward consequences of counterclockwise rotation and superior displacement.[18] There is significant distraction force wasted in rotating the proximal segment cephalad before gaining the desired vertical height of the deficient ramus in the caudal direction. Since 2012, we have been using a check plate attached to the coronoid to engage the zygomatic arch during active distraction in order to focus the vertical/oblique distraction force downward onto the mandibular ramus instead of upward toward the TMJ and cranial base.[50] Our computed tomography (CT) data show improved TMJ morphology when using the check plate. This modification to traditional MDO with a

vertical/oblique vector prevents impaction of the TMJ into the cranial base, prevents cephalic rotation of the proximal segment about the TMJ, and optimizes the position of the subsequent regenerate.[50]

McCarthy and colleagues enumerated several critical lessons in their 22-year review of early MDO in patients younger than 10 years of age with Pruzansky type I/IIA mandibles undergoing unilateral MDO.[30] In a subjective photographic assessment of satisfactory versus unsatisfactory outcomes of patients at skeletal maturity with history of MDO before 10 years of age, the investigators found overcorrection from the midline (>44%) and younger age at time of initial distraction (4.7 vs 7.5 years) to significantly correlate with improved outcomes (our own experiences suggest patients undergoing MDO before 3 years of age benefit from spontaneous descent of the ipsilateral maxillary dentoalveolus with distraction). Moreover, the use of comprehensive orthodontia including postoperative splints further aided successful distraction. In a retrospective outcome analysis of vector selection and overcorrection in MDO, the New York group suggested the oblique vector offered an ideal balance between the horizontal and vertical vectors by simultaneously lengthening

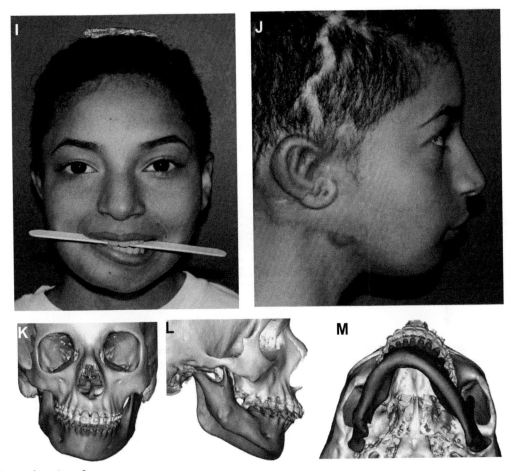

Fig. 1. (*continued*)

the ramus and translating the gonion.[32] They concluded that, although a subset of patients who undergo early MDO require secondary surgery (eg, orthognathic correction) at skeletal maturity, they often maintain satisfactory outcomes if initially overcorrected despite a varying degree of relapse, and invariably benefit from improved appearance-related psychosocial development during childhood. Moreover, patients undergoing early MDO benefit from increased bone stock for secondary orthognathic surgery.

Our experience with early MDO largely mirrors these McCarthy and colleagues' data.[36] Zhang and colleagues[36] compared the need for secondary orthognathic correction in skeletally mature patients with HFM at the Children's Hospital of Philadelphia who either did or did not undergo early MDO over a 25-year study period. The 2 cohorts were matched according to Pruzansky grade, with patients in both cohorts showing similar hypoplasia grades. The mean age at time of MDO was ~9 years, older than the

recommended age per the McCarthy and colleagues data, although patient age at time of distraction did not ultimately correlate to need for orthognathic correction.[30] Approximately 35% of these patients outgrew their initial corrections and underwent repeat MDO at ~10.6 years of age. Of the patients who underwent early costochondral rib grafting only, all 3 out of 3 required secondary orthognathic correction, suggesting that rib growth may not mirror the unaffected side, resulting in recurrence of asymmetry. Interestingly, degree of mandibular deformity as determined by Pruzansky grade did not correlate with need for orthognathic correction in patients who did or did not undergo early MDO. Importantly, the incidence of secondary orthognathic surgery at skeletal maturity did not differ between the 2 cohorts, suggesting early MDO provides functional, aesthetic, and psychosocial benefits, but does not obviate later orthognathic correction in every patient to further refine facial asymmetry. In addition, the enhanced body image and psychosocial

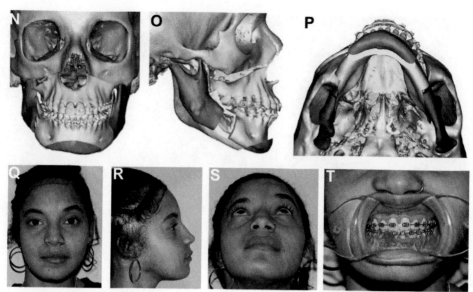

Fig. 1. (*continued*)

impact of a developing child with improved facial asymmetry cannot be overstated, although validated quality-of-life studies are lacking.[51–53]

Despite these long-term data from high-volume centers, there lacks consensus among practitioners regarding the efficacy of early MDO. In a prospective, longitudinal study, Meazzini and colleagues[54] reported a near-100% recurrence rate of mandibular asymmetry occurring 5.8 years after early MDO. In a controversial review of long-term stability after early MDO published in 2009, Mommaerts and coworkers critically evaluated the existing literature and concluded: (1) study designs were poor and failed to stratify results based on Pruzansky type; (2) there was no validation of measurements to determine facial symmetry; (3) 0 of 13 studies showed predictable, long-term stability following early MDO, but instead showed significant relapse; (4) repeated MDO was necessary to improve recurrent facial asymmetry; (5) early MDO did not reduce rates of secondary maxillary deformity; and (6) repeat MDO represents a costlier endeavor than single-stage orthognathic surgery at time of skeletal maturity.[55,56] The investigators concluded that, "there is no convincing evidence supporting the effectiveness of early mandible osteodistraction in hemifacial microsomia patients. Patients need to be informed that additional distraction procedures or definitive secondary surgery at maturity most likely will be required."

Since the publication of Mommaerts and coworkers' review 11 years ago, long-term outcomes data continue to suggest that most patients with HFM require orthognathic correction at the time of skeletal maturity independent of early intervention performed. Ascenço and colleagues[57] reported a 90% recurrence rate of facial asymmetry following unilateral MDO in 33 patients, who subsequently required a referral for orthognathic correction ~3.8 years from time of intervention. Suh and colleagues[42] showed relapse and return to baseline asymmetry in 26 patients over an 11-year follow-up period; however, the investigators failed to overcorrect and accepted leveling of the oral commissure as a clinical end point during activation. In a systematic review by Pluijmers and colleagues,[58] the investigators suggested surgical outcomes in HFM to be patient dependent and not treatment specific, although long-term outcomes lacked radiographic data related to relapse, and clinical end points of correction again failed to emulate those suggested by McCarthy and colleagues. Recent multi-institutional data from 3 large European craniofacial centers suggest that patients undergoing surgical interventions targeting the mandible earlier in life undergo significantly more procedures to correct asymmetry later on, independent of Pruzansky type.[59]

Despite these conflicting reports, the authors believe early MDO is a critical tool to generate bone (and to a lesser extent soft tissue) in order to improve facial asymmetry, at least in the short term. Early distraction does not eliminate the need for definitive orthognathic surgery at skeletal maturity or produce a lesser maxillary deformity; instead, we argue that MDO offers an opportunity to generate new bone, lengthen a hypoplastic

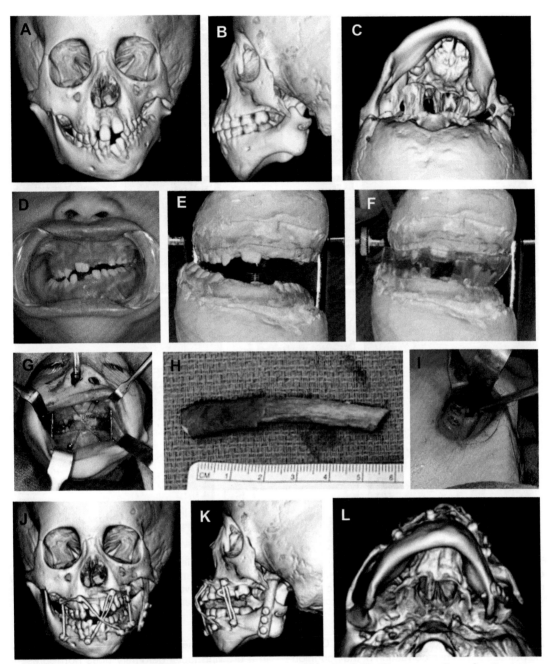

Fig. 2. Costochondral rib grafting of Pruzansky type III mandible. (*A–C*) 3D CT reconstruction of patient at age 6 years born with left HFM with absence of a functional condyle, vertically shortened ramus, and hypoplastic left mandible. (*D–F*) Preoperative evaluation revealed an upward occlusal cant to the left. She was planned with dental impressions and stone models to create a splint that would shift her mandibular midline vertically and create a posterior open bite to allow room for an osteocartilaginous rib construct. (*G*) Intraoperative maxillomandibular fixation using a bone hook under the chin to maximally pull the mandible forward and shift it to the right with insertion of custom-fabricated splint. Intermaxillary fixation screws and 4 wires were used in a crisscross pattern mesially and a vertical pattern distally. (*H*) Rib construct consisting of 5-mm to 7-mm cap with intact periosteum and perichondrium. (*I*) After bluntly developing a space up to the cranial base, the rib construct is slid into position to create a pseudoarthrosis and secured to the native mandible using 3 12-mm predrilled midface screws over washers. Excess bone can be trimmed inferiorly after securing the construct. (*J–L*) Post-operative 3D CT showing appropriately positioned rib construct. The patient remained in maxillomandibular fixation for 3 weeks, at which point she was allowed to move freely. The custom splint remained in place for 12 months postoperatively.

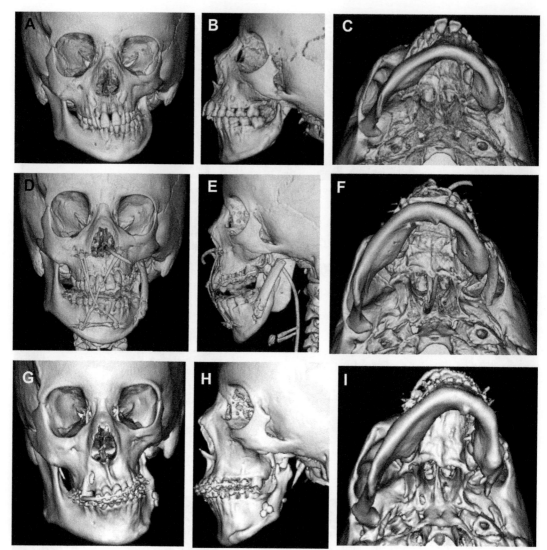

Fig. 3. Need for distraction following costochondral rib grafting. (*A–C*) Patient at 8 years of age presenting with left HFM and Pruzansky type III mandible. (*D–F*) Immediate postoperative imaging of costochondral rib grafting at 9 years of age. (*G–I*) At 18 years of age, the patient shows minimal growth of the rib construct, necessitating MDO to further increase bone stock before completion orthognathic surgery.

mandible, and improve facial asymmetry. Clinical end points such as overcorrection of the pogonion beyond the craniofacial midline and inferior displacement of the affected side oral commissure compared with the unaffected side are critical factors leading to lasting results. Comprehensive presurgical and postsurgical treatment with an orthodontist can not only manage maxillary dental eruption but also maintain an open posterior bite using splints to allow for maxillary growth and eventual closure of the posterior gap. When adhering to these principles of early distraction, we believe there may be patients who need orthognathic surgery to a lesser extent at skeletal

maturity. The need to perform additional surgery in a growing facial deformity does not represent a failure; instead, secondary orthognathic surgery simply represents an opportunity to further refine form and function in the patients with evolving HFM.

SEVERE MANDIBULAR HYPOPLASIA

The management of severe mandibular hypoplasia characterized by Pruzansky grade IIB and/or III mandibles is more straightforward. Sir Harold Gillies[60] first described the autologous costochondral rib graft for TMJ reconstruction in 1920. The

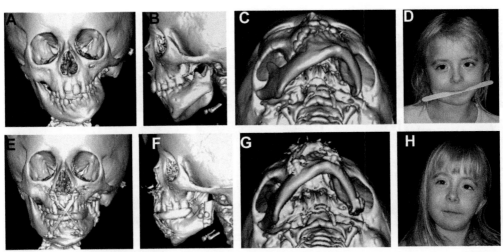

Fig. 4. Costochondral rib grafting of Pruzansky type III mandible followed by vertical distraction and completion orthognathic surgery. (*A–D*) Patient with Pruzansky type III left mandible. (*E–H*) She underwent costochondral rib grafting at age 7 years and was maintained in intermaxillary fixation for 2 weeks thereafter. (*I–M*) At age 8 years, she underwent vertical MDO of her native mandible, and again at age 13 years in order to correct a slight left upward occlusal cant and for planned overcorrection. (*N–R*) She underwent sliding osseous genioplasty to address lip incompetence at age 18 years. (*S, T*) At age 19 years, she underwent completion 2-jaw surgery (*U–Y*) with demonstration of excellent postoperative occlusal relationships.

authors believe costochondral rib grafting remains the gold standard treatment in this patient population, although multiple other autologous grafts have been attempted, including the clavicle and sternoclavicular joint, fibula, iliac bone, and metatarsal bone.[25,61,62] We use costochondral rib graft when there is ramus deficiency and prefer to use the fibula when there is ramus and body deficiency. However, various investigators report unpredictability with costochondral rib grafting for mandibular and TMJ reconstruction, citing graft overgrowth, lack of growth, graft resorption, and ankylosis.[63–69] We have previously published our technique for rib grafting, which is summarized here.[37]

The goals of costochondral grafting for reconstruction in children with Pruzansky type IIB and III mandibles include (1) reconstruction of a new ramus and pseudocondyle; (2) generation of a pseudarthrosis by placing the rib graft in a pocket abutting the cranial base; (3) alignment of the maxillomandibular dental midlines with the midsagittal plane; and (4) correction without overcorrection of the mandibular cant, consequently restoring facial asymmetry with the assumption of ongoing rib growth. Surgical management begins in the orthodontic clinic with preoperative fabrication of an occlusal splint based on predicted final mandibular position and large posterior open bite. Alternatively, the splint may be created intraoperatively using polymethylmethacrylate or virtually planned

using three-dimensional CT technology. We have previously described our technique for costochondral rib grafting, which broadly consists of (1) rib harvest, (2) neofossa creation, and (3) postoperative orthodontic splint therapy (**Fig. 2**).[37]

In our experience, there has been no evidence of graft resorption on postoperative CT imaging, no malunion/nonunion at the level of the rib-mandible junction, 1 patient with TMJ ankylosis, and no requirement for additional interventions in 81.8% of patients.[37] Long-term follow-up suggests that most patients ultimately require additional bone generated via MDO, because the affected mandible rarely grows normally (**Fig. 3**). Consequently, we recommend distraction of the ramus/condyle unit (at the level of the native, nonreconstructed bone) on the affected and potentially unaffected sides. In our series, all patients ultimately undergo completion orthognathic surgery. The patient who developed rib graft ankylosis underwent stacked graft reconstruction, only 1 of which had a cartilaginous cap. We have since abandoned stacked grafts for single costochondral grafts with a small cartilage cap. Importantly, of 5 patients with preoperative tracheostomies, only 1 patient remained cannulated following costochondral rib grafting.

Despite our limited rate of postoperative ankylosis (1 out of 33, 3%), reported rates in the literature range from 19% to 38%, with several investigators suggesting ossification of the

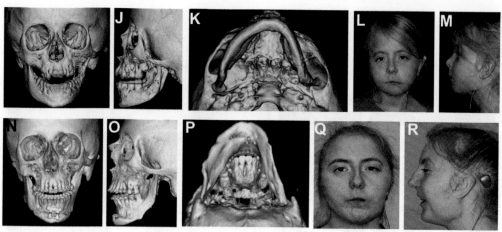

Fig. 4. (continued)

cartilage cap.[63,65,70] We argue that our rare experience with ankylosis can be attributed to (1) small but adequate cartilage cap size of ∼ 0.7 cm, (2) preservation of a periosteal and perichondral sleeve, (3) blunt dissection abutting the cranial base resulting in a pseudoarthrosis rather than a surgically created glenoid fossa, and (4) brief period of immobilization with early joint loading. Moreover, we believe autologous rib grafting before 5 years of age may result in unpredictable outcomes, including increased risk for splitting and poor fixation. In our anecdotal experience with rib grafting of a 2.2-year-old child, he subsequently required further MDO.

Long-term follow-up suggests that most patients undergoing rib grafting eventually require MDO. Although there are a few patients in whom rib grafting alone provides a long-term correction, most fail to grow adequately on the affected side and benefit from subsequent distraction. Distraction of the costochondral rib graft reconstruction requires osteotomy through the native mandible mesial to the graft-mandible junction. Although the literature reports significant variability in distraction outcomes following rib grafting, we believe the location of the osteotomy is crucial in obtaining reliable results.[4,45,71,72] Early reports of distraction osteotomies across the grafted rib were associated with 62.5% complication rates, including 33% nonunions.[45,71] Wan and colleagues[72] reported higher complication rates in patients undergoing distraction osteotomy at the mandible-rib graft junction compared with the native mandible and across the rib graft, which was theoretically substantiated by embryologic differences between endochondral rib and membranous mandible junctional stability. We believe secondary MDO with osteotomy across the native

mandible's membranous bone anecdotally results in more predictable regenerate outcomes with fewer complications (**Fig. 4**).

ORTHOGNATHIC CONSIDERATIONS AT SKELETAL MATURITY

In skeletally mature patients with HFM, conventional 2-jaw movements as previously described by Obwegeser,[23] including BSSO and Le Fort 1 osteotomy with genioplasty, successfully level the occlusal plane and optimize the occlusal relationships.[24] Mandibular osteotomies through regenerate rather than native bone are inherently nontraditional because they may not be based on traditional BSSO landmarks. However, the advent of virtual surgical planning has led to significant contributions in the planning and execution of these challenging maxillomandibular movements. Le Fort 1 segment movements include (1) ipsilateral maxillary vertical elongation with contralateral impaction, (2) horizontal maxillary arch expansion, (3) anterior advancement, and (4) anterior or posterior rotation. Compensatory changes of the contralateral (ie, unaffected) hemimandible include bowing-out and elongation of the mandibular body and ramus. A ramal osteotomy on the contralateral side consequently reduces this asymmetry. Following BSSO, the repositioned mandible results in minimal lateral displacement of the contralateral mandibular body with maximal inferior and lateral displacement of the affected hemimandible (see **Figs. 1** and **4**).

Distraction osteogenesis has provided an immeasurable advancement in the treatment of complex mandibular HFM phenotypes. Without prior distraction, patients undergoing orthognathic correction may present with insufficient bone

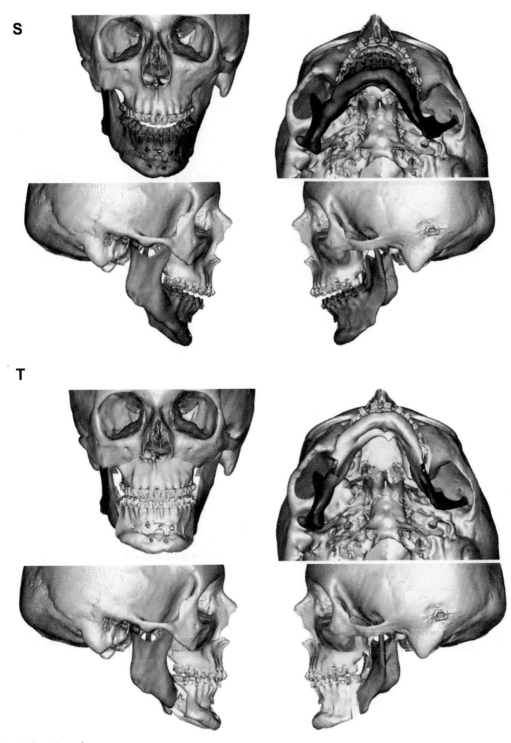

Fig. 4. (*continued*)

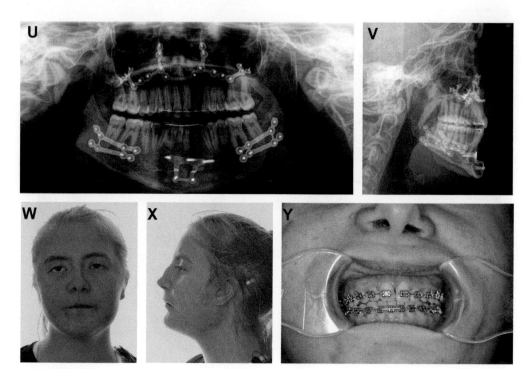

Fig. 4. (continued)

volume to perform osteotomy and mandibular repositioning, prompting the need for an avascular bone graft, which invariably risks infection and malunion. Contrastingly, the authors believe the combination of costochondral rib grafting, interval MDO, and definitive orthognathic surgery through the vascularized regenerate leads to easier, more predictable results compared with those obtained in the pre-MDO era.

CLINICS CARE POINTS

- We primarily use internal, semiburied devices in order to avoid cutaneous scarring and to decrease the likelihood of hardware failure.

- At the time of operative skeletal intervention (eg, mandibular distraction, rib grafting, and orthognathic surgery), we perform fat grafting ad seriatim, which significantly improves the soft tissues over time and frequently obviates more complex augmentation procedures, such as free tissue transfers.

- Since 2012, we have been using a check plate attached to the coronoid to engage the zygomatic arch during active distraction in order to focus the vertical/oblique distraction force downward onto the mandibular ramus instead of upward toward the TMJ and cranial base.

- Long-term follow-up suggests that most patients with Pruzansky type III mandibles ultimately require additional bone generated via MDO, because the affected mandible rarely grows normally following costochondral rib grafting.

- Following rib grafting, we believe secondary MDO with osteotomy across the native mandible's membranous bone anecdotally results in more predictable regenerate outcomes with fewer complications.

- Without prior distraction, patients undergoing orthognathic correction may present with insufficient bone volume to perform osteotomy and mandibular repositioning, prompting the need for an avascular bone graft, which invariably risks infection and malunion.

DISCLOSURE

The authors have nothing to disclose.

REFERENCES

1. Kaban LB, Moses MH, Mulliken JB. Surgical correction of hemifacial microsomia in the growing child. Plast Reconstr Surg 1988;82(1):9–19.

2. Posnick JC. Surgical correction of mandibular hypoplasia in hemifacial microsomia: a personal perspective. J Oral Maxillofac Surg 1998;56(5): 639–50.

3. Ilizarov GA, Devyatov AA, Kamerin VK. Plastic reconstruction of longitudinal bone defects by means of compression and subsequent distraction. Acta Chir Plast 1980;22(1):32–41.

4. Snyder CC, Levine GA, Swanson HM, et al. Mandibular lengthening by gradual distraction. Preliminary report. Plast Reconstr Surg 1973;51(5):506–8.

5. McCarthy JG, Schreiber J, Karp N, et al. Lengthening the human mandible by gradual distraction. Plast Reconstr Surg 1992;89(1):1–8 [discussion 9-10].

6. Cakir-Ozkan N, Eyibilen A, Ozkan F, et al. Stereologic analysis of bone produced by distraction osteogenesis or autogenous bone grafting in mandible. J Craniofac Surg 2010;21(3):735–40.

7. Fisher E, Staffenberg DA, McCarthy JG, et al. Histopathologic and biochemical changes in the muscles affected by distraction osteogenesis of the mandible. Plast Reconstr Surg 1997;99(2):366–71.

8. Hollier LH, Rowe NM, Mackool RJ, et al. Controlled multiplanar distraction of the mandible. Part III: laboratory studies of sagittal (anteroposterior) and horizontal (mediolateral) movements. J Craniofac Surg 2000;11(2):83–95.

9. Mackool RJ, Hopper RA, Grayson BH, et al. Volumetric change of the medial pterygoid following distraction osteogenesis of the mandible: an example of the associated soft-tissue changes. Plast Reconstr Surg 2003;111(6):1804–7.

10. McCarthy JG. The role of distraction osteogenesis in the reconstruction of the mandible in unilateral craniofacial microsomia. Clin Plast Surg 1994; 21(4):625–31.

11. McCarthy JG, Katzen JT, Hopper R, et al. The first decade of mandibular distraction: lessons we have learned. Plast Reconstr Surg 2002;110(7):1704–13.

12. Roth DA, Gosain AK, McCarthy JG, et al. A CT scan technique for quantitative volumetric assessment of the mandible after distraction osteogenesis. Plast Reconstr Surg 1997;99(5):1237–47 [discussion 1248-50].

13. Singh DJ, Glick PH, Bartlett SP. Mandibular deformities: single-vector distraction techniques for a multivector problem. J Craniofac Surg 2009;20(5): 1468–72.

14. van Strijen PJ, Breuning KH, Becking AG, et al. Stability after distraction osteogenesis to lengthen the mandible: results in 50 patients. J Oral Maxillofac Surg 2004;62(3):304–7.

15. Williams JK, Rowe NM, Mackool RJ, et al. Controlled multiplanar distraction of the mandible, Part II: laboratory studies of sagittal (anteroposterior) and vertical (superoinferior) movements. J Craniofac Surg 1998;9(6):504–13.

16. Cohen SR, Simms C, Burstein FD, et al. Alternatives to tracheostomy in infants and children with obstructive sleep apnea. J Pediatr Surg 1999;34(1):182–6 [discussion 187].

17. Denny A, Kalantarian B. Mandibular distraction in neonates: a strategy to avoid tracheostomy. Plast Reconstr Surg 2002;109(3):896–904 [discussion 896-905].

18. Flores RL. Neonatal mandibular distraction osteogenesis. Semin Plast Surg 2014;28(4):199–206.

19. Polley JW, Figueroa AA, Liou EJ, et al. Longitudinal analysis of mandibular asymmetry in hemifacial microsomia. Plast Reconstr Surg 1997;99(2):328–39.

20. Molina F. Mandibular distraction osteogenesis: a clinical experience of the last 17 years. J Craniofac Surg 2009;20(Suppl 2):1794–800.

21. Polley JW, Figueroa AA. Distraction osteogenesis: its application in severe mandibular deformities in hemifacial microsomia. J Craniofac Surg 1997;8(5): 422–30.

22. Rune B, Selvik G, Sarnas KV, et al. Growth in hemifacial microsomia studied with the aid of roentgen stereophotogrammetry and metallic implants. Cleft Palate J 1981;18(2):128–46.

23. Poswillo D. Otomandibular deformity: pathogenesis as a guide to reconstruction. J Maxillofac Surg 1974;2(2–3):64–72.

24. Obwegeser HL. Correction of the skeletal anomalies of oto-mandibular dysostosis. J Maxillofac Surg 1974;2(2–3):73–92.

25. Dingman RO, Grabb WC. Reconstruction of both mandibular condyles with metatarsal bone grafts. Plast Reconstr Surg 1964;34:441–51.

26. Converse JM, Horowitz SL, Coccaro PJ, et al. The corrective treatment of the skeletal asymmetry in hemifacial microsomia. Plast Reconstr Surg 1973; 52(3):221–32.

27. Munro IR, Phillips JH, Griffin G. Growth after construction of the temporomandibular joint in children with hemifacial microsomia. Cleft Palate J 1989; 26(4):303–11.

28. Murray JE, Kaban LB, Mulliken JB. Analysis and treatment of hemifacial microsomia. Plast Reconstr Surg 1984;74(2):186–99.

29. Lauritzen C, Munro IR, Ross RB. Classification and treatment of hemifacial microsomia. Scand J Plast Reconstr Surg 1985;19(1):33–9.

30. Weichman KE, Jacobs J, Patel P, et al. Early distraction for mild to moderate unilateral craniofacial microsomia: long-term follow-up, outcomes, and

Recommendations. Plast Reconstr Surg 2017; 139(4):941e–53e.

31. Birgfeld C, Heike C. Craniofacial microsomia. Clin Plast Surg 2019;46(2):207–21.

32. Grayson BH, McCormick S, Santiago PE, et al. Vector of device placement and trajectory of mandibular distraction. J Craniofac Surg 1997;8(6):473–80 [discussion 472-81].

33. Kitai N, Murakami S, Takashima M, et al. Evaluation of temporomandibular joint in patients with hemifacial microsomia. Cleft Palate Craniofac J 2004; 41(2):157–62.

34. Molina F, Ortiz Monasterio F. Mandibular elongation and remodeling by distraction: a farewell to major osteotomies. Plast Reconstr Surg 1995;96(4): 825–40 [discussion 822-41].

35. Padwa BL, Zaragoza SM, Sonis AL. Proximal segment displacement in mandibular distraction osteogenesis. J Craniofac Surg 2002;13(2):293–6 [discussion 297].

36. Zhang RS, Lin LO, Hoppe IC, et al. Early mandibular distraction in craniofacial microsomia and need for orthognathic correction at skeletal maturity: a comparative long-term follow-up study. Plast Reconstr Surg 2018;142(5):1285–93.

37. Tahiri Y, Chang CS, Tuin J, et al. Costochondral grafting in craniofacial microsomia. Plast Reconstr Surg 2015;135(2):530–41.

38. Argamaso RV. Glossopexy for upper airway obstruction in Robin sequence. Cleft Palate Craniofac J 1992;29(3):232–8.

39. Cohen MM Jr. The Robin anomalad - its nonspecificity and associated syndromes. J Oral Surg 1976; 34(7):587–93.

40. Rachmiel A, Manor R, Peled M, et al. Intraoral distraction osteogenesis of the mandible in hemifacial microsomia. J Oral Maxillofac Surg 2001;59(7): 728–33.

41. McCarthy JG, Hopper RA, Hollier LH Jr, et al. Molding of the regenerate in mandibular distraction: clinical experience. Plast Reconstr Surg 2003;112(5): 1239–46.

42. Suh J, Choi TH, Baek SH, et al. Mandibular distraction in unilateral craniofacial microsomia: longitudinal results until the completion of growth. Plast Reconstr Surg 2013;132(5):1244–52.

43. van Strijen PJ, Breuning KH, Becking AG, et al. Complications in bilateral mandibular distraction osteogenesis using internal devices. Oral Surg Oral Med Oral Pathol Oral Radiol Endod 2003;96(4): 392–7.

44. Verlinden CR, van de Vijfeijken SE, Tuinzing DB, et al. Complications of mandibular distraction osteogenesis for acquired deformities: a systematic review of the literature. Int J Oral Maxillofac Surg 2015;44(8):956–64.

45. Stelnicki EJ, Stucki-McCormick SU, Rowe N, et al. Remodeling of the temporomandibular joint following mandibular distraction osteogenesis in the transverse dimension. Plast Reconstr Surg 2001;107(3):647–58.

46. McCormick SU, McCarthy JG, Grayson BH, et al. Effect of mandibular distraction on the temporomandibular joint: Part 1, Canine study. J Craniofac Surg 1995;6(5):358–63.

47. McCormick SU, Grayson BH, McCarthy JG, et al. Effect of mandibular distraction on the temporomandibular joint: Part 2, Clinical study. J Craniofac Surg 1995;6(5):364–7.

48. Dec W, Peltomaki T, Warren SM, et al. The importance of vector selection in preoperative planning of unilateral mandibular distraction. Plast Reconstr Surg 2008;121(6):2084–92 [discussion 2084-93].

49. Gunbay T, Akay MC, Aras A, et al. Effects of transmandibular symphyseal distraction on teeth, bone, and temporomandibular joint. J Oral Maxillofac Surg 2009;67(10):2254–65.

50. Shakir S, Naran S, Lowe KM, et al. Balancing distraction forces in the mandible: Newton's third law of distraction. Plast Reconstr Surg Glob Open 2018;6(9):e1856..

51. Kearns GJ, Padwa BL, Mulliken JB, et al. Progression of facial asymmetry in hemifacial microsomia. Plast Reconstr Surg 2000;105(2):492–8.

52. Dufton LM, Speltz ML, Kelly JP, et al. Psychosocial outcomes in children with hemifacial microsomia. J Pediatr Psychol 2011;36(7):794–805.

53. Khetani MA, Collett BR, Speltz ML, et al. Health-related quality of life in children with hemifacial microsomia: parent and child perspectives. J Dev Behav Pediatr 2013;34(9):661–8.

54. Meazzini MC, Mazzoleni F, Gabriele C, et al. Mandibular distraction osteogenesis in hemifacial microsomia: long-term follow-up. J Craniomaxillofac Surg 2005;33(6):370–6.

55. Bartlett SP. No evidence for long-term effectiveness of early osteodistraction in hemifacial microsomia. Plast Reconstr Surg 2010;125(5):1567–8.

56. Nagy K, Kuijpers-Jagtman AM, Mommaerts MY. No evidence for long-term effectiveness of early osteodistraction in hemifacial microsomia. Plast Reconstr Surg 2009;124(6):2061–71.

57. Ascenço AS, Balbinot P, Junior IM, et al. Mandibular distraction in hemifacial microsomia is not a permanent treatment: a long-term evaluation. J Craniofac Surg 2014;25(2):352–4.

58. Pluijmers BI, Caron CJ, Dunaway DJ, et al. Mandibular reconstruction in the growing patient with unilateral craniofacial microsomia: a systematic review. Int J Oral Maxillofac Surg 2014;43(3):286–95.

59. Pluijmers BI, Caron C, van de Lande LS, et al. Surgical correction of craniofacial microsomia: evaluation of interventions in 565 patients at three major

craniofacial units. Plast Reconstr Surg 2019;143(5): 1467–76.

60. Gillies H. Plastic surgery of the face. London: Oxford University Press; 1920.

61. Ware WH, Taylor RC. Cartilaginous growth centers transplanted to replace mandibular condyles in monkeys. J Oral Surg 1966;24(1):33–43.

62. Snyder CC, Benson AK, Slater PV. Construction of the temporomandibular joint by transplanting the autogenous sternoclavicular joint. Southampt Med J 1971;64(7):807–14.

63. Guyuron B, Lasa CI Jr. Unpredictable growth pattern of costochondral graft. Plast Reconstr Surg 1992; 90(5):880–6 [discussion 887-9].

64. Lindqvist C, Jokinen J, Paukku P, et al. Adaptation of autogenous costochondral grafts used for temporo-mandibular joint reconstruction: a long-term clinical and radiologic follow-up. J Oral Maxillofac Surg 1988;46(6):465–70.

65. Lindqvist C, Pihakari A, Tasanen A, et al. Autogenous costochondral grafts in temporo-mandibular joint arthroplasty. A survey of 66 arthroplasties in 60 patients. J Maxillofac Surg 1986;14(3):143–9.

66. MacIntosh RB, Henny FA. A spectrum of application of autogenous costochondral grafts. J Maxillofac Surg 1977;5(4):257–67.

67. Mulliken JB, Ferraro NF, Vento AR. A retrospective analysis of growth of the constructed condyle-ramus in children with hemifacial microsomia. Cleft Palate J 1989;26(4):312–7.

68. Ware WH, Brown SL. Growth centre transplantation to replace mandibular condyles. J Maxillofac Surg 1981;9(1):50–8.

69. Ware WH, Taylor RC. Growth center transplantation to replace damaged mandibular condyles. J Am Dent Assoc 1966;73(1):128–37.

70. Saeed N, Hensher R, McLeod N, et al. Reconstruction of the temporomandibular joint autogenous compared with alloplastic. Br J Oral Maxillofac Surg 2002;40(4):296–9.

71. Corcoran J, Hubli EH, Salyer KE. Distraction osteogenesis of costochondral neomandibles: a clinical experience. Plast Reconstr Surg 1997;100(2): 311–5 [discussion 316-7].

72. Wan DC, Taub PJ, Allam KA, et al. Distraction osteogenesis of costocartilaginous rib grafts and treatment algorithm for severely hypoplastic mandibles. Plast Reconstr Surg 2011;127(5):2005–13.

Cleft Lip and Palate
LeFort I Distraction with Halo and Hybrid Internal Maxillary Distractors

Alvaro A. Figueroa, DDS, MS[a],*, Aaron D. Figueroa, DDS, FACS[b],
Richard G. Burton, DDS, MS, FACS[b], Christina Tragos, MD[a]

KEYWORDS

• Distraction osteogenesis • Hybrid distractors • Rigid external distraction • Internal distraction
• Cleft maxillary hypoplasia • Le Fort I • Maxillary advancement

KEY POINTS

- Distraction osteogenesis is a viable treatment option for patients with a cleft associated with severe maxillary retrusion.
- External and internal devices can be utilized.
- The external distraction device is utilized in cases with severe maxillary hypoplasia secondary to a cleft condition greater than 8 to 10 mm, with paranasal and malar deficiencies associated with severe scarring, existing pharyngeal flap, or previously failed advancement with a traditional approach.
- The main advantages of external maxillary distraction include large advancements and ease of vector control and adjustability during the activation process. The technique does not require a second surgical procedure for its removal. The requirement of an external halo and framework is its main disadvantage, although when properly utilized, it is an effective treatment option for otherwise challenging cases.
- Hybrid internal maxillary distractors are utilized in moderate cases of cleft-related maxillary hypoplasia. Virtual surgical planning and 3-dimensional design and manufacturing facilitates accuracy in device placement and vector selection. The hybrid intraoral distractor described in this article does not require a second operation for removal. A high maxillary osteotomy is difficult to use as the plate supporting the distractor, is anchored high in the maxillary/ malar bones, limiting it's placement.

INTRODUCTION

The conventional treatment of dentofacial deformities in patients with cleft includes both orthodontic treatment and orthognathic surgery (OGS). The key surgical procedures required for the correction of these conditions include the Le Fort I osteotomy, sagittal split mandibular ramus osteotomies, and on occasion a genioplasty utilizing rigid fixation techniques. With these approaches, successful and predictable correction is usually obtained. However, the use of these techniques in patients with severe maxillary hypoplasia, either related to clefts or syndromic deformities, may fall short of expectations, as this particular group of patients includes additional challenges.

In patients with a cleft presenting with severe maxillary hypoplasia, marked mandibular excess, deficiency or asymmetry, a 2-jaw approach must

[a] Division of Plastic Surgery, Department of Surgery, Rush Craniofacial Center, Rush University Medical Center, 1725 West Harrison Street, Suite 425 POB 1, Chicago, IL 60612, USA; [b] Oral and Maxillofacial Surgery, Hospital Dentistry Institute, University of Iowa Hospitals and Clinics, 200 Hawkins Drive, Iowa City, IA 52242, USA
* Corresponding author. Figueroa Orthodontics, 1075 Gage Street, Winnetka, IL 60093.
E-mail address: alvarofigueroadds@gmail.com

Clin Plastic Surg 48 (2021) 391–405
https://doi.org/10.1016/j.cps.2021.02.002

be undertaken. The advantage of this surgical-orthodontic approach is that with 1 operation, the reconstructive team can provide the patient with close to ideal occlusion and markedly improved function and aesthetics. At the time of OGS, the surgeon has the added advantage of access to the nasal cavity to address the deviated septum, large turbinates, and residual nasal floor defects. In addition, the alveolar segments (when separated) can be approximated in such a way to facilitate the closure of nasolabial fistulas with locally elevated flaps while concurrently reconstructing the alveolar cleft with bone graft. The 2-jaw OGS approach can limit the extent of the maxillary advancement. However, it is recognized that patients undergoing OGS in which multiple segments are used present a higher risk to stability and surgical complications.[1] These complications may include instability of bony translation or loss of individual teeth or bone segment loss secondary to vascular compromise. It has been reported that the risks for complications after Le Fort I maxillary surgery are about 4% in patients without a cleft. However, for patients with orofacial clefts and other deformities, this increases to about 25%.[2] The maxillary advancement in patients with a cleft can be unstable, and the tendency for long-term relapse is high compared with that in noncleft patients.[3–6] In addition, patients with orofacial clefts have mandibles that are of normal size or slightly smaller.[7] For this reason, in many patients in whom the maxilla is extremely hypoplastic, the surgeon may choose to sagittally correct both the maxilla and mandible during OGS, thereby increasing the complexity of the operation.

Conventional orthognathic surgical procedures in this challenging group of patients should be done with the utmost care, and alternative treatments should be explored. In 1992, McCarthy and colleagues[8] introduced the use of distraction osteogenesis (DO) in the craniofacial skeleton. Since that time, the technique has been applied to all of the bones of the craniofacial skeleton as detailed in this issue of Clinics in Plastic Surgery. It is now the treatment of choice for patients with craniofacial conditions such as Crouzon syndrome and Apert syndrome[9–16] as well as hemifacial microsomia.[8,17–20] In addition, the technique has been successfully applied to patients with severe maxillary hypoplasia secondary to orofacial clefts.[21–26]

Molina and Ortiz-Monasterio[27] were the first to report maxillary distraction osteogenesis by means of elastic traction with an orthopedic face mask. Although this approach appeared promising, the results were disappointing. An external cranially fixed halo (rigid external distractor –RED) was developed as a point of anchorage to advance the maxilla and midface. The maxilla is connected with surgical wires through the dentition by an intraoral splint with removable traction hooks to the halo device. This distraction system utilizes both bone and dental anchorage[28] and provides stable maxillary advancement in patients with severe hypoplasia of the lower midface. In addition the technique is relatively simple, with low morbidity, predictable, and has shown stable long-term results.[21,22,25,29]

The benefits of distraction for correction of severe maxillary hypoplasia in patients with a cleft are well appreciated, but the benefits and limitations of internal versus external devices remain topics of active debate. Hybrid internal maxillary distractors (HIMXDs) can be used to correct deficiencies at or just above the Le Fort I level. They can be more technically demanding to place because of limitations in bone stock and surgical exposure. The benefits of the HIMXDs include: greater rigidity of the hybrid device leading to an earlier return to function and ease of maintaining the devices during the consolidation phase Furthermore, the device described in this article does not require a secondary procedure for removal. Cases requiring major advancements and significant control in 3 dimensions are better suited for RED. Recommendations for case selection are summarized in **Table 1**.

The surgical protocol for maxillary distraction utilizing a RED device and HIMXDs will be described.

PRESURGICAL ORTHODONTIC ALIGNMENT OF THE DENTITION AND THE FABRICATION OF A TOOTH-SUPPORTED INTRAORAL SPLINT
Presurgical Orthodontics

Ideally, all patients are prepared like any other patient undergoing OGS. Orthodontic treatment aligns the dentition and restores dental arch form. In patients with primary or transitional dentition, it may not be possible to ideally prepare the dental arches because of the presence of deciduous teeth. If early maxillary advancement is deemed necessary because of airway or psychosocial issues, the orthodontic alignment can be completed afterward. However, patients with a cleft who undergo early maxillary distraction are unlikely to undergo subsequent anterior maxillary growth and will often require finishing distraction or OGS at the time of facial maturity. Ideally, orthodontic alignment and arch coordination should be done before this procedure. The authors' preference is to delay maxillary distraction in patients with a cleft until facial growth is completed.

Table 1
Indications for the use of rigid external distractor and hybrid internal maxillary distractor

Recommendations	RED Yes	RED No	HIMXD Yes	HIMXD No
1. Intact neurocranium	✓		n/a	n/a
2. Adequate dentition	✓		✓	
3. Maxillary edentulous patients	✓			✓
4. Primary and transitional dentition	✓			✓
5. Small mouth aperture	✓			✓
6. Ideally well aligned arches with orthodontic appliances	✓		✓	
7. Requires a dental borne splint and/or orthodontic appliances for fixation of the device	✓		✓	
8. Requires an occlusal splint		✓	?	
9. Mandible with normal size and position	✓		✓	
10. Maxillary deficiency with overjet of 8–10 mm or more	✓		✓	
11. Maxillary deficiency with overjet of 10 mm or more	✓			✓
12. Maxillary deficiency with severe malar and infraorbital deficiency	✓			✓
13. Severe palatal and lip scarring from previous surgeries	✓		✓	
14. Pharyngeal flap	✓		✓	
15. Severe airway issues related to maxillary hypoplasia	✓		✓	
16. Ideal time late adolescence, can be done in growing patients with the understanding that repeat surgery might be required	✓		✓	
17. Virtual surgical planning recommended	?		✓	
18. Can be done before finishing OGS	✓		✓	
19. Can be done in combination with OGS	✓		✓	

Presurgical Planning

Thorough facial and intraoral examination with speech velopharyngeal evaluation is performed in all patients. Traditional cephalometry (with hand tracing), digital cephalometry, or 3-dimensional virtual surgical planning can be used. The planning radiograph or 3-dimensional scan is obtained with the lips in repose and the teeth in full occlusion. If the patient has vertical maxillary hypoplasia, the clinician should determine the degree of vertical overclosure, as a radiographic record taken in an overclosed position will disrupt accurate presurgical planning in several ways (**Fig. 1**A). First, the predicted maxillary advancement will be greater than what will be required. Second, the upper lip form will be abnormal in the study photographs and radiographs. Third, an incorrect mandibular occlusal plane measurement will be recorded, leading to an inappropriate maxillary distraction vector. If the patient exhibits overclosure, the radiographic record is taken with the mandible in rest position and the lips in repose. To assure accuracy of the mandibular position, a central relation registration bite is obtained and used while the necessary facial photographs and radiographs are taken (**Fig. 1**B). The radiographs are traced to determine the mandibular occlusal plane and the distraction vector of the maxilla. The maxillary occlusal plane is drawn and compared with the mandibular plane relative to Frankfort Horizontal Plane. The difference between the two is the desired vector (**Fig. 1**C). It is also critical to know the location of the approximate center of mass of the bone segment to be distracted.[30,31] In the sagittal plane, force vectors passing above, through, or below the center of mass will rotate the segment in a clockwise, straight, or counterclockwise direction respectively. In the maxilla, the approximate centers of mass and resistance are located above the mesial root of the first molar.[30–32] The position of the eyelets on the external traction hooks is lateral to the alar cartilages bilaterally and at or above the level of the nasal aperture or palatal plane. It is important to record tooth shown in repose and the maxillary dental midline relative to the skeletal midline. If they are different, the distractor device needs to be differentially activated to correct the midline. When utilizing the HIMXD, the midline

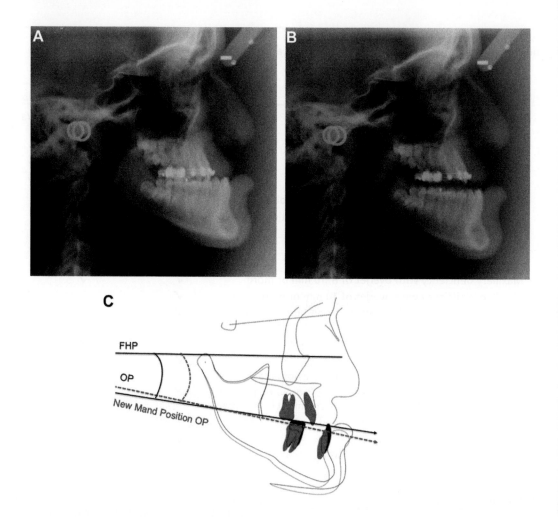

FHP to New Mand Position OP° (-) FHP to OP° = Distractor Vector°

Fig. 1. Cephalometric radiographs in occlusion (A) and at rest (B). Note improved soft tissue relation at rest. Calculation of the maxillary distraction vector (C).

can be corrected at the time of device placement with fine adjustment in yaw position, then at the end of activation with differential final extension of the right and left devices. The RED and HIMXD systems allow for correction of the inferior pitch, as well as yaw. The RED system also has the capacity for a degree of roll correction. These adjustments are done by differentially activating the distraction screws, repositioning the horizontal distractor bar toward the right or left, then differentially altering the superior or inferior position of the distraction screws mounted on the horizontal bar combined with the use of interarch elastics (**Fig. 2**).

Intraoral Splint

For both external and internal distraction devices, the authors use 0.040″ stainless steel wire

conformed to the labial and palatal aspects of the dental arch and soldered to the first molar bands (**Fig. 3**A–C). If desired, additional teeth can be incorporated for added retention of the appliance. In younger patients undergoing RED distraction, maxillary second primary molars can be used to support the splint if they have adequate root support and are stable. The RED splint has 2 square tubes just medial to the oral commissures that are used to secure 2 removable rectangular hooks, which connect the intraoral splint to distraction screws mounted onto the RED system.[33,34] The height of the traction hooks is such that they are level to or above the palatal plane for vector control (see **Fig. 2**; **Fig. 3**D).

The splint for the HIMXD has multiple hooks on right and left posterior aspects of the labial wire for eventual fixation of the inferior arm of the

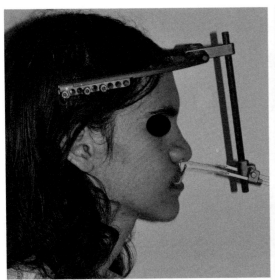
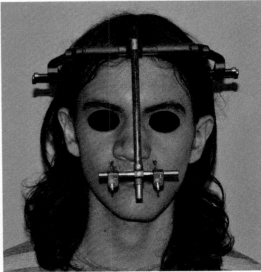

Fig. 2. Patient wearing a RED appliance on profile (*left*) and frontal views (*right*). Note proper placement of appliance in all planes of space. Note the horizontal bar supporting the distraction screws. To adjust the distraction vectors, the horizontal bar can be moved up, down, right, and left. The distraction screws have vertical and lateral adjustments also.

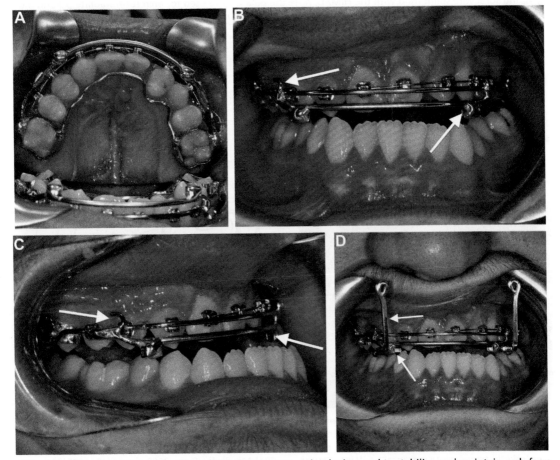

Fig. 3. Intraoral wire splint used with the RED device. Note palatal wire used to stabilize and maintain arch form (*A*). Note the facemask hooks and the rectangular tubes to receive the external distraction hooks (*arrows*) (*B, C*). Distraction external hooks in position (*upper arrow*) into the rectangular tubes (*lower arrow*) (*D*).

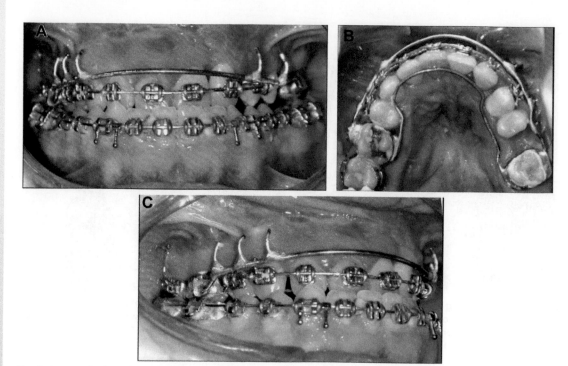

Fig. 4. Intraoral wire splint used with the HIMXD; note the palatal wire used for arch form stability (*A*) and multiple soldered hooks to wire the lower arms of the distractor (*B, C*).

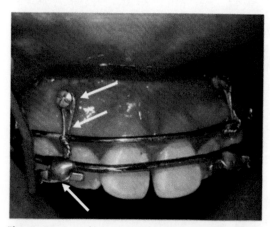

Fig. 5. Bone anchor screws (*upper arrow*) between the roots of the lateral incisors and canines. Anterior part of the intraoral splint secured with suspension wires (*middle arrow*). Note extraoral hook into square tube of the splint (*lower arrow*).

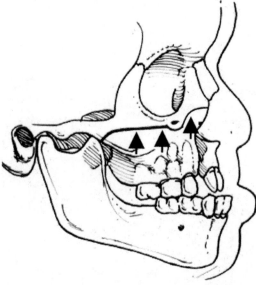

Fig. 6. Diagram illustrating a high Le Fort I osteotomy extending to the malar bone and lateral nasal wall to improve malar and paranasal deficiencies. (*From* Figueroa AA, Polley JW. Clinical controversies in oral and maxillofacial surgery: Part two. External versus internal distraction osteogenesis for the management of severe maxillary hypoplasia: external distraction. J Oral Maxillofac Surg. 2008 Dec;66(12):2598-604; with permission.)

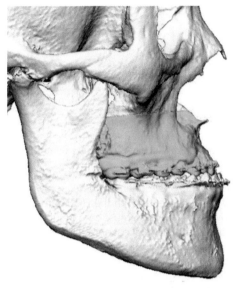
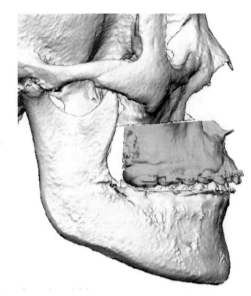

Fig. 7. 3-dimensional planning a case for maxillary advancement using HIMXD device. Left preoperative, and right planned maxillary position with correction of anterior crossbite.

distractor device[35] (**Fig. 4**). The palatal wire is required to maintain the arch form during the distraction process. The HIMXD can also be secured with wires to an occlusal splint secured to the maxillary teeth used for stability and guidance during the distraction process (See **Fig. 9** right).

SURGERY (RIGID EXTERNAL DISTRACTOR)
Securing the Intraoral Splint

At the time of surgery, the surgeon additionally secures the intraoral splint by placing 2 orthodontic bone anchorage screws (BAS) between the root apices of the maxillary lateral incisor and canine bilaterally and suspends it anteriorly with surgical wires (**Fig. 5**).

Osteotomy

A complete Le Fort I osteotomy with septal and pterygomaxillary disjunction is completed. When the RED technique is used, the maxilla is not down fractured, as it is usually done during conventional OGS, but the surgeon must assure that the maxillary bone is completely free. In cases in which RED is used, a complete downfracture will result in the vertical displacement of the maxilla with no bone to bone contact in the osteotomy. When using the RED system, it is difficult to correct the vertical maxillary displacement secondary to the downfracture. The height of the osteotomy can be modified to include the base of the malar bones circumventing the inferior orbital foramen. In this way, the paranasal, malar, and infraorbital

regions can be significantly improved, and the dental roots can be avoided in younger patients (**Fig. 6**). In patients for whom the HIMXD device is used, a complete typical downfracture can be performed, as the maxilla will be firmly held in close bone contact with the cranial aspect of the osteotomy by the distractor attached to the bone above the osteotomy and below the dentition or dental splint. The downfracture allows removal of

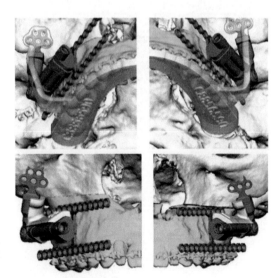

Fig. 8. Initial position of virtual distractors after osteotomy (top). Drill guides in place for accurate positioning and bending of the supporting plate (bottom). 3-dimensional virtual plan allows accurate placement and vector of the distractors.

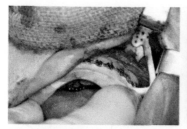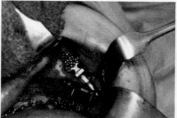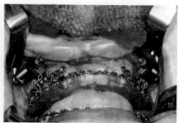

Fig. 9. Intraoperatively occlusal supported left drill guide in place (*left*). Plate supporting HIMXD (*center*). Distractors in place (*right*). Note wiring of the distractor directly to the orthodontic appliances and occlusal splint (*right*).

potential bony interferences and intraoperative correction of a significant midline deviation. A high maxillary osteotomy is difficult to use as the plate supporting the distractor, is anchored high in the maxillary/ malar bones, limiting it's placement.

Distractor Placement

Rigid external distractor

After closure of the intraoral incision, the halo is aligned in the sagittal and transverse planes assuring sufficient clearance from the skull. The halo is secured to the cranium using specialized safety cranial pins, usually 3 to 4 per side. It is not necessary to shave any hair, as the assistant can digitally separate the hair as the pin is secured in place.

The pins are initially turned manually and once the halo position is confirmed, the screws are carefully hand tightened with the RED surgical kit screwdriver. The surgeon must be careful to position these pins on the thickest part of the temporal/ parietal bones, usually about 3 to 5 cm above the earlobe. The halo is usually positioned slightly upward to the Frankfort plane (15–20°). The vertical anterior bar used to secure the distraction screws is placed midline and 3 to 5 cm anterior to the facial plane (see **Fig. 2**). The remainder of the distraction system is assembled in the clinic 3 to 7 days after surgery. In this way, the anesthesiologist does not have any interference with masking and ventilation of the patient in the postoperative period.

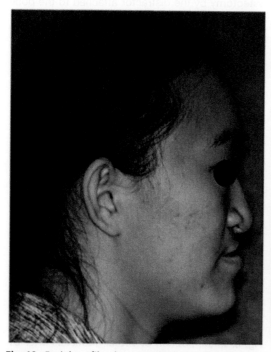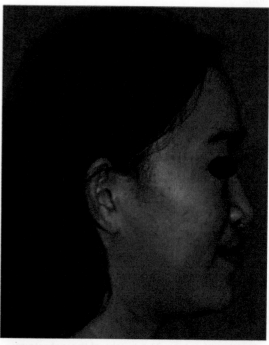

Fig. 10. Facial profile photographs from a female patient with repaired bilateral cleft lip and palate with secondary maxillary hypoplasia treated with distraction using HIMXD. Note significant profile changes and improved maxillary position and occlusion after treatment. **Figs. 7–9** illustrate her planning and intraoperative photographs.

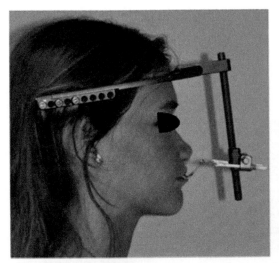
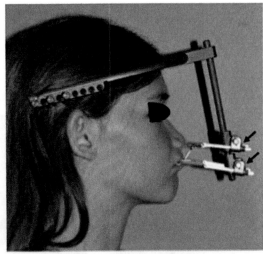

Fig. 11. Patient undergoing maxillary advancement with RED. Note single horizontal bar at the beginning of distraction and a double bar toward the end to exert additional force.

Hybrid internal maxillary distractors

For the internal system, careful virtual surgical planning is preferred, as it will assist in vector planning and accurate placement of the bone and dental arms of the device using positioning and drilling surgical guides. A guiding occlusal splint can be used to avoid bone and dental interferences during distraction and to guide the dentition into the planned occlusion[36] (**Figs. 7–10**).

Postoperative Management

Patients are placed on a liquid diet 24 hours after surgery and a progressive soft diet afterward. After

the desired latency period is completed, the distraction part of the RED device is assembled in the clinical setting without discomfort to the patient. The removable traction hooks are attached to the square tubes on the intraoral splint with light gauge orthodontic wire or heavy orthodontic elastomeric O rings (see **Figs. 3** and **5**). Soft surgical wire (24 gauge) is twisted and utilized to connect the traction hooks to the distraction screws mounted to the halo. The distraction screws are moved up or down on the vertical bar until the appropriate vector is obtained (see **Fig. 2**). With the HIMXD system, the devices are ready to start

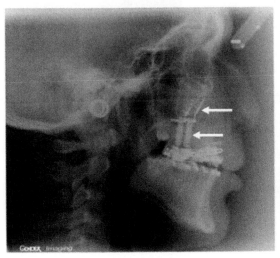
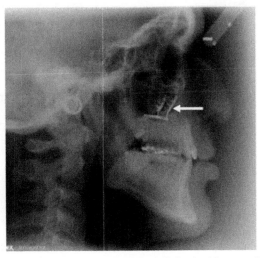

Fig. 12. Lateral radiographs of a patient undergoing maxillary advancement with HIMXD (*left, double arrows*) and after distractor removal (*right*). Note the supporting plate left behind (*single arrow*).

the active phase of distraction at the time of placement so that no additional visits are required until initiation of distraction.

The rate of activation is usually between 1 to 2 mm per day, depending on the severity of maxillary hypoplasia. Most patients are corrected within 2 weeks, and afterward they enter the phase of consolidation that is usually 8 to 12 weeks, depending on the stability of the maxilla. If the maxilla is mobile and the patient would like the

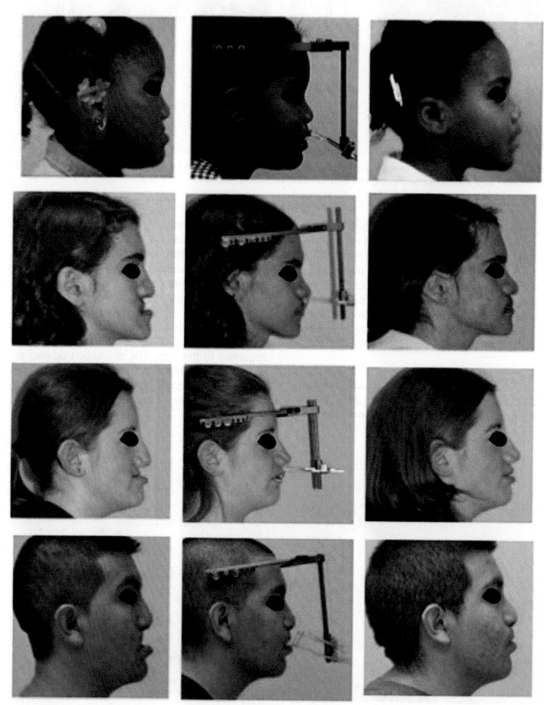

Fig. 13. Profile photographs from 4 patients with clefts who underwent maxillary advancement with RED. Note severity of the maxillary deficiency and marked improvement after treatment.

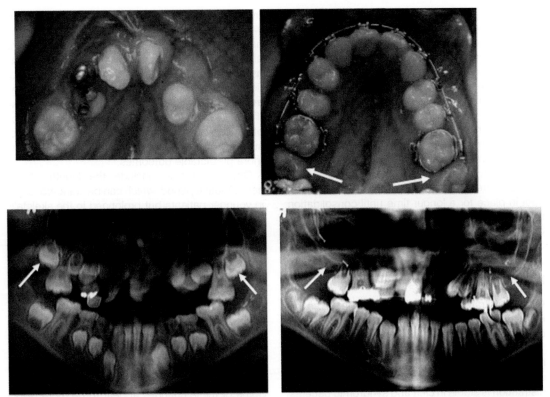

Fig. 14. Maxillary intraoral occlusal photos of a patient with a repaired bilateral cleft lip and palate and severe maxillary hypoplasia before (*top left*) and after (*top right*) undergoing maxillary advancement with RED. Note collapsed and crowded arch before treatment and eruption of second M (*arrows*) after distraction and orthodontics. The pretreatment panoramic radiograph (*bottom left*) demonstrates lack of space for the maxillary second M (*arrows*), and after treatment (*bottom right*) the second M have spontaneously erupted with the development of additional bone space posterior to them (*arrows*).

halo removed, the patient is returned to the operating room to remove the halo, and the maxilla is fixated with resorbable or titanium plates. Resorbable plates are recommended for younger patients, as they are growing and likely will require additional surgical treatment. On occasion, some patients demonstrate resistance to advancement toward the end of the distraction period; in these situations, a second bar with distraction screws is mounted on the vertical bar of the distractor, and 2 additional distraction screws are mounted and directly connected to the intraoral splint with surgical wires. This provides a 4-point traction system that is significantly stronger, which can overcome soft tissue resistance (**Fig. 11**).

Once it is determined that the maxilla is consolidated, the halo system is removed in the clinical setting without the need for local anesthesia. In apprehensive young children, it is advisable to remove the halo in the operating room under light sedation. The HIMXD devices also do not require additional general anesthesia for removal. The distractors are removed in the office setting from their intraoral attachments, and the set screw is removed from the vestibular access, allowing for removal of the device with the exception of the zygomatic bone plate, which can be left in place (**Fig. 12**). The devices can be removed in the operating room if it is necessary to perform minor improvements in occlusion and maxillary position. This allows for refracturing the Le Fort I osteotomy for final positioning with rigid fixation.

Retention

Once the halo and the traction hooks attached to the intraoral splint are removed, an orthopedic face mask is attached to the intraoral splint. This face mask is used at night to promote additional retention. The face mask is used with elastic force of 400 to 500 g and applied for 6 to 8 weeks or until the clinician notes that the maxilla is stable in its new position. At this point, the intraoral splint can be removed and orthodontic treatment with Class

III elastics is continued to finalize the occlusion. In patients in whom the maxillary advancement is extreme, clinicians might note mobility of the maxillary bone even after 3 months of halo and face mask consolidation. If the motion of the maxilla is uncomfortable for the patient, the surgeon may elect to place rigid fixation plates to further secure the maxillary bone. It is of interest that in patients with delayed consolidation of the maxilla, the motion of the bone is usually in the vertical and transverse planes, and there is minimal or no tendency for anterior/posterior movement. If HIMXD system is used, the intact device can be kept in place for a longer time until consolidation is complete and patients do not require a period of face mask retention. After removal, the patient continues with final orthodontic treatment.

DISCUSSION

Fig. 13 illustrates 4 patients with clefts in whom the RED system had been used to correct severe cleft-related maxillary hypoplasia.

The long-term stability after maxillary distraction in patients with a cleft and patients with syndromic conditions has been well documented.[22] Maxillary distraction is stable in cleft and syndromic patients through bone generation in the pterygomaxillary osteotomy. This area is known to be critical to stability after maxillary and midface advancements. The bony generate in this area has been characterized as dense lamellar bone through histologic and radiographic analysis.[22,37] The generation of new bone in the posterior maxillary region not only provides stability but also an additional bony foundation for dental eruption (**Fig. 14**).

As experienced is gained with distraction techniques, application of the system to conditions challenging for conventional OGS may be better appreciated by the surgical team. In addition, the technique has been used in combination with conventional orthognathic surgery in severely affected patients with a cleft. In some instances, because of directional movement limitations of the distraction technique, it becomes necessary to finalize treatment with conventional OGS. The benefit of combining the 2 techniques resides in the attainment of most correction through distraction and with the conventional OGS, the surgeon refines the position of the bones and the occlusion, usually with minor, safe, predictable and skeletally stable movements.

It is the opinion of the authors that several challenges remain for patients requiring distraction for the correction of maxillary and midface hypoplasia. Some of these challenges are technical, while others are related to the patient's response to treatment. Case selection concerning patients who will benefit from OGS, distraction, or combination approaches is critical. Device selection is also important.[38] Internal systems are appealing as they are concealed, but they have some limitations concerning surgical placement, adjustment, and degree of advancement. Internal devices like the HIMXD, can be oriented with the assistance of 3-dimensional design and manufacturing, assuring accurate and simplified placement and more predictable outcomes.[36]

Other challenges include the length of the consolidation period, which can be standard length in younger patients but prolonged in the skeletally mature patient. If the maxilla is significantly advanced, the time required for consolidation can be long and impractical. For this reason, close cooperation between clinicians and researchers to decrease this important stage in the distraction process is critical. Recent advancements in the use or delivery of bone morphogenetic proteins, growth factors, and the use of ultrasound and laser therapy may address this concern.[39–43]

The authors believe that more studies are needed regarding the soft tissue response to the gradual movement of bone within the lower midface. Some of these changes appear to be more favorable utilizing distraction techniques, such as an improved lip and nose position after maxillary distraction when compared with conventional orthognathic surgery.[44,45] In addition, the response of the velopharyangeal tissues appears to be more favorable through maxillary distraction compared with acute advancement during OGS.[46,47]

Finally, little is known about the patient's emotional and psychological response to gradual midface distraction compared with acute maxillary repositioning. How much do the distraction devices interfere in the psychosocial well-being of the patient[48] and what is the impact of patient participation in the improvement of their condition on their psychosocial well-being and development when dealing with a challenging facial difference? At the time of this publication, this questions remain unanswered but are important areas of future investigation.

SUMMARY

Distraction osteogenesis has been applied throughout craniofacial skeleton with remarkable success. The technique of RED for maxillary distraction in patients with a cleft or craniofacial syndromes can be simple, predictable, and stable. The clinical knowledge available at this time indicates that distraction is a viable intervention for patients with severe maxillary hypoplasia that in the past was a challenge for traditional OGS techniques. For conditions of lesser severity, hybrid internal maxillary distractors can be a useful option. With current 3-dimensional planning and manufacturing technology, precise placement, ease of application, adjustability, and predictability of results can be achieved. The use of distraction techniques does not preclude the combination of traditional surgical techniques with the distraction approach. Although the benefits of distraction are well established, opportunities remain to improve the clinical management of patients with a cleft and syndromic conditions using this technique. These include the development of new hardware, improvements in surgical design and technique, reduction of the consolidation period through cytokines, biomodulation (laser, ultrasound, and vibration) and the understanding of soft tissue response to gradual distraction and psychosocial aspects of the technique on the overall well-being of patients.

CLINICS CARE POINTS

- Maxillary distraction is a treatment alternative for severe maxillary hypoplasia secondary to orofacial clefts.
- External and internal devices for maxillary distraction are available.
- External devices are indicated for moderate-to-severe conditions, while internal devices are used for moderate conditions.
- Hybrid (bone-tooth supported) external and internal distractors offer better occlusal control compared with bone-supported devices.
- External devices offer a greater degree of advancement and adjustability of the distraction vector.
- Computer-aided design and manufacturing and 3-dimensional virtual surgical planning allow for improved internal distractor selection and placement.
- Although external distractors are easily applied, adjusted, and removed, some clinicians object to their use as they are external.
- Cases with maxillary/mandibular discrepancies with concomitant mandibular asymmetry are well managed with orthognathic surgery. If the antero-posterior discrepancy is severe, maxillary advancement with distraction can be done first, followed by finishing orthognathic surgery.

DISCLOSURE

The authors have nothing to disclose.

REFERENCES

1. Thomas PM, Sarver DM, Tucker MR. Prevention and management of complications. In: Proffit WR, Sarver DM, editors. Contemporary treatment of dentofacial deformity. St Louis (MO): Mosby; 2003. p. 677–709.
2. Kramer FJ, Baethge C, Swennen G, et al. Intra- and perioperative complications of the Le Fort I osteotomy: a prospective evaluation of 1000 patients. J Craniofac Surg 2004;15(6):971–7 [discussion 78-9].
3. Erbe M, Stoelinga PJ, Leenen RJ. Long-term results of segmental repositioning of the maxilla in cleft palate patients without previously grafted alveolo-palatal clefts. J Craniomaxillofac Surg 1996;24(2):109–17.
4. Hochban W, Ganss C, Austermann KH. Long-term results after maxillary advancement in patients with clefts. Cleft Palate Craniofac J 1993;30(2):237–43.
5. Cheung LK, Samman N, Hui E, et al. The 3-dimensional stability of maxillary osteotomies in cleft palate patients with residual alveolar clefts. Br J Oral Maxillofac Surg 1994;32(1):6–12.
6. Posnick JC, Dagys AP. Skeletal stability and relapse patterns after Le Fort I maxillary osteotomy fixed with miniplates: the unilateral cleft lip and palate deformity. Plast Reconstr Surg 1994;94(7):924–32.
7. da Silva Filho OG, Normando AD, Capelozza Filho L. Mandibular growth in patients with cleft lip and/or cleft palate–the influence of cleft type. Am J Orthod Dentofacial Orthop 1993;104(3):269–75.
8. McCarthy JG, Karp N, Thorne CH, et al. Lengthening the human mandible by gradual distraction. Plast Reconstr Surg 1992;89(1):1–8..
9. Satoh K, Mitsukawa N, Hosaka Y. Dual midfacial distraction osteogenesis: Le Fort III minus I and Le Fort I for syndromic craniosynostosis. Plast Reconstr Surg 2003;111(3):1019–28.
10. Fearon J. Halo distraction of the Le Fort III in syndromic craniosynostosis: a long-term assessment. Plast Reconstr Surg 2005;115(6):1524–36.
11. Polley JW, Figueroa AA, Charbel FT, et al. Monobloc craniomaxillofacial distraction osteogenesis in a newborn with severe craniofacial synostosis: a preliminary report. J Craniofac Surg 1995;6(5):421–3.
12. Figueroa AA, Polley JW, Ko E. Distraction osteogenesis for treatment of severe cleft maxillary deficiency with the RED technique. In: Samchukov ML, Cherkaskin AM, editors. Craniofacial distraction osteogenesis. St. Louis: Mosby; 2001. p. 485–93.
13. Meling TR, Due-Tonnessen BJ, Hogevold HE, et al. Monobloc distraction osteogenesis in pediatric

patients with severe syndromal craniosynostosis. J Craniofac Surg 2004;15(6):990–1000 [discussion 01].

14. Way BLM, Khonsari RH, Karunakaran T, et al. Correcting exorbitism by monobloc frontofacial advancement in Crouzon-Pfeiffer syndrome: an age-specific, time-related, controlled study. Plast Reconstr Surg 2019;143(1):121e–32e.

15. Witherow H, Dunaway D, Evans R, et al. Functional outcomes in monobloc advancement by distraction using the rigid external distractor device. Plast Reconstr Surg 2008;121(4):1311–22.

16. Witherow H, Dunaway D, Ponniah A, et al. Monobloc distraction in an infant, using the rigid external distractor: problems and solutions–a case report. J Craniomaxillofac Surg 2008;36(1):15–20.

17. Figueroa AA, Polley JW. Mandibular distraction osteogenesis. Op Tech Otolaryn Head Neck Surg 2002;13(1):17–28.

18. Molina F. Mandibular distraction osteogenesis: clinical analysis of the first 10 years. In: Samchukov ML, Cherkaskin AM, editors. Craniofacial distraction osteogenesis. St. Louis: Mosby; 2001. p. 196–205.

19. Ortiz Monasterio F, Molina F, Andrade L, et al. Simultaneous mandibular and maxillary distraction in hemifacial microsomia in adults: avoiding occlusal disasters. Plast Reconstr Surg 1997;100(4): 852–861..

20. Sant'Anna EF, Lau GW, Marquezan M, et al. Combined maxillary and mandibular distraction osteogenesis in patients with hemifacial microsomia. Am J Orthod Dentofacial Orthop 2015;147(5): 566–77.

21. Figueroa AA, Polley JW, Ko EW. Maxillary distraction for the management of cleft maxillary hypoplasia with a rigid external distraction system. Semin Orthod 1999;5(1):46–51.

22. Figueroa AA, Friede H, Ko EW. Long-term skeletal stability after maxillary advancement with distraction osteogenesis using a rigid external distraction device in cleft maxillary deformities. Plast Reconstr Surg 2004;114(6):1382–1392..

23. Harada K, Baba Y, Ohyama K, et al. Maxillary distraction osteogenesis for cleft lip and palate children using an external, adjustable, rigid distraction device: a report of 2 cases. J Oral Maxillofac Surg 2001;59(12):1492–1496..

24. Hierl T, Hemprich A. Callus distraction of the midface in the severely atrophied maxilla–a case report. Cleft Palate Craniofac J 1999;36(5):457–61.

25. Polley JW, Figueroa AA. Management of severe maxillary deficiency in childhood and adolescence through distraction osteogenesis with an external, adjustable, rigid distraction device. J Craniofac Surg 1997;8(3):181–5 [discussion 86].

26. Polley JW, Figueroa AA. Rigid external distraction: its application in cleft maxillary deformities. Plast Reconstr Surg 1998;102(5):1360–72 [discussion 73-4].

27. Molina F, Ortiz Monasterio F, de la Paz Aguilar M, et al. Maxillary distraction: aesthetic and functional benefits in cleft lip-palate and prognathic patients during mixed dentition. Plast Reconstr Surg 1998; 101(4):951–63.

28. Cope JB, Samchukov ML, Cherkashin AM. Historical development and evolution of craniofacial distraction osteogenesis. In: Samchukov ML, Cope JB, editors. Craniofacial distraction osteogenesis. St Louis (MO): Mosby; 2001. p. xxvii-xxxvi.

29. Polley JW, Figueroa AA. Maxillary distraction osteogenesis with rigid external distraction. Atlas Oral Maxillofac Surg Clin North Am 1999;7(1):15–28.

30. Ahn JG, Figueroa AA, Braun S, et al. Biomechanical considerations in distraction of the osteotomized dentomaxillary complex. Am J Orthod Dentofacial Orthop 1999;116(3):264–70.

31. Figueroa AA, Polley JW, Figueroa AD. Biomechanical considerations for distraction of the monobloc, le fort III, and le fort I segments. Plast Reconstr Surg 2010;126(3):1005–13.

32. Nanda R, Upadhyay M. Skeletal and dental considerations in orthodontic treatment mechanics: a contemporary view. Eur J Orthod 2013;35(5):634–43.

33. Figueroa AA, Polley JW. Orthodontics in cleft lip and palate management. In: Mathes SJ, editor. Plastic surgery. 2nd edition. Philadelphia: Saunders; 2006. p. 271–310.

34. Figueroa AA, Polley JW. Management of the severe cleft and syndromic midface hypoplasia. Orthod Craniofac Res 2007;10(3):167–79.

35. Figueroa AA, Polley JW, Figueroa AL. Introduction of a new removable adjustable intraoral maxillary distraction system for correction of maxillary hypoplasia. J Craniofac Surg 2009;20(Suppl 2):1776–86.

36. Combs PD, Harshbarger RJ 3rd. Le Fort I maxillary advancement using distraction osteogenesis. Semin Plast Surg 2014;28(4):193–8.

37. Kusnoto B, Figueroa AA, Polley JW. Radiographic evaluation of bone formation in the pterygoid region after maxillary distraction with a rigid external distraction (RED) device. J Craniofac Surg 2001; 12(2):109–17 [discussion 18].

38. Figueroa AA, Polley JW. Clinical controversies in oral and maxillofacial surgery: part two. External versus internal distraction osteogenesis for the management of severe maxillary hypoplasia: external distraction. J Oral Maxillofac Surg 2008;66(12): 2598–604.

39. El-Bialy TH, Royston TJ, Magin RL, et al. The effect of pulsed ultrasound on mandibular distraction. Ann Biomed Eng 2002;30(10):1251–61.

40. Cheung LK, Zheng LW. Effect of recombinant human bone morphogenetic protein-2 on mandibular

distraction at different rates in an experimental model. J Craniofac Surg 2006;17(1):100–8 [discussion 09-10].

41. Raschke MJ, Bail H, Windhagen HJ, et al. Recombinant growth hormone accelerates bone regenerate consolidation in distraction osteogenesis. Bone 1999;24(2):81–8.

42. Sarmadi S, Tanbakuchi B, Hesam Arefi A, et al. The effect of photobiomodulation on distraction osteogenesis. J Lasers Med Sci 2019;10(4):330–7.

43. Taha SK, El Fattah SA, Said E, et al. Effect of laser bio-stimulation on mandibular distraction osteogenesis: an experimental study. J Oral Maxillofac Surg 2018;76(11):2411–21.

44. Wen-Ching Ko E, Figueroa AA, Polley JW. Soft tissue profile changes after maxillary advancement with distraction osteogenesis by use of a rigid external distraction device: a 1-year follow-up. J Oral Maxillofac Surg 2000;58(9):959–69 [discussion 69-70].

45. Harada K, Baba Y, Ohyama K, et al. Soft tissue profile changes of the midface in patients with cleft lip and palate following maxillary distraction osteogenesis: a preliminary study. Oral Surg Oral Med Oral Pathol Oral Radiol Endod 2002;94(6):673–7.

46. Guyette TW, Polley JW, Figueroa A, et al. Changes in speech following maxillary distraction osteogenesis. Cleft Palate Craniofac J 2001;38(3):199–205.

47. Ko EW, Figueroa AA, Guyette TW, et al. Velopharyngeal changes after maxillary advancement in cleft patients with distraction osteogenesis using a rigid external distraction device: a 1-year cephalometric follow-up. J Craniofac Surg 1999;10(4):312–20 [discussion 21-2].

48. Cheung LK, Loh JS, Ho SM. The early psychological adjustment of cleft patients after maxillary distraction osteogenesis and conventional orthognathic surgery: a preliminary study. J Oral Maxillofac Surg 2006;64(12):1743–50.

Cleft Lip and Palate
Le Fort I Distraction Using an Internal Device

Waleed Gibreel, MBBS[a], Jordan R. Wlodarczyk, MD, MS[a,b],
Erik M. Wolfswinkel, MD[a], Stephen Yen, DMD, PhD[a,c],
Mark M. Urata, MD, DDS[a,b,c,d], Jeffrey A. Hammoudeh, MD, DDS[a,b,c,d],*

KEYWORDS

- Craniofacial distraction • Le Fort I distraction • Internal distraction • External distraction
- Midface hypoplasia • Cleft lip and palate

KEY POINTS

- Distraction osteogenesis should be considered in advancement of the maxilla greater than 10 mm.
- Internal distraction is a safe and efficacious modality for the correction of midface hypoplasia after cleft lip and palate repair.
- Internal distraction devices have the advantage of reducing the amount of physical and psychological stress placed on patients, families, and caregivers.
- Internal distraction can facilitate larger movements of the maxilla than traditional advancement and fixation without significant relapse or nonunion.
- New innovation in internal distraction devices has addressed previous disadvantages of internal distraction, such as limitations on distraction distance and inability to adjust distraction vector.

INTRODUCTION

Maxillary hypoplasia is a common dentofacial deformity in patients with cleft lip and palate (CLP). During growth and at the time of facial maturity, patients commonly develop class III malocclusion, a concave facial profile with a retruded midface, and a narrow maxillary arch. Class III malocclusion in patients with CLP may result in impairment of the patient's speech, mastication, lip function, swallowing, breathing, and facial esthetics. Approximately 48% to 65% of patients with a cleft require orthognathic surgery at skeletal maturity,[1] although the reported percentage is variable and ranges from 14% to 75%.[2,3]

Before the successful clinical application of craniofacial distraction,[4] maxillary advancement (Le Fort I) with fixation was the mainstay surgical treatment of lower midface retrusion. Currently, conventional orthognathic surgery with fixation, Le Fort I distraction, or a combination of the two are the surgical modalities commonly used for the treatment of maxillary hypoplasia in patients with a cleft.[5] The use of craniofacial skeleton distraction osteogenesis (DO) has significantly expanded since the initial clinical report by McCarthy and coworkers,[4] who successfully elongated the hypoplastic mandible of a patient with hemifacial microsomia. A plethora of clinical and basic science reports have validated McCarthy and coworkers[4] innovative work on craniofacial DO and

[a] Division of Plastic and Maxillofacial Surgery, Children's Hospital Los Angeles, 4650 West Sunset Boulevard, Mailstop 96, Los Angeles, CA 90033, USA; [b] Division of Plastic and Reconstructive Surgery, Keck School of Medicine, Los Angeles, CA, USA; [c] Division of Dentistry and Orthodontics, Children's Hospital Los Angeles, Los Angeles, CA, USA; [d] Division of Oral and Maxillofacial Surgery, University of Southern California, Los Angeles, CA, USA
* Corresponding author. Division of Plastic and Maxillofacial Surgery, Children's Hospital Los Angeles, 4650 West Sunset Boulevard, Mailstop 96, Los Angeles, CA 90033.
E-mail address: jhammoudeh@chla.usc.edu

Clin Plastic Surg 48 (2021) 407–417
https://doi.org/10.1016/j.cps.2021.02.003
0094-1298/21/Published by Elsevier Inc.

long-term studies have confirmed the ability to obtain a successful and a stable maxillary advancement through maxillary distraction.[4–25]

MAXILLARY ADVANCEMENT WITH FIXATION VERSUS MAXILLARY DISTRACTION

Le Fort I maxillary advancement with plate fixation is the preferred single-step treatment of maxillary hypoplasia.[5] When deciding between traditional Le Fort I advancement and fixation and Le Fort I distraction for correction of class III occlusion, the magnitude of anterior/posterior (AP) maxillary movement must be considered, especially in patients with CLP. Patients with CLP present a unique challenge to the orthodontist and orthognathic surgeon. The surgical repair of the CLP produces dense scar tissue formation in the surgically treated areas, which contributes to a tight soft tissue envelope against which the maxilla is advanced. In addition, the presence of prior midface surgery, such as Le Fort I or III advancement and surgically assisted rapid palatal expansion, increases the difficulty advancing the maxilla. Additionally, any pharyngeal surgery for velopharyngeal insufficiency (sphincter pharyngoplasty and pharyngeal flap) performed in patients with a cleft invariably results in scar tissue formation at the posterior aspect of the palate. This has been demonstrated to increase the difficulty in reliably advancing the maxilla more than 6 to 7 mm.[26] One of the advantages of maxillary DO is in its ability to slowly stretch the soft tissue envelope during skeletal advancement. The most frequent use of maxillary DO at the Le Fort I level is the sagittal (anterior) advancement of the maxilla to overcome these restrictive forces. This gradual expansion of the soft tissues and soft tissue histogenesis allows for a greater stability of the skeletal advancement and a superior esthetic result.

There is a known incidence of maxillary AP relapse following conventional Le Fort I advancement and fixation. Maxillary advancement greater than 10 mm has been demonstrated to have a higher rate of relapse especially in patients with CLP.[11] Multiple reports in this patient population have confirmed a direct association between the degree of AP maxillary advancement and the degree of midfacial relapse, with a wide reported incidence of 10% to 50%.[6,9,10,26–31] The higher rate of AP maxillary relapse in patients with CLP is multifactorial and has been attributed to: excessive scar tissue, limited blood supply, more complex maxillomandibular deformity, and poor bone quality.[4]

At our institution we reviewed our experience treating patients with or without CLP who underwent Le Fort I maxillary advancement. Our data revealed that the average maxillary advancement for all patients without distraction was 6.3 mm with a corresponding AP relapse of 1.8 mm, indicating a 28.6% relapse. A history of cleft and the magnitude of maxillary advancement were directly correlated with increased skeletal relapse, whereas bone graft at the osteotomy site demonstrated a protective effect on relapse. Our results revealed that patients with cleft have an average of 1.25 mm greater AP relapse when compared with patients without cleft. Our findings also demonstrated that each additional millimeter in maxillary advancement was associated with an additional 0.298 mm of relapse. The degree of relapse was not associated with cleft phenotype (unilateral CLP, bilateral CLP, and isolated cleft palate).[26] Other studies have echoed our findings, specifically Cheung and colleagues,[32] who demonstrated AP plane relapse rate of 22% and 22.5% in patients with a unilateral and bilateral cleft.

In the era preceding DO, patients with class III malocclusion secondary to maxillary hypoplasia necessitating a maxillary advancement of more than 10 mm frequently underwent a bimaxillary surgery (Le Fort I with advancement and bilateral sagittal split osteotomy with mandibular setback). This manipulation of the maxilla and mandible worked to "split the difference" in the negative overjet, therefore avoiding a large maxillary advancement and its associated high rate of relapse. When this approach is followed, maxillary advancement is limited to less than 10 mm of AP advancement and the remaining difference, if any, is addressed via mandibular setback. Alternatives to splitting the difference (two jaw surgeries) include maxillary advancement via DO. This is usually performed in patients with a cleft requiring AP maxillary advancement greater than 10 mm.[33] Maxillary distraction in these situations has been associated with a far lower relapse rate.[34–36]

EXTERNAL VERSUS INTERNAL (SEMIBURIED) DISTRACTION DEVICE

Currently, two main surgical approaches exist for maxillary DO: internal distraction using subcutaneously placed distraction devices, and external (halo) distraction device with cranial fixation.[4,20–25] The rigid external distraction (RED) device was the first external distractor used for midface DO and is still used today to translate the maxilla and midface. The RED device requires concurrent use of a cranial halo that is secured to the skull with pins (**Fig. 1**A). The halo is attached to a midline vertical bar, which has mobile horizontal bars that can move along (up and down) the length of the vertical bar to provide anchorage for the wires that are attached to the distractor plates or orthodontic anchors (**Fig. 1**A,B).[22,33]

The main advantage of using a RED device is the ability to change the vector along multiple vectors of distraction during the activation phase and (theoretically) unlimited distraction length. Additional advantages include the ease of use and relative ease of device removal after completion of consolidation. Despite the previously mentioned advantages, the RED device has several risks, such as site infection, device dislodgement, intracranial pin migration, pin site alopecia (**Fig. 1**C), and susceptibility to trauma.[33] Moreover, wearing a RED device for 8 to 12 weeks is cumbersome and it is difficult to wear in school or in public.[33] These limitations led to the development of internal (semiburied) maxillary distraction devices.

In 1995, Cohen and colleagues[23,25] reported on the use of DO to advance the maxilla using

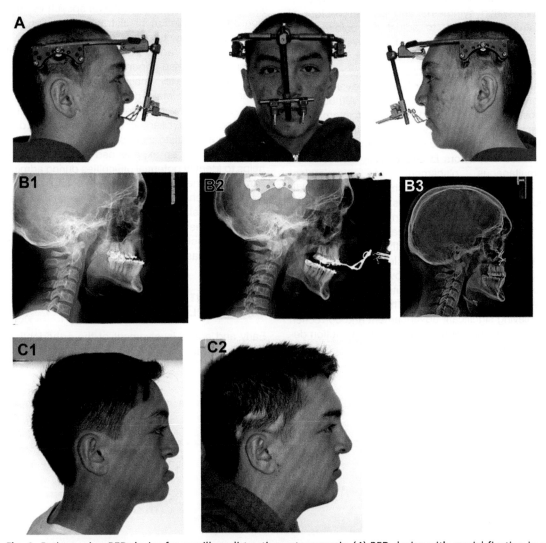

Fig. 1. Patient using RED device for maxillary distraction osteogenesis. (*A*) RED device with cranial fixation in a patient with unilateral cleft lip and palate. (*B1*) Preoperative lateral cephalograms of patient with unilateral cleft lip and palate with preoperative orthodontics. (*B2*) Postoperative lateral cephalogram of patient with unilateral cleft lip and palate with activation phase of RED device. (*B3*) Postoperative lateral cephalogram of patient with unilateral cleft lip and palate post-RED device activation and internal fixation. (*C1*) Preoperative lateral profile of patient with unilateral cleft lip and palate. (*C2*) Postoperative lateral profiles of patient with unilateral cleft lip and palate after RED device distraction and Le Fort I fixation (note pin site alopecia).

internal devices in humans. Internal distraction devices have the advantage of reducing the amount of physical and psychological stress placed on patients, families, and caregivers. These internal distractors are more socially acceptable and allow earlier return to work and easier socialization. Internal distractors were initially limited by the size of the lengthening screws to advance the maxilla and the stability of the devices as they are lengthened. The advent of the telescoping lengthening screws has compensated for this problem (**Fig. 2**).[33] Some of the challenges of the internal distractor devices include: difficulty in placing the right and left devices within symmetric and parallel vectors of distraction, inability to adjust the unidirectional vector of distraction during the activation phase, discomfort related to the stretch of the buccal tissues by the distractor rods, and the need for a second operation for hardware removal after the consolidation phase is complete.[33] Although the most frequently cited drawback of internal distractors is the inability to adjust the vector of distraction during activation, vector control with midface distractors is successfully achieved via simultaneous placement of microimplant anchored class III relationship elastics.[37] Additionally, as a result of this limitation, internal distraction for our institution often functions to advance the maxilla to a location that makes the final advancement and rigid fixation during a secondary surgery more feasible and stable rather than provide the entire movement required to achieve occlusion. Despite the previously described limitations we have had success achieving significant advancement and correction of class III occlusion using internal distraction devices (**Fig. 3**).

PATIENT EVALUATION

All patients should be evaluated by a multidisciplinary team consisting of a speech pathologist, social worker, dietician, anesthesiologist, orthodontist, and a surgeon. Compliance and the ability of the patients and parents to tolerate a complex distraction protocol should be thoroughly assessed before initiation of treatment. Any degree of velopharyngeal incompetence (VPI) is evaluated and accurately documented before operation. With the speech pathologist's input, patients with VPI are informed that their VPI will either remain unaffected or, most likely, get worse after completion of distraction. Interval speech evaluation after completion of distraction functions to evaluate the "new baseline" speech function.

Preoperative and postoperative nutritional consultation is also important for discussing dietary strategies for maintaining optimum and balanced caloric intake during the distraction process for ideal wound healing. All patients are informed of the need to adhere to a soft diet throughout the distraction process.

Evaluation by an experienced anesthesiologist helps to identify potential difficulties during administration of anesthesia. Nasotracheal intubation is particularly challenging in patients with choanal stenosis/atresia, turbinate hypertrophy, or septal deviation. The presence of previous pharyngeal flap or sphincter pharyngoplasty can add to the difficulty of nasotracheal intubation.

ORTHODONTIC CONSIDERATIONS AND SURGICAL PLANNING

Early and active involvement of the orthodontist, frequent and serial evaluation, and close

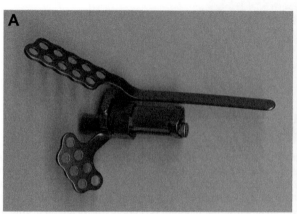
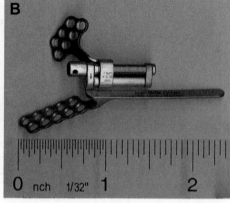

Fig. 2. (*A*) KLS Martin (Jacksonville, FL) internal distraction device. (*B*) KLS Martin internal distraction device (alternate view).

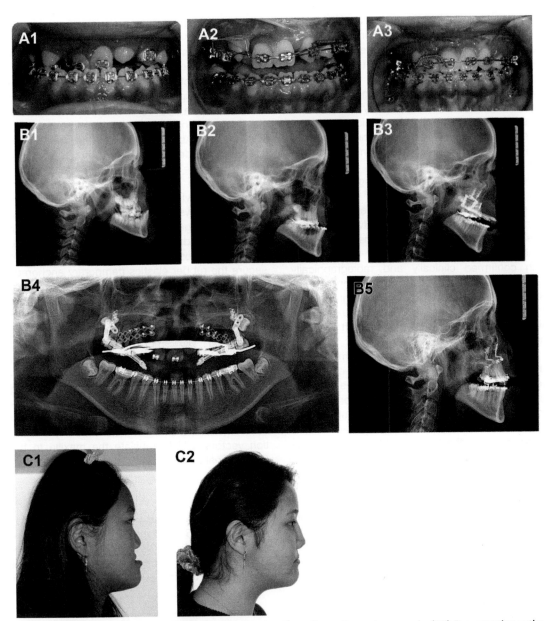

Fig. 3. Patient using internal distraction device for maxillary distraction osteogenesis. (*A1*) Preoperative orthodontics before internal distraction. (*A2*) Preoperative orthodontics before internal distraction (alternate view). (*A3*) Postoperative orthodontics post internal distraction. (*B1*) Preoperative lateral cephalograms of patient with unilateral cleft lip and palate before orthodontics. (*B2*) Preoperative lateral cephalograms of patient with unilateral cleft lip and palate with preoperative orthodontics. (*B3*) Postoperative panorex of patient with unilateral cleft lip and palate with activation phase of internal distraction device. (*B4*) Postoperative lateral cephalogram of patient with unilateral cleft lip and palate with activation phase of internal distraction device. (*B5*) Postoperative lateral cephalogram of patient with unilateral cleft lip and palate post internal distraction device activation and internal fixation. (*C1*) Preoperative lateral profile of patient with unilateral cleft lip and palate. (*C2*) Postoperative lateral profiles of patient with unilateral cleft lip and palate after completion of internal distraction and final Le Fort I maxillary fixation.

communication between the orthodontist and surgeon are crucial to executing a successful treatment plan. Predistraction orthodontics, orthodontic manipulation during the activation and consolidation phases, and postdistraction orthodontic management are all phases to be considered when planning maxillary distraction (see **Fig. 3**A1–A3).[33,38]

The goal of Le Fort I distraction is the restoration of class I occlusion. The final position of the maxilla required to restore occlusion is determined by the orthodontic and surgical team. A treatment plan for orthodontic preparation with the goals of leveling, aligning, and coordinating the maxillary and mandibular arches is crafted by the orthodontic team executed with close clinical follow-up. Determining the final position of the maxilla and final occlusion is done with a combination of physical examination, dental models, photographs, three-dimensional computed tomographic imaging, and cephalometric analysis.[33] Continuity of the maxillary arch should be ensured before performing maxillary distraction. Alveolar clefts, when present, should be reconstructed with bone graft and the continuity of the maxillary arch confirmed clinically and radiographically before maxillary distraction. The presence of an alveolar cleft or unidentified fracture through the grafted site can lead to an unstable maxilla (two-piece maxilla with separation at the cleft site) during osteotomy and device activation.

When using internal distractors, the importance of advancing the maxilla as a single piece cannot be overemphasized. It should also be remembered that the maxilla is wider posteriorly and application of internal distractors and subsequent activation invariably leads to collapse and compression of the two unstable maxillary segments as the two segments advance anteriorly and medially. A transpalatal support bar or palatal expander should be used during maxillary distraction because it helps reduce the chance of bone separation at the site of the cleft and can also keep the two maxillary segments stable in the event of unwanted bone separation at the alveolar cleft site (Fig. 4).[33] Even if fracture across the grafted alveolus does not occur during surgery,

fracture can occur during activation because the bone stock at the site of the grafted alveolus may not be strong enough to withstand the distraction forces.

Regardless of the method of maxillary distraction, the transported bone has a tendency to move around a point of rotation in the region of the first molar/premolar region in a counterclockwise fashion. As the maxilla is translated forward an open bite develops unless there is a way to counteract the forces creating this opening. Placing bone anchors/plates or temporary anchorage devices in the anterior maxilla and mandible allows placement of interarch elastic traction to mitigate this problem. The elastics can also be used during the consolidation phase to maintain the position of the bone. The method to secure the rubber elastics (temporary anchorage devices, miniplates, bonded brackets, or surgical hooks) is preoperatively planned with the orthodontist.

With the expanding use of virtual surgical in craniofacial DO, more predictable maxillary advancement and vector control is achieved with internal maxillary DO. Through virtual determination of the new maxillary position, maxillary cutting guides and device positioning guides are fabricated to facilitate a precise execution of maxillary osteotomies and accurate orientation of distraction vectors, which translate the maxilla to the desired final position.[33]

SURGERY

The maxilla is exposed via a standard vestibular incision about 5 to 10 mm from the depth of the gingivolabial sulcus. Dissection is carried down to bone using electrocautery. Subperiosteal dissection is carried out to expose the anterior

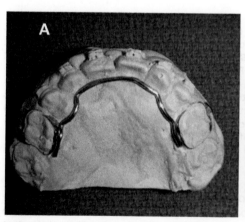
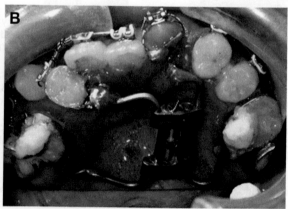

Fig. 4. (A) Transpalatal support bar or palatal expander for maxillary distraction. (B) Palatal expander for maxillary distraction.

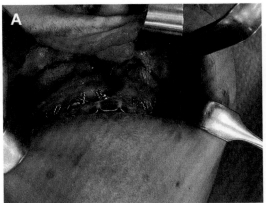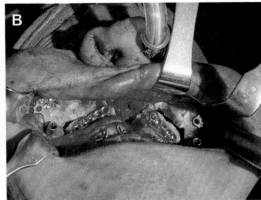

Fig. 5. (*A*) Before internal distractor device placement for Le Fort I maxillary distraction. (*B*) Post internal distractor device placement for Le Fort I maxillary distraction.

nasal spine, lateral rims of the pyriform aperture, nasomaxillary and zygomaticomaxillary buttresses, and lateral wall of the maxillary sinus. A standard Le Fort I osteotomy is made extending from the lateral nasal wall and nasomaxillary buttress, across the anterior maxillary sinus wall, zygomaticomaxillary buttress, and through the lateral wall of the maxillary sinus. The nasal septum is subsequently separated from the maxilla from the anterior nasal spine to the posterior nasal spine. Pterygomaxillary separation is then performed and the maxilla is gently separated and adequate mobility is ensured. Any difficulty with full mobilization of the maxilla should prompt evaluation of osteotomy sites to ensure completion of osteotomies. We believe that use of force to down-fracture or mobilize the maxilla should be avoided because this can lead to propagation of fracture lines at sites of incomplete osteotomies. With gentle maxillary down-fracture, areas of bone interferences are removed and the maxilla is placed in its natural position ensuring maximum bone contact at the osteotomy sites. It is important to anteriorly stretch the soft tissue envelope by mobilizing the maxilla.

Two internal distractors are then applied, one on each side of the maxilla, in as parallel position as possible for a symmetrically oriented vector (**Fig. 5**). The plates above and below the activation rod are conformed to the underlying bone and secured using monocortical screws; care is taken to place the screws cephalad to tooth roots. Before fixation of the device, the activation system is adjusted to the initial setting (no extension). Activation arms are then connected to the activation rod and the device is activated to ensure symmetric maxillary translation that follows the planned trajectory. The device is again dialed back to the initial setting before wound closure to reposition the maxilla to the original position and ensure the appropriate bone-to-bone contact and callus formation required for bone generation.

POSTOPERATIVE MANAGEMENT

After a latency period of 5 to 7 days, activation is started at a rhythm of 0.5 mm every 12 hours to achieve a total distraction of 1 mm/day. Turning the activation arms is simple; however, patients and families require education on how to perform this task. Most devices have a rachet mechanism to ensure only clockwise rotation to prevent asymmetric distraction or incorrect use of the device. Patients are typically discharged from the hospital the day after surgery. Patients are seen in clinic every 3 to 4 days to monitor the progress of activation and address any difficulties that the families or patients may encounter. The intraoral part of the device should be kept clean and meticulous oral hygiene is encouraged. Turning the pins and activation arms should not be painful; however, as progression of distraction continues, and the soft tissue envelope stretches, mild discomfort during active distraction is common. This is easily managed by over-the-counter analgesics 30 minutes before distraction. The presence of significant pain could signify the presence of incomplete osteotomy, premature bone consolidation,[33] or device failure/dislodgment. The end point of distraction is usually predicted preoperatively; however, as a general rule it is preferable to overdistract 2 to 4 mm in anticipation of some relapse, especially in patients with a cleft. Once activation is completed, the two activation arms are removed and the remainder of the device is left in place during the consolidation period.

The consolidation period varies and depends on the degree of bone advancement. The consolidation period requires intramembranous bone calcification along the distraction gap from the periphery to the center. In general, the consolidation period is 3 to 6 months with internal devices. However, the longer the bone is lengthened, the longer the time period required for the fibrous interzone zone to calcify and be stable enough to withstand the forces of relapse. The most reliable way to assess new bone formation and union at the osteotomy sites is through computed tomography analysis. Usually bone deposition is appreciable at the region of pterygoid plates.[33] Maxillary stability is obtained with adequate bone formation at the region of pterygoid plates even in the absence of adequate bone formation at the anterior maxillary osteotomy site.

Given the single vector of distraction associated with internal devices, achieving a perfect occlusion is challenging. Some patients are placed in guiding rubber elastics to refine the occlusion and the esthetic result. In patients with a cleft associated with severe maxillary retrusion, a Le Fort I reosteotomy and fixation is performed after completion of consolidation and at the time of distractors removal to achieve the desired final occlusion. This method uses maxillary distraction to stretch the soft tissue envelope and then finalizes the occlusion with less final bony movement during the Le Fort I reosteotomy with rigid fixation to achieve final occlusion.

COMPLICATIONS

Perioperative complications associated with Le Fort I maxillary distraction using an internal device include excessive bleeding, damage to the maxillary tooth roots, and infection. During the activation phase complications include discomfort related to the device and activation arms, upper lip mucosal erosion, abnormal bony contact of the Le Fort I segment with the superior midface preventing further anterior translation, device dislodgement, device malfunction, and loss of distraction vector.[33,39] Relapse is a significant concern with any large maxillary advancement. However, the amount of relapse in patients who have undergone maxillary distraction is significantly less than those who undergo advancement and fixation alone, particularly with advancements greater than 10 mm.[34–36]

SPEECH OUTCOMES FOLLOWING MAXILLARY DISTRACTION

Le Fort I advancement carries the soft palate forward, which in patients with poor compliance of their palatal soft tissue can lead to VPI and hypernasal speech.[40] In patients with a cleft and signs of VPI, the speech tends to worsen after maxillary advancement. Even in patients without preoperative VPI, Le Fort I advancement can lead to the development of VPI with the risk increasing with the greater magnitude of maxillary advancement. In patients with a cleft, baseline velar anatomy, more specifically, a physiologically short soft palate, is a predictor of postoperative VPI after maxillary advancement.[40] It has been hypothesized that the potential negative effects on velopharyngeal competence associated with conventional Le Fort I advancement and fixation may be mitigated by maxillary DO.[36] Prospective comparison between patients undergoing moderate (4–10 mm) maxillary advancement by conventional Le Fort I advancement and fixation versus DO found no difference in velopharyngeal function between the groups.[41] However, none of the patients in this study had a maxillary advancement greater than 10 mm. Therefore, it is hard to extrapolate the study findings to patients requiring larger (greater than 10 mm) AP maxillary advancement. In addition, it is generally rare to perform maxillary distraction at a Le Fort I level for maxillary advancement less than 10 mm.

Recent studies have evaluated speech outcomes in patients with CLP undergoing maxillary advancement and compared their outcomes between the two modalities of maxillary advancement (conventional Le Fort I advancement and fixation, and DO). In the conventional Le Fort I advancement and fixation group, speech deterioration was noted in 0% of patients with 1- to 5-mm maxillary advancement and 44% in patients with 6- to 8-mm maxillary advancement. Among patients who underwent maxillary advancement via DO, speech deterioration was noted in 0% of patients with a magnitude of 9- to 10-mm maxillary advancement, 50% of patients with 11- to 12-mm maxillary advancement, and 100% of patients with 13- to 16-mm maxillary advancement.[3] This study highlights the ability of DO to achieve a larger degree of AP maxillary advancement with a decreased negative impact on the speech. This study also shows that any maxillary distraction exceeding 10 mm is associated with some degree of speech deterioration. A third study similarly demonstrated a greater degree of maxillary stability and a statistically significant benefit to speech outcomes using Le Fort I distraction compared with traditional orthognathic surgery.[36] In this last study, the onset of VPI in patients undergoing Le Fort I distraction greater than 10 mm was observed to a lesser degree than reported previously. Because most patients with a cleft who undergo distraction require a maxillary advancement greater than 10 mm, patients and families should be counseled regarding the possibility of speech deterioration or worsening of VPI at the completion of surgery.

SUMMARY

DO is a power tool for maxillary advancement in patients with a cleft. Long-term skeletal stability is achieved with Le Fort I maxillary distraction. Although not suggested for most patients requiring orthognathic surgery for cleft skeletal malformations, the technique has been helpful in obtaining stable results for large advancements of the facial skeleton compared with conventional Le Fort I advancement and fixation of the maxilla.

CLINICS CARE POINTS

- Approximately 48% to 65% of cleft lip and/or palate patients require orthognathic surgery at skeletal maturity.

- The higher rate of AP maxillary relapse in patients with cleft lip and palate has been attributed to many factors, such as excessive scar tissue, poor blood supply, more complex maxillomandibular deformity, and poor bone quality.

- Maxillary advancement greater than 10 mm in all patients and 6 to 7 mm in cleft lip and palate patients has been demonstrated to have a higher rate of relapse.

- Distraction osteogenesis facilitated by an internal distraction device is a powerful tool for maxillary advancement in patients with cleft lip and palate.

- Distraction osteogenesis has the ability to slowly stretch the soft tissue envelope with the skeletal advancement and prevent nonunion and relapse. One may consider overdistraction to account for relapse versus in preparation for final occlusion correction surgery.

- Internal distraction devices have the advantage of reducing the amount of physical and psychological stress placed on patients, families, and caregivers. These internal distractors are more socially acceptable and allow earlier return to work.

- The advent of the telescoping lengthening screws found in newer internal distraction devices has compensated for previous limitations on distraction distance.

- Simultaneous placement of microimplant anchored class III relationship elastics can work to adjust the vector of distraction in the activation phase of internal distraction.

FINANCIAL DISCLOSURE STATEMENT

J.A. Hammoudeh has two existing royalties with KLS for contributions to a mandibular hardware endoprosthetic design and a maxillary distractor design.

REFERENCES

1. Daskalogiannakis J, Mehta M. The need for orthognathic surgery in patients with repaired complete unilateral and complete bilateral cleft lip and palate. Cleft Palate Craniofac J 2009;46(5):498–502.
2. Roy AA, Rtshiladze MA, Stevens K, et al. Orthognathic surgery for patients with cleft lip and palate. Clin Plast Surg 2019;46(2):157–71.
3. Chung J, Lim J, Park H, et al. Correlation between speech outcomes and the amount of maxillary advancement after orthognathic surgery (Le Fort I conventional osteotomy and distraction osteogenesis) in patients with cleft lip and palate. J Craniofac Surg 2019;30(6):1855–8.
4. McCarthy JG, Schreiber J, Karp N, et al. Lengthening the human mandible by gradual distraction. Plast Reconstr Surg 1992;89(1):1–8 [discussion: 9–10].
5. Hirjak D, Reyneke JP, Janec J, et al. Long-term results of maxillary distraction osteogenesis in nongrowing cleft: 5-years experience using internal device. Bratisl Lek Listy 2016;117(12):685–90.
6. Rachmiel A, Even-Almos M, Aizenbud D. Treatment of maxillary cleft palate: distraction osteogenesis vs. orthognathic surgery. Ann Maxillofac Surg 2012;2(2):127–30.
7. Austin SL, Mattick CR, Waterhouse PJ. Distraction osteogenesis versus orthognathic surgery for the treatment of maxillary hypoplasia in cleft lip and palate patients: a systematic review. Orthod Craniofac Res 2015;18(2):96–108.
8. Cheung LK, Chua HD. A meta-analysis of cleft maxillary osteotomy and distraction osteogenesis. Int J Oral Maxillofac Surg 2006;35(1):14–24.
9. Cheung LK, Chua HD, Bendeus M. Distraction or osteotomy for the correction of maxillary cleft deformities: which is better? Ann R Australas Coll Dent Surg 2004;17:57–63.
10. Cheung LK, Chua HD, Hagg MB. Cleft maxillary distraction versus orthognathic surgery: clinical morbidities and surgical relapse. Plast Reconstr Surg 2006;118(4):996–1008.

11. Combs PD, Harshbarger RJ 3rd. Le Fort I maxillary advancement using distraction osteogenesis. Semin Plast Surg 2014;28(4):193–8.

12. Figueroa AA, Polley JW, Friede H, et al. Long-term skeletal stability after maxillary advancement with distraction osteogenesis using a rigid external distraction device in cleft maxillary deformities. Plast Reconstr Surg 2004;114(6):1382–92 [discussion: 93–4].

13. Kanno T, Mitsugi M, Hosoe M, et al. Long-term skeletal stability after maxillary advancement with distraction osteogenesis in nongrowing patients. J Oral Maxillofac Surg 2008;66(9):1833–46.

14. Mitsukawa N, Satoh K, Morishita T. Le Fort I distraction using internal devices for maxillary hypoplasia in patients with cleft lip, palate, and alveolus: complications and their prevention and management. J Craniofac Surg 2010;21(5):1428–30.

15. Olmez S, Dogan S, Pekedis M, et al. Biomechanical evaluation of sagittal maxillary internal distraction osteogenesis in unilateral cleft lip and palate patient and noncleft patients: a three-dimensional finite element analysis. Angle Orthod 2014;84(5):815–24.

16. Picard A, Diner PA, Galliani E, et al. Five years experience with a new intraoral maxillary distraction device (RID). Br J Oral Maxillofac Surg 2011;49(7):546–51.

17. Proffit WR, Turvey TA, Phillips C. The hierarchy of stability and predictability in orthognathic surgery with rigid fixation: an update and extension. Head Face Med 2007;3:21.

18. Rachmiel A, Aizenbud D, Peled M. Long-term results in maxillary deficiency using intraoral devices. Int J Oral Maxillofac Surg 2005;34(5):473–9.

19. Wiltfang J, Hirschfelder U, Neukam FW, et al. Long-term results of distraction osteogenesis of the maxilla and midface. Br J Oral Maxillofac Surg 2002;40(6):473–9.

20. Figueroa AA, Polley JW. Management of severe cleft maxillary deficiency with distraction osteogenesis: procedure and results. Am J Orthod Dentofacial Orthop 1999;115(1):1–12.

21. Molina F, Ortiz Monasterio F, de la Paz Aguilar M, et al. Maxillary distraction: aesthetic and functional benefits in cleft lip-palate and prognathic patients during mixed dentition. Plast Reconstr Surg 1998;101(4):951–63.

22. Polley JW, Figueroa AA. Management of severe maxillary deficiency in childhood and adolescence through distraction osteogenesis with an external, adjustable, rigid distraction device. J Craniofac Surg 1997;8(3):181–5 [discussion: 6].

23. Cohen SR, Burstein FD, Stewart MB, et al. Maxillary-midface distraction in children with cleft lip and palate: a preliminary report. Plast Reconstr Surg 1997;99(5):1421–8.

24. Figueroa AA, Polley JW, Cohen M. Reactivation of a mandibular lengthening device for maximal distraction. J Craniofac Surg 1995;6(5):412–3.

25. Cohen SR, Rutrick RE, Burstein FD. Distraction osteogenesis of the human craniofacial skeleton: initial experience with new distraction system. J Craniofac Surg 1995;6(5):368–74.

26. Fahradyan A, Wolfswinkel EM, Clarke N, et al. Impact of the distance of maxillary advancement on horizontal relapse after orthognathic surgery. Cleft Palate Craniofac J 2018;55(4):546–53.

27. Kloukos D, Fudalej P, Sequeira-Byron P, et al. Maxillary distraction osteogenesis versus orthognathic surgery for cleft lip and palate patients. Cochrane Database Syst Rev 2016;(9):CD010403.

28. Louis PJ, Waite PD, Austin RB. Long-term skeletal stability after rigid fixation of Le Fort I osteotomies with advancements. Int J Oral Maxillofac Surg 1993;22(2):82–6.

29. Saltaji H, Major MP, Alfakir H, et al. Maxillary advancement with conventional orthognathic surgery in patients with cleft lip and palate: is it a stable technique? J Oral Maxillofac Surg 2012;70(12):2859–66.

30. Saltaji H, Major MP, Altalibi M, et al. Long-term skeletal stability after maxillary advancement with distraction osteogenesis in cleft lip and palate patients. Angle Orthod 2012;82(6):1115–22.

31. Baek SH, Lee JK, Lee JH, et al. Comparison of treatment outcome and stability between distraction osteogenesis and LeFort I osteotomy in cleft patients with maxillary hypoplasia. J Craniofac Surg 2007;18(5):1209–15.

32. Cheung LK, Samman N, Hui E, et al. The 3-dimensional stability of maxillary osteotomies in cleft palate patients with residual alveolar clefts. Br J Oral Maxillofac Surg 1994;32(1):6–12.

33. Drew SJ, Kapadia H. LeFort distraction in the cleft patient. Oral Maxillofac Surg Clin North Am 2020;32(2):269–81.

34. Ganoo T, Sjostrom M. Outcomes of maxillary orthognathic surgery in patients with cleft lip and palate: a literature review. J Maxillofac Oral Surg 2019;18(4):500–8.

35. Bertrand AA, Lipman KJ, Bradley JP, et al. Consolidation time and relapse: a systematic review of outcomes in internal versus external midface distraction for syndromic craniosynostosis. Plast Reconstr Surg 2019;144(5):1125–34.

36. Kumar A, Gabbay JS, Nikjoo R, et al. Improved outcomes in cleft patients with severe maxillary deficiency after Le Fort I internal distraction. Plast Reconstr Surg 2006;117(5):1499–509.

37. Francis C, Rommer E, Mancho S, et al. Vector control in internal midface distraction using temporary anchorage devices. J Craniofac Surg 2012;23(7 Suppl 1):2000–3.

38. Yen S, Hammoudeh J, Edwards SP, et al. Orthodontic considerations for cleft orthognathic surgery. Oral Maxillofac Surg Clin North Am 2020;32(2):249–67.

39. Hwang DS, Choi HS, Kim UK, et al. Complications following orthognathic surgery for patients with cleft lip/palate. J Craniofac Surg 2019;30(6):1815–9.

40. McComb RW, Marrinan EM, Nuss RC, et al. Predictors of velopharyngeal insufficiency after Le Fort I maxillary advancement in patients with cleft palate. J Oral Maxillofac Surg 2011;69(8): 2226–32.

41. Chua HD, Whitehill TL, Samman N, et al. Maxillary distraction versus orthognathic surgery in cleft lip and palate patients: effects on speech and velopharyngeal function. Int J Oral Maxillofac Surg 2010;39(7):633–40.

Alveolar Distraction

Elçin Esenlik, DDS, PhD[a],*, Evellyn M. DeMitchell-Rodriguez, BS[b]

KEYWORDS

- Cleft lip and palate • Alveolar distraction • Closing the cleft gap • Alveolar grafting

KEY POINTS

- Alveolar distraction is used for lengthening, widening, or augmenting the alveolus in patients with a wide or complex alveolar cleft.
- Alveolar distraction can approximate the alveolar segments to reduce the size of the bony deficiency and the fistula.
- A smaller alveolar cleft and smaller fistula leads to more predictable outcomes to bony reconstruction.

INTRODUCTION

Congenital or acquired alveolar bone defects often are encountered in the dental practice. The former generally are associated with craniofacial anomalies, such as cleft lip and palate. These bony deficiencies have stereotypical characteristics, such as maxillary halves with deficient bone, lack of nasal floor support, and a hypoplastic maxilla. Acquired alveolar defects may be caused by trauma, periodontal diseases, tooth extraction, congenital tooth agenesis, and tumor resection and can present in a more variable pattern. Alveolar defects can be primarily in the horizontal dimension and often are associated with vertical resorptions, which require bone augmentation.[1] In modern dentistry, restoration of the missing teeth and atrophic alveolus in patients with or without cleft has shifted from large obturators and bulky removable prostheses to providing a bony platform for implant restorations and an esthetic soft tissue lining of the smile.

Several augmentation methods have been developed for increasing the volume of alveolar bone for patients without a cleft. Autologous or allogenic grafting is a common technique used to establish a bony platform for dental rehabilitation in patients with atrophic alveolus of various etiologies.[2] Although successfully treated cases have been reported in the literature, there are limitations of these grafting procedures. For example, the bone grafted area may resorb due to poor stabilization, limited bone contact, soft tissue tension, and vascularization problems due to the large volume of the graft material.[1,3] As an alternative treatment to grafting, alveolar distraction osteogenesis (ADO) has been suggested to increase bone volume in patients with and without cleft. The common indications for the general population in dental practice and specific indications for the cleft lip and palate population are summarized from an orthodontist's perspective.

GOALS OF ALVEOLAR DISTRACTION

ADO has become increasingly popular in orthodontics after rapid canine retraction with the distraction procedure was introduced by Liou and colleagues[4] for shortening the treatment duration. Several types of distractors and distraction types have been introduced for different purposes, including lengthening, widening, and augmenting the alveolus. Indications and conditions include

- Rapid canine distalization[4]
- Atrophic alveolus due to congenital missing or lost teeth and edentulous jaws[5,6]
- Management of ankylosed teeth[7]

The authors have no conflict of commercial or financial conflicts of interest and any funding sources.
[a] Faculty of Dentistry, Department of Orthodontics, Akdeniz University, Dumlupinar cad, Konyaaltı, Antalya 07058, Turkey; [b] Hansjörg Wyss Department of Plastic Surgery, NYU Langone Health, 550 1st Avenue, New York, NY 10016, USA
* Corresponding author.
E-mail address: elcinesenlik@gmail.com

Clin Plastic Surg 48 (2021) 419–429
https://doi.org/10.1016/j.cps.2021.02.004
0094-1298/21/© 2021 Elsevier Inc. All rights reserved.

- Alveolar/partial jaw deficiencies after tumor resections or trauma[6]
- Approximation of cleft segments in patients with cleft lip and palate[8]

The goals of ADO include

- To improve the shape of the alveolar arch in 3 dimensions (3-D)
- To expand the alveolar bone volume for subsequent orthodontic treatment
- To restore the vertical height of the alveolus before dental rehabilitation (implant placement and prosthetic restoration)

Multiple alveolar distraction procedures have been described to treat bony and soft tissue deficiencies of the jaws. These procedures are summarized as vertical, horizontal, and sagittal distraction techniques as well as alveolar distraction in patients with a cleft. A 3-D understanding of the bony and soft tissue deficiencies associated with the defect is critical to planning an effective treatment plan.

VERTICAL ALVEOLAR DISTRACTION

Vertical alveolar distraction (VAD) is used to treat local alveolar atrophy caused by traumatic tooth loss, previous failed grafting, or an ankylosed tooth.[1,7] VAD was first reported as a case series by Chin and Toth[5] in 1996, in which different distraction methods were described. Included in this study was a patient who had suffered a traumatic injury and required bone and mucosa augmentation in the anterior mandible. The investigators distracted the atrophic edentulous bone vertically, which allowed them to insert implants for dental rehabilitation. Now, after 2 decades of use, the method is considered an excellent solution for bone and soft tissue regeneration in areas with significant bone atrophy.

A systematic review of VAD concluded that survival rate of the dental implants in cases utilizing vertical distraction was similar to those without any augmentation technique.[6] Generated bone height can be up to 15 mm in certain cases.[1] Although VAD has shown to be a useful tool for bone and soft tissue augmentation, overcorrection at a 10% to 20% rate is recommended, because a degree of relapse may occur during consolidation period.[9] Additionally, although this technique has been reported in more than 300 cases in the literature, long-term data are lacking. Of the available studies that discuss long-term results, the alveolar marginal bone demonstrates approximately 15% to 20% resorption at 5-year follow-up.[10]

HORIZONTAL ALVEOLAR DISTRACTION

Horizontal alveolar distraction (HAD) is used for expanding the atrophic alveolar crest. This widening has been performed conventionally using different bone grafting procedures. Similar to conventional vertical augmentation techniques, these routine surgeries have resulted in severe bone resorption.[11] Therefore, alveolar distraction technique has been suggested by dental practitioners who experienced bone resorption and difficulty inserting osseointegrated implants. Osseointegrated implants cannot be inserted successfully in patients exhibiting an alveolar ridge less than 5 mm[12] and the narrow alveolus hinders the orthodontic tooth movement due to the insufficient bone coverage of the teeth. HAD has been used since 2004 and has been shown superior to conventional grafting due to less infection risk and minimal resorption postoperatively.[11]

Both VAD and HAD are preferred in select cases due to the decreased overall treatment time compared with conventional staged bone grafting techniques. Sufficient bone generation by the distraction allows for stable implant restoration without the need for graft surgery. The relapse or resorption of the generated bone has been found to be limited.[13] Long-term data and prospective randomized clinical trial assessment, however, are lacking.

SAGITTAL ALVEOLAR DISTRACTION

ADO in the sagittal plane has been commonly preferred in patients with cleft lip or palate for reducing the cleft gap and in patients who have undergone partial resection of the maxilla or mandible due to a tumor resection.[6] Patients with cleft lip or palate may have deficiencies in any of the 3 planes that require vertical, horizontal, or sagittal distraction, and the geometry of bony deficiency must be correctly diagnosed in 3-D in order to formulate an effective treatment plan.

ALVEOLAR DISTRACTION FOR PATIENTS WITH CLEFT
Nature of the Problem

In patients with a cleft, alveolar defects requiring VAD or HAD present unique challenges because an oral cleft commonly is associated with oronasal communication and a soft tissue deficiency. There is a wide variation in the extent of the cleft deformity from mild to severe and many alveolar defects easily can be managed using traditional surgical and orthodontic techniques. Complex alveolar defects associated with a large fistula, wide bony gap, rudimentary premaxilla, or a malformed cleft segment may benefit from more specialized interventions.[3] Different techniques have been suggested for the reconstruction of these defects, such as buccal or tongue flaps as well as obturators to cover the remaining cleft defect.[14,15] Although secondary alveolar bone grafting is the gold standard for reconstruction n of the maxillary bony cleft, the presence of a hypoplastic maxilla, significant vertical discrepancy of the alveolar segments and minimum contact surface between the cleft segments, malposition of the segments in more than 1 dimension, and soft tissue deficiency are considered risk factors for grafting surgery. Additionally, cases of flared or deviated hypoplastic premaxilla with large cleft gaps also pose challenges for traditional grafting techniques due to blood supply and deficiency of the soft and hard tissues and often lead to grafting failures or unideal reconstructions. Moreover, previous surgeries and failed grafting procedures leave more scar and resorptive bone margins behind, making future procedures more challenging for clinicians.[8] In such cases, ADO has been suggested as an alternative method to increase the success rate of the grafting procedure and increase the bone volume.

The orthodontic treatment of a patient with a cleft also is challenged by additional variables not related directly to diagnosis of cleft lip and palate. For example, the Decayed, Missing, and Filled Teeth (DMFT) index rate has been reported to be significantly higher than in noncleft controls, regardless of the sample origin. Furthermore, tooth anomalies, malpositions, and malformed roots frequently are observed in these patients.[16] These anomalies and alveolar bone deficiencies can create challenges to orthodontic treatment, because the use of routine orthodontic anchorage systems may not be feasible. In these cases, alveolar distraction is recommended to obtain better surgical and orthodontic results.

Clinical Relevance

ADO has been implemented in select patients with a cleft due to the ability to decrease the size of the alveolar gap, which can increase the success rate of subsequent bone grafting.[8] Liou and Chen[8] suggested the use of alveolar distraction when the cleft gap is wider than a canine tooth. Because large cleft gaps and the presence of large oronasal fistulas are particularly challenging to repair, commonly requiring repetitive surgeries,[14] ADO may be an important treatment options in this challenging subset of patients. There is no consensus on the treatment of oronasal fistulas located in the alveolar region in the literature.[17] It was stated that the closure of the fistulas can be done at the time a bone graft is done, which provides stability and maxillary continuity.[18] In cases of a large fistula located at the hard palate near the alveolus, the fistula can be reduced by the distraction, resulting in a smaller defect that can be closed more easily. Liou and Chen[8] reported their 21 cases in which they performed alveolar distraction procedure for approximation of the cleft segments. They obtained an average of 12-mm distraction with a range of 10 mm to 20 mm, and their 5-year follow-up showed stable results.[8]

Another advantage of alveolar distraction is providing vertical alignment of the cleft segments when needed. This can be achieved by either performing VAD following sagittal transposition as reported by Rachmiel and colleagues[19] or by remodeling the soft callus after the distraction period. Because VAD can align the alveolar segments properly in the vertical plane, bone graft survival is improved through the formation of better contact surface between the alveolar segments.

ADO also expands the mucoperiosteal lining associated with the transported bone, decreasing soft tissue tension at the time of bone graft, and improving graft take.[18] The restoration of a single-piece maxilla facilitates future orthognathic surgery. Furthermore, sagittal transposition of the lesser segment medially delivers osseous tissue to the deficient nasolabial area, providing better structural support of the soft tissues as well as an augmented bony foundation for orthodontic tooth movement, resulting in a more pleasant prosthetic restoration. Finally, improvement of the maxillary arch can be facilitated by this approach (from V shape to ovoid arch form) as well, if there is a lack of bone in the anterior region.[20] Even though providing a curvilinear arch form is not easily established, case-specific devices and postdistraction orthodontics are utilized to obtain a good platform. Although ADO has been shown beneficial, randomized controlled trial studies that compare success rates of traditional alveolar grafting to ADO methods currently are lacking.

Presurgical Orthodontic Preparation

Presurgical orthodontics include aligning the teeth to establish a robust anchorage, creating a sufficient interdental space for the osteotomy site and making a case-specific appliance for the distraction. Maxillary teeth are aligned first, as much as the alveolus remodeling capacity allows. Next, a stainless steel rectangular arch wire should be engaged to the brackets. This arch should be as large as possible to provide stability for future alveolar transposition. This arch wire also can be used to expand the maxillary arch just after the activation period in the event that the transport segment collapses palatally. A transpalatal arch bar made of stainless steel can be used for guiding the transport segment direction and to prevent medial and palatal collapse.[9,20,21] Erverdi and colleagues[20] describe using metal crowns if the number of the teeth are not sufficient for the anchorage.

In certain complex cases, there may be multiple occlusal planes due to differing vertical positions of the alveolar segments. In these cases, the use of segmental arches is recommended in order to avoid excessive tooth movement; thus, aligning the teeth is done separately for each segment. Following the leveling, interdental space is enlarged orthodontically at the planned osteotomy site for avoiding any periodontal injuries and root damage. It has been suggested that a 3-mm gap should be released orthodontically between teeth and the osteotomy line.[21] If the incisor tooth adjacent to the cleft is rotated or extremely retruded and enough bone coverage of the teeth on the cleft side exists, it can be derotated orthodontically to create an accessible surgical area.

Periodontal health is of great importance to ensure the success of soft tissue distraction. As in traditional grafting procedures, oral hygiene should be optimized preoperatively and postoperatively to avoid bone resorption. Another important aspect to consider is elimination of possible primary contacts of the transporting segment because of the overerupted or inclined teeth at the maxillary or mandibular arches on the planned route. To avoid this risk, a removable acrylic plate can be made for the mandibular arch to prevent premature contact of the tooth apices during activation and to establish a smooth platform for the transportation.

DISTRACTION PROCEDURE

The age of 9 years to 10 years is the suggested age for alveolar distraction for cleft approximation in order to graft the area before canine eruption.[8] In cases that require tertiary bone graft (after canine eruption), ADO can be performed at any time prior to the bone graft procedure.[22] Alveolar distraction involves osteotomy, latent phase, transport (active distraction), and consolidation periods similar to distraction in other craniofacial areas.

The latency period in alveolar distraction should be between 4 days to 7 days.[20,21,23] The length of this period is determined according to the extent of soft tissue healing. The rate of activation should be 0.5 mm or 1 mm per day,[21] with a frequency up to twice a day. The distraction procedure is continued until the transport segment reaches the targeted area by closing the alveolar gap in cleft population or planned final tissue expansion in the noncleft population. Caution should be used, because the amount of distractor activation tends to be more than the estimated amount, and the actual increase in width might not be the same as the amount of activation.[24] Therefore, an amount of activation exceeding the size of the alveolar cleft should be planned for, and the distractor device should have enough capacity to fulfill this increased need.

The distracted segment should be translated without inclination toward the greater segment (or premaxilla) to maximize surface apposition between the alveolar segments and to minimize displacement between the segments. In certain cases, early contact can occur due to bone irregularities or soft tissue prominences along the advancing surface. Under these circumstances, the transported segment may be tilted during activation to optimize reduction of the alveolar cleft. Therefore, the final position of the alveolar segment should be determined by: best reduction of the maxillary cleft an occlusion. If the alveolar gap is larger than 2 mm, a bone grafting procedure is suggested and if it is less than 2 mm, then gingivoperiosteoplasty may be considered.[8] Gingivoperiosteoplasty is more efficacious when performed at the time of infancy. An important factor during the activation period is the soft tissue expansion of the mucosal lining during the distraction process. Otherwise, soft tissue dehiscence can occur, resulting in an open wound that could risk the success procedure.

When activation is completed, the distractor is converted to a passive mode as a consolidation device. After a consolidation between 3 months and 4 months,[21,25] alveolar bone graft is performed and postdistraction orthodontics is completed to move the teeth distally into the generated bone.

TYPES OF DISTRACTORS

The choice of distractor (custom-made or manufactured) depends on the clinical circumstances, including the type of bone defect, dentition, and experience of the clinicians. Alveolar distractors can be classified as tooth-borne, bone-borne, or hybrid based on the anchorage type. Liou and Chen,[8] who reported the first alveolar distraction for approximating the cleft segments, used tooth-borne distractors, which were attached to the dentition only. Erverdi and colleagues[20] also designed a tooth-borne distractor that they referred to as "archwise distraction" for the cleft approximation.[21] Clinicians who use tooth-borne devices report that arch wire guidance can transport the alveolar segment to achieve an anatomic curvilinear movement along the dental arch.[19,20,23] In contrast, Mitsugi and colleagues[22] prefer bone-borne devices for sagittal distraction because tooth-borne devices impose a burden on the teeth and caused an unstable fixation, which is unfavorable for controlled bone transport. They reported 22 cleft cases that underwent ADO with fabricated bone-borne distractors and reported a degree of curvilinear transport was achieved through guidance of the arch wire.[22] Rachmiel and colleagues[18] also used bone-borne distractors for both sagittal and vertical distraction in a patient with severe cleft defect.

Rapid palatal expansion screws (hyrax-type) commonly are used for custom-made devices, which can reduce cost of care. This screw can be inserted parallel to the palatal surface or along the vestibular side of the teeth. Various designs using these expansion screws have been introduced according to the anchorage site and the planned route of the transport segment.[19,23] Zemann and colleagues[21] reported 6 cases that underwent alveolar distraction and achieved curvilinear transport of the segment using an expansion screw at the buccal side and a transpalatal bar. Other clinicians prefer to combine tooth-borne devices and temporary anchorage devices (TADs).[21] Both expansion screw devices and fabricated intraoral distractors should be oriented properly to avoid any protrusions through the buccal side or the palatal side, which can cause tongue irritation.

CASE PRESENTATIONS

The following cases reports are successful applications of ADO using bone-borne or a combination of tooth-borne and bone-borne devices in patients with a cleft.

Case 1

An 18-year-old man with unilateral cleft lip and palate presents with a large oronasal fistula and an alveolar cleft on the left side (**Fig. 1**A–C). Alveolar distraction was planned to reduce the alveolar cleft following presurgical orthodontics. After inserting brackets and arch wires, maxillary teeth were aligned and an extremely rotated left incisor tooth was derotated. The lesser segment was expanded by using arch wires (**Fig. 1**D–F). After 11 months of fixed orthodontic treatment, a fabricated alveolar distractor was applied to the lesser segment. The activation rate was 0.5 mm/d with

twice-daily activation for a period of 3 weeks. The same distractor was used during the consolidation period of 4.5 months (**Fig. 1**G, H). Alveolar bone graft was performed after consolidation was completed. A gingival recession occurred at the maxillary first premolar (**Fig. 1**I). Postoperative panoramic radiograph showed narrowing of the alveolar cleft and new bone at the cleft site compared with the presurgical panoramic radiograph (**Fig. 1**J, K). Orthognathic surgery was planned for the maxillomandibular discrepancy.

Case 2

A 14-year-old boy with a right unilateral complete cleft lip and palate presents with a congenitally absent maxillary lateral tooth, a large alveolar cleft, and associated fistula (**Fig. 2**A, B). The patient had undergone a secondary alveolar bone grafting previously but this procedure failed. Due to the large bony defect, alveolar distraction of the lesser segment was planned before the second grafting surgery. A Liou Cleft Distractor (KLS Martin, Jacksonville, Florida) was used to transport the alveolar segment (**Fig. 2**C–E). After 22 days of activation, at a rate of 0.5 mm/d, and a 5-month consolidation period (**Fig. 2**F, G), the patient underwent secondary alveolar bone graft. New bone was generated at the alveolar cleft 9 months after the surgery (**Fig. 2**H). At 2-year follow-up of the distraction, panoramic radiograph showed stable results (**Fig. 2**I).

Case 3

A 19-year-old man with bilateral cleft lip and palate underwent a previous and unsuccessful alveolar bone graft. He presented with a diminutive and edentulous premaxilla, which was deviated to the right side and associated with a large left-sided oronasal fistula (**Fig. 3**A). A combined of tooth and bone-borne distractor was created to decrease the size of the alveolar cleft on the left side (**Fig. 3**B–D). After an activation period of approximately 2 weeks and completion of consolidation, alveolar bone graft was performed (**Fig. 3**E, F). Five-year follow-up examination showed stable results (**Fig. 3**G).

Case 4

A 21-year-old man with unilateral cleft lip and palate presents with a large alveolar cleft and associated palatal fistula with loss of the maxillary upper incisors, canines, and second molars (**Fig. 4**A–C). Alveolar distraction was planned to transport the mesial ends of both alveolar segments to the midline in order to reduce the cleft defect (**Fig. 4**D). A bilateral and simultaneous distraction was planned, and

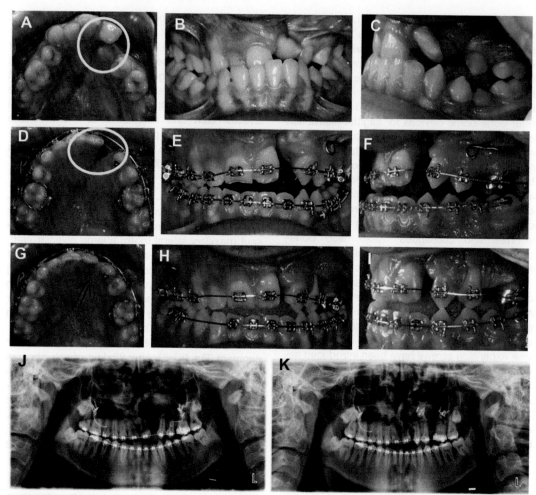

Fig. 1. Case 1. (*A–C*) Preorthodontic view of a unilateral cleft lip and palate with transverse deficiency. (*D–F*) Aligning the teeth presurgically, the fistula became larger. Yellow circle shows the collapsed lesser segment (*A*). Yellow circle shows the fistula (*D*). (*G–I*) After alveolar distraction, the cleft gap was closed. Please note that some gingival recession and gingival bulge occurred postoperatively. Black arrow shows the closed fistula (*G*). (*J*) Predistraction panoramic view. A large cleft gap is seen. (*K*) The cleft gap has closed and new bone is seen between the second premolar and the first molar teeth.

Liou Cleft Distractors were inserted between the premolars on the right and second premolar and molar teeth on the left. A transpalatal bar was used to guide the alveolar segments (**Fig. 4**E, F). An alveolar osteotomy was followed by a 3-week activation period. Alveolar bone graft was performed 8 months after the completion of AVO. Alveolar bone graft was followed by 2 jaw surgeries as well as prosthetic rehabilitation (**Fig. 4**G–K). Five year-follow-up radiographs demonstrates stable bone formation with limited resorption at the anterior alveolus (**Fig. 4**L).

POSTDISTRACTION ORTHODONTICS

Postdistraction orthodontics includes refinement of occlusion using elastics and TADs as well as maintaining the directed transport segment in its new position. This period presents 3 main advantages to clinicians: facilitating the tooth movement into the new generated bone; improving bone maturation of the generate through orthodontic transposition of the teeth, increasing or reforming the residual bone; and (when required) correcting the displaced transported segment, or molding the generate. The molding of the generate can be crucial to manage complications, such as collapsed or dislocated alveolar segments. Pichelmayer and Zemann[26] reported a case of undergoing a distraction protocol in which maxillary arch was expanded by using a fixed expansion plate after collapsing the segment transversally following the VAD.

The distraction device generally is kept in place for 3 months to 4 months to maintain the new generated

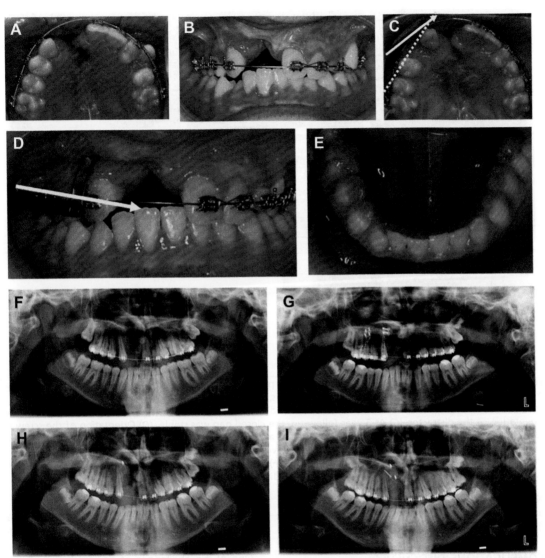

Fig. 2. Case 2. (*A, B*) Predistraction photographs after orthodontic preparation. (*C–E*) The angulation of the distractor is seen to obtain a curvilinear route. Some bonded material is added at the occlusal surface of the lower molar teeth for bite jumping. The fistula and cleft gap were both reduced. Yellow arrow shows the transversal angulation of the distractor and dotted line shows the occlusal plane (*C*). The yellow arrow shows the vertical angulation of the distractor (*D*). (*F*) Presurgical panoramic radiograph. (*G*) Third month of the consolidation period. (*H*) At the ninth month after active distraction period, new generated bone can be seen mesial and distal to the right canine. (*I*) At 2 years after distraction, stable results can be seen.

bone. During this period, tooth movement easily can be done because the newly formed bone is not mature yet. Aligning ectopic erupted teeth is facilitated at this time. Although there are different opinions about the timing of tooth movement into the new generated bone, the authors' protocol entails transposition 6 weeks after distraction.[8,27] The authors believe this protocol accelerates tooth movement because the regenerate is soft.

In addition to aligning the teeth, stimulating the generated bone through orthodontic techniques

(appositional stimulation) is an important issue to focus on. Bone regeneration can be augmented by orthodontic tooth transposition into the bony generate, thereby increasing atrophic or insufficient alveolar bone volume.[28] Liou and Chen[8] demonstrated an improved alveolar height by closing the space with orthodontic tooth movement following an insufficient bone graft. Therefore, the alveolar height obtained by the distraction can be improved by these same methods. Namely, the residual bone can be

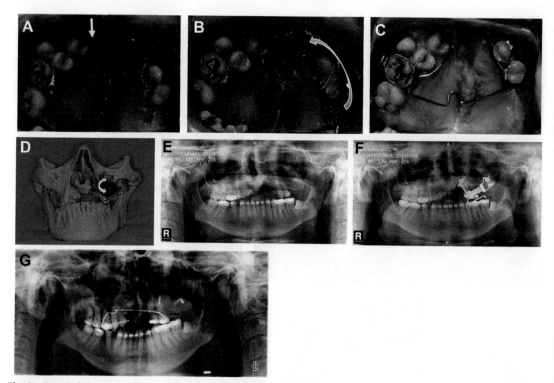

Fig. 3. Case 3. (*A*) A patient with a bilateral cleft lip and palate with a large fistula. Yellow arrow shows the rudimentary premaxilla (*A*). (*B*) After distraction osteogenesis, the cleft gap was reduced and the fistula was minimalized. Yellow arrow shows te curvature of the distracted bone (*B*). The curvilinear movement was achieved by orientation of the distractor. (*C*) At 5-year follow-up, the closed gap was stable. (*D*) Orientation of the screw is seen. It is not located parallel to the vestibular surface and occlusal plane. Yellow arrow shows the transversal angulation of the device and black arrow shows the vertical angulation of it (*D*). (*E*) A large cleft gap and many lost teeth are seen in presurgical panoramic film. (*F*) Panoramic view just after the active distraction period. A bone-borne and tooth-borne device is seen. (*G*) The distracted bone was maintained at 5-year follow-up.

remodeled by the postdistraction orthodontics, and this period can benefit from refinement of the dentoalveolar structures.

COMPLICATIONS/DIFFICULTIES

Although the alveolar distraction method has many advantages, it can be a technically challenging procedure. Major complications include fracture of the transport segment or surrounding bones, nonunion of the bone segments, and infection. Minor complications include displacement of the transported segment, soft tissue breakdown, periodontal recession, gingivitis, injured teeth adjacent to the osteotomy site, loss of anchorage, and debonding of the tooth-borne distractor during activation.[29,30] Soft tissue problems can be caused by soft tissue irritation/trauma due to the distraction device, inadequate soft tissue stretching according during activation, and periodontal infections secondary to poor patient compliance.

Patients with a cleft may have congenital absence of 1 or more teeth that make the alveolus irregular and can lead to vertical discrepancies between the alveolar segments. In those cases, the presurgical orthodontic preparation may take longer. The alveolar cleft may expand, after presurgical orthodontics is completed.

One of the challenges of device during placement is that there may be an insufficient vestibular height to accommodate the device. The same device is left intraorally during the activation and consolidation period. Therefore, adequate vestibular lining and oral hygiene are critical to limiting soft tissue complications associated with alveolar distraction. Another challenge can be lack of skeletal anchorage to fix the distractor device. Patients with cleft commonly have hard tissue deficiencies of the maxilla. Obtaining a 3-D skeletal model of the patient before the operation and simulating device placement can allow a clinician to determine the secure areas to anchor surgical guides that can be customized if needed. This allows shorter operation time and a more predictable operation. Virtual surgical planning also can be considered.

Despite successful cases reported in the literature, some clinicians contend that ADO is a difficult

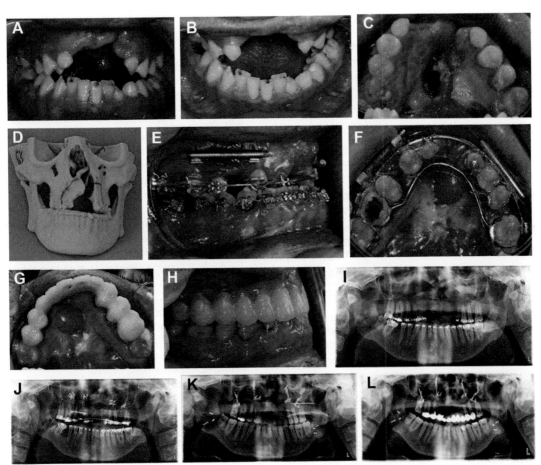

Fig. 4. Case 4. (*A–C*) A patient with unilateral cleft lip and palate with missing teeth at the anterior area and a large fistula. (*D*) Transported segments are planned on the 3-D model. (*E, F*) Bilateral alveolar distraction with bone-borne distractors. (*G, H*) At 5-year follow-up of alveolar distraction. (*I*) Presurgical radiograph of the patient with a large cleft defect. (*J*) Transported segments are seen following the distraction. (*K*) At 2-year follow-up of alveolar distraction. (*L*) At 5-year follow-up of alveolar distraction.

and unpredictable method due to the possibility of displacement of the transport segment and difficultly In controlling activation. Most of the distraction devices move linearly, and the need for an arched path of distraction can be seen as challenge. Distracted alveolar segments tend to deviate more palatally.[30] These medial deviations can be managed by using expansion appliances. However inferior deviations of the alveolar segment, it may be difficult to intrude, necessitating an additional procedure.

Additional surgeries are required after ADO to restore the bone deficiency of the alveolar cleft and/or approximation of the segments to graft the area or to close the residual fistula. Approximating of the cleft segments may not guarantee a successful bone graft. The significant number of variables that must be considered is the greatest hurdle for the popularization of this technique.[7] The authors believe ADO has a critical role in the treatment of large and complex alveolar clefts; however, it should be performed with a skilled orthodontic and surgical team with a high volume and high complexity practice in cleft care.

SUMMARY

ADO is a versatile technique that can be used as a staged treatment plan to close large and complex alveolar clefts. This approach is used widely for alveolar augmentation in 3-D in both noncleft and cleft populations. The technique reduces the size of the alveolar cleft, transports additional soft tissue lining to the area of the alveolar cleft, and generates new bone within the alveolus. These changes simplify future alveolar bone grafts, increase the likelihood of success, provide a bony platform for orthodontic treatment, and facilitate dental rehabilitation. A majority of cases require customized case-specific devices and route planning. This technique should be considered in patients with severe clefts; and, due to the complexity of the technique and the target patient population, ADO should be performed only by skilled orthodontic/surgical teams with a significant experience in cleft care.

CLINICS CARE POINTS

- The effectiveness of ADO in bone and soft tissue lengthening is well established.
- This technique is used for approximating the cleft segments and narrowing large fistulas to facilitate the alveolar bone grafting.
- The complication seen most frequently during alveolar distraction is palatal displacement of the transported segment.
- Appropriate distraction route planning is critical to success and case-specific distractor/distraction designs commonly are necessary.

ACKNOWLEDGMENTS

The authors thank Dr Y. Findik, DDS, PhD; Dr T. Baykul, DDS, PhD; and Dr A. Aydin, MD, from Süleyman Demirel University, Isparta, for surgical part of the cases.

REFERENCES

1. Carlino F, Pantaleo G, Borri A, et al. Alveolar distraction in elderly patients by implant:borne devices for functional-aesthetic dental rehabilitation of the jaws. Aging Clin Exp Res 2017;29(Suppl 1):197–204.
2. Dahlin C, Simion M, Hatano N. Long-term follow-up on soft and hard tissue levels following guided bone regeneration treatment in combination with a xenogeneic filling material: a 5-year prospective clinical study. Clin Implant Dent Relat Res 2010;12:263–70.
3. Posnick JC, Tompson B. Cleft-orthognathic surgery: complications and long-term results. Plast Reconstr Surg 1995;96(2):255–66.
4. Liou EJ, Chen PK, Huang CS, et al. Interdental distraction osteogenesis and rapid orthodontic tooth movement: a novel approach to approximate a wide alveolar cleft or bony defect. Plast Reconstr Surg 2000;105:1262–72.
5. Chin M, Toth BA. Distraction osteogenesis in maxillofacial surgery using internal devices: review of five cases. J Oral Maxillofac Surg 1996;54:45–53.
6. Pérez-Sayáns M, Martínez-Martín JM, Chamorro-Petronacci C, et al. 20 years of alveolar distraction: a systematic review of the literature. Med Oral Patol Oral Cir Bucal 2018;23:e742–51.
7. Agabiti I, Capparè P, Gherlone EF, et al. New surgical technique and distraction osteogenesis for ankylosed dental movement. J Craniofac Surg 2014;25:828–30.
8. Liou EJ, Chen KT. Intraoral distraction of segmental osteotomies and miniscrews in management of alveolar cleft. Semin Orthod 2009;15:257–67.
9. Keestra JA, Barry O, Jong L, et al. Long-term effects of vertical bone augmentation: a systematic review. J Appl Oral Sci 2016;24:3–17.
10. Ettl T, Gerlach T, Schüsselbauer T, et al. Bone resorption and complications in alveolar distraction osteogenesis. Clin Oral Investig 2010;14:481–9.
11. Takahashi T, Funaki K, Shintani H, et al. Use of horizontal alveolar distraction osteogenesis for implant placement in a narrow alveolar ridge: a case report. Int J Oral Maxillofac Implants 2004;19:291–4.
12. Albrektsson T, Zarb G, Worthington P, et al. The long-term efficacy of currently used dental implants: a review and proposed criteria of success. Int J Oral Maxillofac Implants 1986;1:11–25.
13. Laster Z, Rachmiel A, Jensen OT. Alveolar width distraction osteogenesis for early implant placement. J Oral Maxillofac Surg 2005;63:1724–30.
14. Denadai R, Seo HJ. Lo LJ Persistent symptomatic anterior oronasal fistulae in patients with Veau type III and IV clefts: a therapeutic protocol and outcomes. J Plast Reconstr Aesthet Surg 2020;73:126–33.
15. Borzabadi-Farahani A, Groper JN, Tanner AM, et al. The nance obturator, a new fixed obturator for patients with cleft palate and fistula. J Prosthodont 2012;21:400–3.
16. Tan ELY, Kuek MC, Wong HC, et al. Secondary dentition characteristics in children with nonsyndromic unilateral cleft lip and palate: a retrospective study. Cleft Palate Craniofac J 2018;55:582–9.
17. Miranda BL, Júnior JLA, Paiva MAF, et al. Management of oronasal fistulas in patients with cleft lip and palate. J Craniofac Surg 2020;31:1526–8.
18. Rachmiel A, Emodi O, Gutmacher Z, et al. Oral and dental restoration of wide alveolar cleft using distraction osteogenesis and temporary anchorage devices. J Craniomaxillofac Surg 2013;41:728–34.
19. Yen SLK, Yamashita DD, Gross J, et al. Combining orthodontic tooth movement with distraction osteogenesis to close cleft spaces and improve maxillary arch form in cleft lip and palate patients. Am J Orthod Dentofacial Orthop 2005;127:224–32.
20. Erverdi N, Küçükkeleş N, Şener C, et al. Interdental distraction osteogenesis for the management of alveolar clefts: archwise distraction. Int J Oral Maxillofac Surg 2012;41:37–41.

21. Zemann W, Pichelmayer M. Maxillary segmental distraction in children with unilateral clefts of lip, palate, and alveolus. Oral Surg Oral Med Oral Pathol Oral Radiol Endod 2011;111:688–92.

22. Mitsugi M, Ito O, Alcalde RE. Maxillary bone transportation in alveolar cleft-transport distraction osteogenesis for treatment of alveolar cleft repair. Br J Plast Surg 2005;58:619–25.

23. Neha N, Tripathi T, Mohanty S, et al. A novel minimally invasive technique of using tooth-borne hyrax expansion screw for distraction osteogenesis of large alveolar cleft defects (HYDIS-TB). Cleft Palate Craniofac J 2018;55:895–902.

24. Yamauchi K, Takahashi T, Nogami S, et al. Horizontal alveolar distraction osteogenesis for dental implant: long-term results. Clin Oral Implants Res 2013;24: 563–8.

25. Rachmiel A, Emodi O, Aizenbud D, et al. Two-stage reconstruction of the severely deficient alveolar ridge: bone graft followed by alveolar distraction

26. Pichelmayer M, Zemann W. Alveolar cleft closure by osseodistraction: pitfalls and troubleshooting. J Craniofac Surg 2012;23:e72–5.

27. El Sharaby FA, El Bokle NN, El Boghdadi DM, et al. Tooth movement into distraction regenerate: when should we start? Am J Orthod Dentofacial Orthop 2011;139:482–94.

28. Gündüz E, Rodríguez-Torres C, Gahleitner A, et al. Bone regeneration by bodily tooth movement: dental computed tomography examination of a patient. Am J Orthod Dentofacial Orthop 2004;125:100–6.

29. Garcia Garcia A, Somoza Martin M, Gandara Vila P, et al. Minor complications arising in alveolar distraction osteogenesis. J Oral Maxillofac Surg 2002;60:496–501.

30. Zhao K, Wang F, Huang W, et al. Clinical outcomes of vertical distraction osteogenesis for dental implantation: a systematic review and meta-analysis. Int J Oral Maxillofac Implants 2018;33:549–64.

osteogenesis. Int J Oral Maxillofac Surg 2018;47: 117–24.

Treacher Collins Mandibular Distraction

Connor J. Peck, BS[a], Joseph Lopez, MD, MBA[a], John T. Smetona, MD[a],
Derek M. Steinbacher, MD, DMD[b],*

KEYWORDS

- Treacher Collins syndrome • Mandibular distraction osteogenesis • Curvilinear distraction
- Curvilinear distraction osteogenesis • Mandibular distraction • Distraction osteogenesis
- Craniofacial distraction

KEY POINTS

- Patients with Treacher Collins syndrome (TCS) and a tracheostomy or severe sleep apnea may be candidates for mandibular distraction osteogenesis, which can expand the oropharyngeal airway and lengthen the mandible.
- Reconstruction of the TCS mandible poses a unique challenge to craniofacial surgeons, because bony deficiencies and deformities are seen along both the body and ramus of the mandible. More recently described techniques, such as curvilinear distraction and counterclockwise distraction, offer surgeons improved surgical options when addressing the TCS mandibular morphology.
- Even with proper implementation of these techniques, the rates of complications and relapse in mandibular reconstruction in patients with TCS tend to be higher than in other craniofacial conditions. Proper surgical management and planning, including the use of virtual surgical planning (VSP) software, can help mitigate risks and improve outcomes.
- Because patients with TCS typically require multiple procedures throughout childhood, surgeons must work closely within a multidisciplinary team in order to optimize long-term functional and quality-of-life outcomes.

BACKGROUND

Treacher Collins syndrome (TCS), also known as mandibulofacial dysostosis, is a rare autosomal dominant genetic disorder with variable expressivity.[1,2] Early descriptions of this condition by the ophthalmologist Edward Treacher Collins reported bilateral and symmetric abnormalities including orbital coloboma and periorbital dysmorphology.[2] The clinical findings in TCS are caused by abnormalities of the first and second branchial arches,[3] which can manifest with a variety of asymmetric craniofacial sequelae ranging from mild to severe. Although the molecular underpinning of TCS remains a subject of study, most cases have been linked to a variety of mutations within the TCOF1 gene on chromosome 5, which are thought to disinhibit the ribosome biogenesis pathway.[4]

CLINICAL FEATURES

The clinical features of TCS, although variable, are distinct from other craniofacial conditions. Patients with TCS present with a convex facial profile, a prominent nasal dorsum, and a retrognathic lower jaw (Fig. 1). A distinct feature is the ocular and periorbital findings, as described by Collins. Patients typically have dysmorphic orbits, downslanting palpebral fissures, and malar hypoplasia, resulting in an enophthalmic or birdlike appearance. Vision loss, congenital cataracts, and microphthalmia can be seen in severe cases.[5] The most common periorbital abnormalities include (1) thin

[a] Section of Plastic Surgery, Department of Surgery, Yale School of Medicine, Boardman Building Room 321, New Haven, CT 06519, USA; [b] Plastic and Craniomaxillofacial Surgery, Yale School of Medicine, Boardman Building Room 321, New Haven, CT 06519, USA
* Corresponding author.
E-mail address: derek.steinbacher@yale.edu

Clin Plastic Surg 48 (2021) 431–444
https://doi.org/10.1016/j.cps.2021.02.005
0094-1298/21/

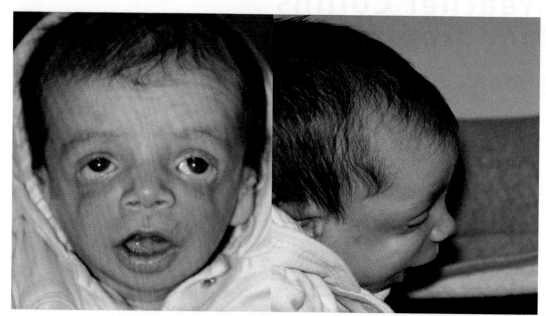

Fig. 1. Infants with TCS present with prominent ocular and periorbital findings in addition to a retrognathic lower jaw.

lower lid skin with lateral canthi malposition, (2) colobomas, (3) periorbital dermoids, (4) attenuated or absent orbicularis oculi muscles, (5) meibomian glands puncta, and (6) atresia of the lacrimal duct. Laxity of the lid margin and absence of lashes are also highly characteristic.

In addition to periorbital dysmorphology, patients with TCS also possess a characteristic dysmorphology of the maxilla and mandible (**Fig. 2**). These features include decreased sella-nasion-B point, decreased height of the lower third of the face, and a steep, clockwise rotation of the occlusal plane leading to an Angle class II anterior open bite malocclusion.[6–9] This dysmorphology stems largely from decreased ramal height, and significant condylar hypoplasia is also seen at

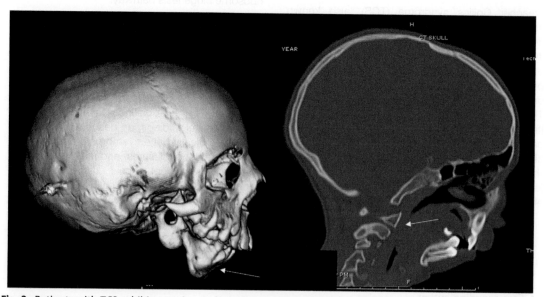

Fig. 2. Patients with TCS exhibit prominent clockwise rotation of the mandibular ramus in relation to the body, resulting in a convex facial profile with prominent microretrognathia (*left arrow*) and resulting airway obstruction (*right arrow*).

higher rates among patients with TCS compared with normal controls.[10,11] Condylar hypoplasia can secondarily result in temporomandibular joint (TMJ) dysfunction.[2] Importantly, these mandibular and maxillary dysmorphologies frequently cause marked glossoptosis with associated upper airway obstruction; obstructive sleep apnea (OSA) can be seen in as many as 95% of patient with TCSs, and, as a result, some require tracheostomy to ensure airway patency.[12–14]

Other common features of TCS include microtia, cleft palate with or without cleft lip, and malar and zygomatic hypoplasia with decreased width of the midface.[14–16] A bony cleft is often observed at the zygomatic arch with limited formation of the residual zygoma, including the glenoid fossa. Other craniofacial skeleton abnormalities include a reduced cranial base angle with decreased anteroposterior length and bitemporal width.[14] Additional but less common craniofacial findings include choanal atresia, complete or submucous cleft palate, and absent parotid glands. Extracranial features can also include cryptorchidism, renal abnormalities, congenital heart disease, and extremity malformation. The summation of these multiple deformities commonly produces significant functional and aesthetic concerns, as well as psychological/social challenges in affected patients.

GENERAL PRINCIPLES ON THE MANAGEMENT OF TREACHER COLLINS SYNDROME

Early management of TCS should be directed toward functional aspects of care, most importantly airway assessment and (when needed) intervention. The degree and type of airway obstruction (choanal atresia, glossoptosis, lower airway obstruction) should be identified through complete endoscopic airway analysis. When indicated, polysomnography can quantify the extent of airway obstruction and provide a baseline of function. Management of airway deficiency depends on the severity of obstruction; in the most severe cases, intubation or tracheostomy may be required at an early age.

Early intervention priorities for patients with TCS include feeding, growth, and ocular evaluation. In patients with severe retrognathia, oral feeding can be a challenge and gastrostomy tube placement may be necessary. Specific education is sometimes needed to aid patients in feeding, especially among patients with cleft palate. Ocular evaluation must be performed to assess the degree of eye involvement. Tarsorrhaphy may be required to prevent permanent corneal damage.

Following, and sometimes concurrent with, early management, children with TCS should undergo multidisciplinary craniofacial assessment to address their functional and aesthetic challenges. Surgical evaluation is an early priority in patients with severe expressions of TCS associated with significant functional compromise.

MANDIBULAR DISTRACTION
Overview

Surgical evaluation of the mandible should be an early area of focus, because the marked mandibular retrusion secondary to loss of posterior facial height and clockwise rotation of the mandible can lead to glossoptosis and upper airway obstruction. The narrow pharynx commonly found in many patients with TCS compounds upper airway obstruction caused by the retropositioned tongue.[17] Prior studies have documented the sites of airway obstruction in TCS and have found that the entire upper airway respiratory tract from nasopharyngeal to laryngeal level may be affected.[18] These studies have found a strong correlation between craniofacial morphology and airway findings, highlighting the importance of both endoscopic airway studies and computed-tomography imaging prior to any intervention.[18–20] The goals of surgical management are centered on either achieving definitive airway control (ie, tracheostomy) or improving airway volume through the use of tongue-lip adhesion, mandibular advancement (orthognathic surgery), or mandibular distraction osteogenesis (MDO).

Mandibular Distraction Osteogenesis Indications and Timing in Patients with Treacher Collins Syndrome

The strict or relative indications for MDO remain a subject of debate. In the past, mandibular distraction was largely reserved for patients requiring decannulation[21,22]. While recent advancements in techniques for TCS have shown promise for intervention prior to tracheostomy or in patients with less severe deformities, MDO is still generally reserved for cannulated patients and/or those with moderate/severe OSA.

Although evaluation and planning for mandibular distraction should begin early, the procedure itself should be delayed until early childhood (age of mixed dentition) if the airway is stable and the OSA symptoms are limited such that they can be managed conservatively.[23] Waiting as long as possible minimizes the risk of multiple distractions before the patient reaches skeletal maturity. Initial distraction around ages 8 to 10 years followed by definitive orthognathic corrective surgery in late adolescence is preferred, when possible. The exact timing of surgery should be guided by the sleep study and functional evaluations performed.

In addition to an assessment of functional and airway status, proper imaging assessment through computed tomography (CT) should be performed to determine the anatomic feasability of MDO.

The extent of bony loss and mandibular deformity all have implications to the patient's candidacy for mandibular distraction. For example, a lack of condyle(s) or deficient TMJ anatomy is a contraindication for MDO, although there are strategies for overcoming these deficiencies in some patients (described later). Severe clockwise rotation of the mandible can also be difficult to definitely correct through distraction. If distraction is pursued in these cases, patients should be informed of increased risks of mandibular relapse.

Preoperative Virtual Surgical Planning

Before the introduction of virtual surgical planning (VSP) and three-dimensional (3D) printing technology to craniofacial surgery, several studies documented the associated detrimental effects of MDO on (1) injury to developing tooth buds, (2) deformational growth effects on the mandible, (3) facial soft tissue scarring, (4) inferior alveolar nerve damage, and (5) mandibular hypomotility caused by TMJ ankyloses.[24] However, the more recent experience of MDO in patients with TCS has been favorable with the introduction of computer-assisted design and computer-assisted manufacturing, which enables surgeons to design osteotomy guides and simulate hardware placement virtually (**Fig. 3**). In our experience, VSP osteotomy guides substantially decrease

the risk of iatrogenic injury to the inferior alveolar nerve or tooth buds, and preoperative simulation also allows finer control of the distraction vector. VSP has also been shown to help craniofacial surgeons perform preplanned mandibular and curvilinear distraction with a high degree of accuracy across a variety of surgical approaches, and has been associated with improved outcomes among patients receiving other forms of mandibular reconstruction.[25–28]

Given the benefits associated with VSP and the inherently challenging morphology seen in patients with TCS, the senior author routinely uses VSP before any TCS-related MDO in order to improve clinical outcomes. The senior author acquires a preoperative maxillofacial CT scan in all surgical patients with TCS and performs virtual simulation of the procedure with an industry partner that provide VSP services.

Technique

As previously discussed, MDO in patients with TCS is challenging, and prior reports have associated MDO with high rates of relapse and an inability to adequately maintain airway patency.[22,29] This problem is likely attributable to the significant deficiency of the TCS mandible in both mandibular height (ramus) and length (body), as well as the well-defined clockwise rotation of the deformity. Because of this rotational morphology, univector distraction lengthening[30] or genioglossus advancement are often limited in their capacity to correct the deficiencies.[31] Thus, treatment of patients with TCS may require more

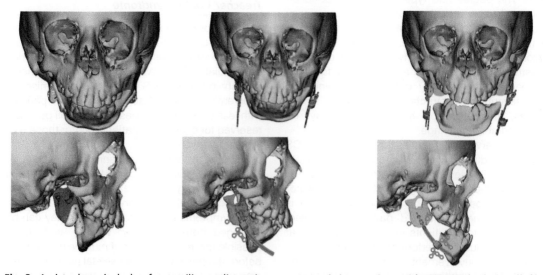

Fig. 3. A virtual surgical plan for curvilinear distraction osteogenesis in a patient with TCS: guide design (*left*), distractor placement (*center*), and distractor end position (*right*). Virtual surgical planning should be used in patients with TCS to simulate the optimal surgical plan and develop osteotomy splints and guides.

creative surgical approaches. Regardless of technique, MDO in patients with TCS should be performed with adequate understanding of the physiology and principles of distraction as well as the anatomic deformity affecting the jaw.[32]

Although univector MDO is the most frequently used technique for patients with TCS,[33,34] the authors preferred approach is curvilinear distraction osteogenesis, which can address both the vertical and horizontal mandibular deficiencies. Although curvilinear distraction is advocated by the senior author, other distraction techniques may be indicated depending on the patient's craniofacial morphology.

Curvilinear Distraction Osteogenesis

Many multiplanar distraction techniques have been developed to overcome the shortcomings associated with standard, univector MDO. At our institution, our preferred technique is curvilinear distraction to reconstruct the jaw deformity associated with TCS in growing patients.[35,36] First introduced by Schendel and coworkers in 2000, curvilinear distraction builds on the premise of a logarithmic growth pattern of the mandible.[37–39] Curvilinear distraction regenerates mandibular bone stock in both the body and ramus, and corrects the clockwise dysmorphology along a natural curved path.[40] This technique has been shown to be an effective treatment of neonatal OSA and TCS.[28,41]

Our surgical approach is similar to that described by Kaban and colleagues.[36] A standard extraoral approach is implemented, with an incision placed 2 cm inferior to the mandibular border, followed by sharp dissection through the platysma and elevation of a wide subperiosteal envelope.[42] A wider subperiosteal dissection is typically required to accommodate the VSP cutting guide. An osteotomy line is drawn after securing the VSP guide (**Fig. 4**) on the inferior aspect of the antegonial notch and angle and pre-planned fixation screw pilot holes are made both proximal and distal to the osteotomy (at least 2 anteriorly and posteriorly). The guide can then be removed, and corticotomies and/or osteotomies performed. After execution of the osteotomy, the distraction device is placed. The curvilinear device can then be assembled and secured (see **Fig. 4**); mobility of the osteotomized segment should be ensured bilaterally. Distraction arms can be posteriorly attached through stab incisions that exit postauricularly.

One challenge when performing distraction in patients with TCS is the lack of a natural skeletal condylar or TMJ. The senior author believes that a condyle or TMJ structure is necessary to perform MDO. One approach for overcoming this limitation is reconstructing the entire costochondral ramus and TMJ. Previously, we reported a procedure in a patient with hemifacial microsomia in which autologous bone graft was used to reconstruct the ramus-condyle unit simultaneously with curvilinear distraction.[43] We used a scalp flap (taking care to avoid tissue needed for ear reconstruction) to create a neo-TMJ, and a costochondral rib graft to reconstruct the mandibular ramus and condyle (**Fig. 5**). This approach created a proximal stop that allowed curvilinear distraction with good effect.

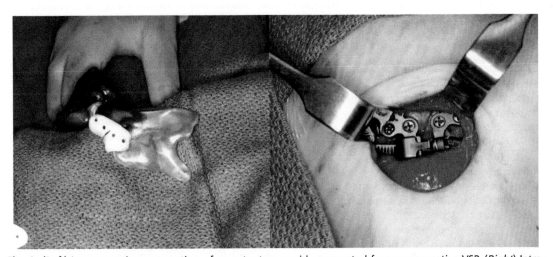

Fig. 4. (*Left*) Intraoperative preparation of an osteotomy guide generated from preoperative VSP. (*Right*) Intraoperative position of the curvilinear distraction device.

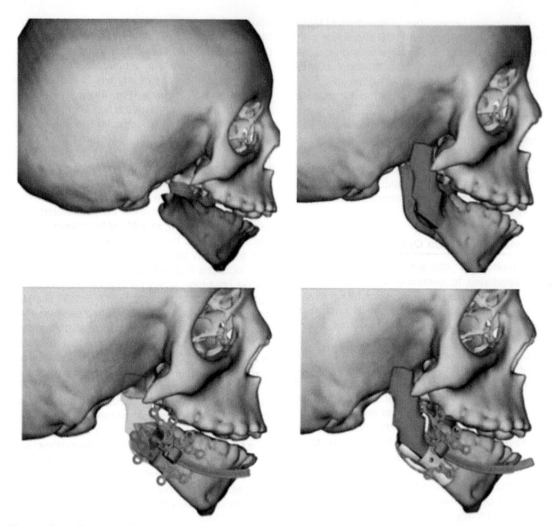

Fig. 5. Three-dimensional planning for simultaneous costochondral ramus-condyle reconstruction and mandibular distraction in a patient with hemifacial microsomia: preoperative condition (*top left*), placement of costochondral rib graft (*top right*), placement of curvilinear distracter (*bottom left*), and operative guide placement (*bottom right*). (*From* Morris R, Beckett J, Steinbacher DM. Simultaneous costochondral ramus-condyle reconstruction and mandibular distraction for hemifacial microsomia. *J Oral Maxillofac Surg.* 2012;70(10):e541-e546; with permission.)

Distraction Protocol

Postoperatively, patients are kept in the hospital overnight for pain control and monitoring. Correct placement of the device is confirmed by plain film radiograph on postoperative day 1. The patient's family are thoroughly educated during the period of distraction to ensure proper understanding of the device.

Distraction is performed according to protocols previously described by the senior author, with consideration of 3 distinct stages following the operation: latency, activation, and consolidation (**Table 1**). The latency period typically lasts 5 to 7 days in young children or 1 to 2 days in infants, and allows for the formation of a preliminary callous at the site of the osteotomy. Following this period, active distraction is performed to slowly expand the bone space and allow for the formation of new bony matrix. We typically perform distraction at a rate of 0.5 to 1.0 mm in older children, and 1.0 to 2.0 mm in infants. Serial weekly radiographs and close biweekly or weekly follow-up is required during this time to ensure adequate family education and monitor active distraction (**Fig. 6**). Completion of activation is achieved at the preplanned interval, at which time distraction arms can be removed. Class III occlusion is the target mandibular position in the growing face. The consolidation phase typically

Table 1
Phases of distraction osteogenesis and overall approach to distraction

Phase	Latency	Activation	Consolidation
Time	4–7 d child 1–2 d infant	Days to weeks	Months (at least 6 wk or 2× activation period)
Considerations	• Obtain radiograph on postoperative day 1 to ensure appropriate device placement • Educate patient and family regarding the device and performing turns	• 0.5–1 mm/d in older children; I–2 mm/d in infants (or until reaching class III occlusion) • Overcorrect to negative overjet • Monitor with weekly radiograph and follow-up	• Activation arms may be removed; device remains in place • Continue to monitor closely for infection and hardware failure • Older children typically require longer consolidation phase than infants

lasts 6 weeks or longer (twice the activation period is a useful reference), and allows for final bony ossification. After consolidation, the device is removed. Exposure of the mandible for device removal incorporates the same incision used during device placement. Scar revision is often performed at this time to optimize aesthetic appearance.

Following device removal, patients may be candidates for decannulation or deescalation of other respiratory support measures depending on the degree of postoperative airway expansion. These decisions should be guided by follow-up sleep studies; possible follow-up airway endoscopy; and coordination with other airway specialists, the patient, and the patient's family.

Outcomes

Distraction osteogenesis in patients with TCS can typically be performed with low surgical morbidity and good overall outcomes (**Figs. 7–9**). Minor surgical complications include surgical site infection (typically treated with antibiotics but may require incision and drainage in more severe cases) and transient facial nerve palsies.[44] Device dislodgement and/or misplacement can occur and can be diagnosed with serial radiographs immediately following placement. Curvilinear distraction of the vertical vector increases risk of iatrogenic damage to the TMJ, either directly by placing the screws too close to the condyle or indirectly by extending the distraction vector into the glenoid fossa.[42] In our experience, these complications can be largely avoided with the use of VSP preoperatively because VSP can control for screw placement and distraction vector. Nonetheless, extra attention should be given to both avoid this potential complication intraoperatively and monitor for its occurrence postoperatively.

One of the most common complications associated with distraction in patients with TCS is

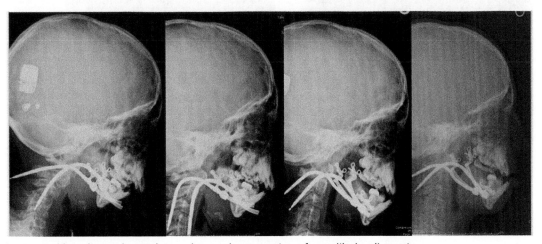

Fig. 6. Weekly radiographs can be used to track progression of mandibular distraction.

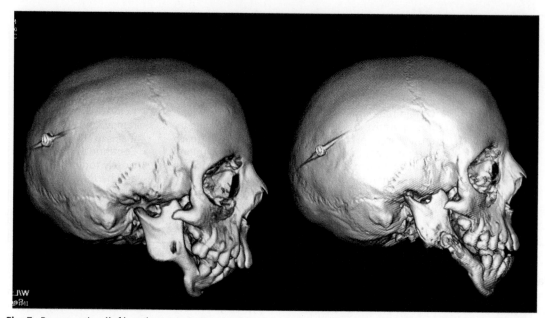

Fig. 7. Preoperative (*left*) and postoperative (*right*) 3D images in a patient with TCS who received MDO.

relapse. High rates of relapse may be secondary to mandibular bony hypoplasia, chronic traction of the strap muscles on the lower jaw, and the limited growth potential of the TCS mandible.[2] Although overcorrection to a class III profile can be performed, it is often insufficient to prevent relapse. Although curvilinear distraction has been associated with relative long-term stability in patients not affected by TCS,[45] the true rate of relapse after

curvilinear distraction in the TCS patient population is still largely unknown. Further research will be required to determine the relapse rate in children with curvilinear MDO compared with standard univector MDO.

Repeat Distraction

The primary strategy for addressing relapse and preventing airway obstruction is repeat

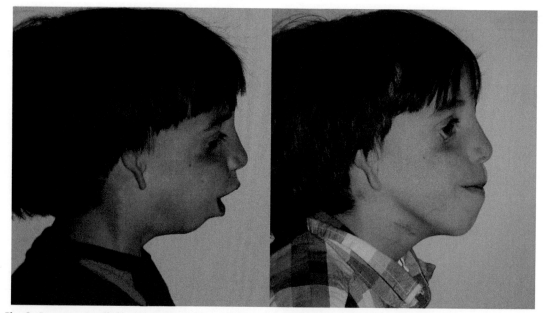

Fig. 8. Preoperative (*left*) and postoperative (*right*) clinical photographs of a patient with TCS following MDO.

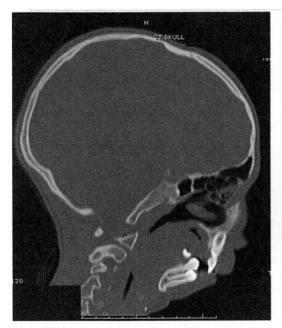 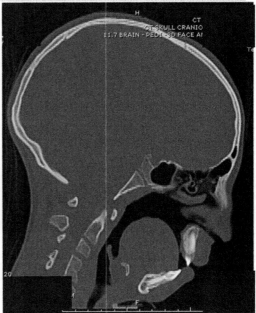

Fig. 9. Predistraction (*left*) and postdistraction (*right*) CT showing significant decrease in airway obstruction.

distraction, which may be anticipated in young patients with severe TCS. Repeat distraction procedures can be used either to prevent or resolve airway sequalae. However, redistraction may be associated with additional morbidity such as inferior alveolar nerve damage, tooth bud injuries, and retardation of future growth. Furthermore, limitations in the quality of the bony generated by the previous distraction procedure may present challenges to surgical planning. Given the limited evidence on the impact and efficacy of redistraction in children with TCS, further studies will be necessary to elucidate the morbidity associated with this procedure.

New and Future Approaches

Although the authors have experienced success with curvilinear distraction among patients with TCS, strategies to overcome the shortcomings of this and other approaches are the subject of ongoing research. New developing techniques have shown promise of further optimizing the results of mandibular distraction in TCS.

Counterclockwise craniofacial distraction osteogenesis as proposed by Hopper and colleagues,[46] which is described in a separate article in this issue, may allow greater airway improvement compared with current standard techniques by enabling en bloc distraction of the entire maxillary-mandibular complex. The authors recently reported a modified version of this

approach in a mixed-dentition patient with TCS with worsening OSA.[47] We implemented a 2-jaw repositioning strategy with intermediate and final splints before active distraction (**Fig. 10**). The first (intermediate) splint was placed following bilateral sagittal split osteotomy of the mandible to rotate the mandible and create a posterior open bite. The second (final) splint was placed following Le Fort III osteotomy, which allowed correction of the posterior open bite and occlusal discrepancy. This strategy allowed early clockwise rotation and correction of the airway deformity, as well as improvement of baseline occlusion (**Fig. 11**).

Another proposed but untested technique has suggested the use of a staged, segmental curvilinear distraction approach.[48,49] This strategy is based on observations that the regenerated bone in the distracted gap in curvilinear distraction forms along a different vector than the curvilinear distraction tract, presumably because of linear bone formation along a fixed strain vector that differs from the designed distraction vector.[50] Thus, this strategy proposes performing several different fixations throughout active osteogenesis in order to create various distraction gaps with different strain vectors, which would allow greater control of the curvature and direction of bone growth.

Although these techniques have yet to be tested in a large number of patients and the long-term stability remains a question, they show great promise in overcoming some of the standard challenges faced when performing distraction in

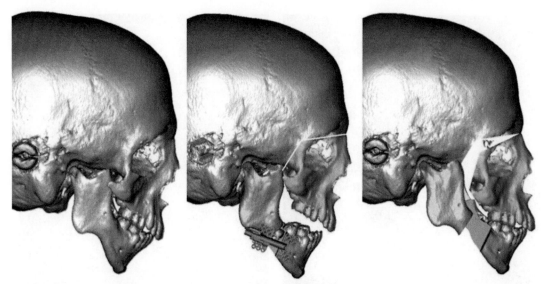

Fig. 10. (*Left*) Preoperative state. (*Center*) Planned intermediate splint position following bilateral sagittal split osteotomy and mandible repositioning. (*Right*) Planned postdistraction positions following Le Fort III osteotomy and movement of the midface using final splint. (*From* Steinbacher DM. Discussion: Counterclockwise Craniofacial Distraction Osteogenesis for Tracheostomy-Dependent Children with Treacher Collins Syndrome. *Plast Reconstr Surg.* 2018;142(2):458-462; with permission.)

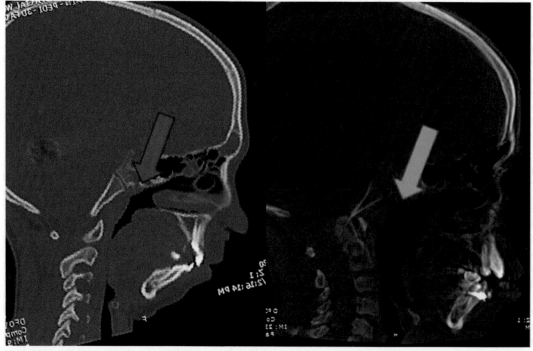

Fig. 11. Predistraction and postdistraction sagittal computed topographic images showing rotation of the maxillary-mandibular complex and significant airway enlargement. (*From* Steinbacher DM. Discussion: Counterclockwise Craniofacial Distraction Osteogenesis for Tracheostomy-Dependent Children with Treacher Collins Syndrome. *Plast Reconstr Surg.* 2018;142(2):458-462; with permission.)

Table 2
Treatment timeline for patients with Treacher Collins syndrome

Age	Birth	Infancy	Childhood	Early Adolescence	Late Adolescence
Studies	• Airway assessment • Sleep study • Eye examination	• Feeding, growth evaluation • Monitor dentition and oral hygiene	• Repeat sleep study • Cephalometric evaluation	• Sleep studies and/or cephalometrics when indicated	• Sleep studies and/or cephalometrics when indicated
Procedures	• Tracheostomy vs MDO (in severe cases)	• Begin removable BAHA • Cleft palate repair: age 1 y	• Initial and/or repeat distractions • Otoplasty first stage	• Repair of orbits, zygoma • Otoplasty second stage • Eyelid repair • Permanent BAHA • Presurgical orthodontics • Repeat distractions when needed	• Orthognathic surgery • Fat grafting and/or microvascular free flaps

patients affected by TCS. Better understanding and further optimization of these and other techniques are areas of future research.

ADDITIONAL SURGICAL PROCEDURES IN TREACHER COLLINS SYNDROME

Mandibular distraction is one of many procedures typically required for the treatment of patients with TCS. As described earlier, patients with TCS can have a host of craniofacial anomalies that present multiple aesthetic and functional challenges. Given the risks inherent to any procedure, especially among younger children, care should be taken to optimize the surgical treatment plan and minimize additional procedures when possible. Thus, mandibular distraction and repeat distractions in patients with TCS must be performed within the context of the long-term view of the treatment plan through the time of facial maturity. Performing mandibular distraction on a growing patient with TCS (or any patient with a craniofacial anomaly) simply because the opportunity presents itself is ill advised and is not necessarily in the best interests of the patient.

Although mandibular distraction alone may allow for a degree of descent and growth of the posterior maxilla, bimaxillary surgery is still typically required at skeletal maturity to close the residual posterior open bite and restore normal facial projection.[51] This surgery is typically performed in late adolescence, after facial growth has finished. Dental extraction and implantation is often required because poor bone stock predisposes to tooth devascularization, which may be compounded by repeated surgical procedures.[52] Palatoplasty should be performed in patients with cleft palate after airway stabilization, with efforts to minimize flap elevation so as to not compromise the potentially limited vasculature in the mucoperiosteum.[53] Malar reconstruction using bone grafting or alloplastic implants is usually performed in late childhood.[54,55] Ear reconstruction using autologous tissue or implants is performed in a staged approach to address the auricular abnormalities.[56] Patients also often require hearing rehabilitation using bone-assisted hearing aid (BAHA) implantation or other devices.[57]

Even after skeletal reconstruction, soft tissue deficits are common in patients with TCS. Fat grafting is our preferred method for augmenting soft tissue in atrophic areas, especially of the midface.[58] These procedures can be performed concurrently with other surgeries in the face and can be progressively implemented in the growing face. Periorbital deficits, especially of the lower lid, can be addressed by skin grafting, fat grafting, Z-plasty, and/or canthopexy.[59]

Treatment Timeline

In order to better plan the care of patients with TCSs, a proposed timeline for the surgical treatment of children is shown in **Table 2**. Although this timeline has not been validated by high-level evidence, our anecdotal experience suggests that this approach can assist craniofacial surgeons in the management of TCS dysmorphology.

SUMMARY

Mandibular distraction in TCS is a clinically challenging procedure given the prominent clockwise rotation of the mandible and the 3D deficiency and dysmorphology of the bone. Recent innovative techniques, such as curvilinear, counterclockwise mandibular distraction, have provided surgeons with an effective tool to address this challenging craniofacial deformity. These interventions can expand the pharyngeal airway and improve functional and aesthetic outcomes.

CLINICS CARE POINTS

- MDO is indicated in patients with TCS associated with moderate/severe OSA. The authors prefer delaying distraction until absolutely necessary, with definitive orthognathic surgery performed during late adolescence.

- Virtual surgical planning and the use of osteotomy guides can greatly mitigate complications such as injury to the inferior alveolar nerve and tooth buds.

- Curvilinear distraction allows greater recreation of ramus height and is the preferred MDO method in severely affected patients with TCS. However, standard unidirectional MDO can also be used.

- A careful evaluation of the mandibular morphology with careful attention to the condyle-TMJ unit is important to determine the feasibility of MDO.

- Repeat distractions are often necessary in patients with Treacher Collins given the high relapse rate in this population. The risks of repeat distraction can be mitigated by proper planning and appropriate surgical timing.

REFERENCES

1. Dixon MJ. Treacher collins syndrome. Hum Mol Genet 1996;5(Supplement_1):1391–3.
2. Chang CC, Steinbacher DM. Treacher collins syndrome. Semin Plast Surg 2012;26(2):83–90.
3. Sharma R, Sharma B, Babber M, et al. Treacher Collins syndrome: a case report and review of ophthalmic features. Taiwan J Ophthalmol 2016; 6(4):206–9.
4. Dixon MJ. Treacher collins syndrome. J Med Genet 1995;32(10):806–8.
5. Hertle RW, Ziylan S, Katowitz JA. Ophthalmic features and visual prognosis in the Treacher-Collins syndrome. Br J Ophthalmol 1993;77(10):642–5.
6. Chong DK, Murray DJ, Britto JA, et al. A cephalometric analysis of maxillary and mandibular parameters in Treacher Collins syndrome. Plast Reconstr Surg 2008;121(3):77e–84e.
7. Steinbacher DM, Bartlett SP. Relation of the mandibular body and ramus in Treacher Collins syndrome. J Craniofac Surg 2011;22(1):302–5.
8. Posnick JC, Tiwana PS, Costello BJ. Treacher Collins syndrome: comprehensive evaluation and treatment. Oral Maxill Surg Clin North America 2004;16(4):503–23.
9. Esenlik E, Plana NM, Grayson BH, et al. Cephalometric predictors of clinical severity in treacher collins syndrome. Plast Reconstr Surg 2017;140(6): 1240–9.
10. Terner JS, Travieso R, Chang C, et al. An analysis of mandibular volume in treacher collins syndrome. Plast Reconstr Surg 2012;129(4):751e–3e.
11. Travieso R, Terner J, Chang C, et al. Mandibular volumetric comparison of treacher collins syndrome and hemifacial microsomia. Plast Reconstr Surg 2012;129(4):749e–51e.
12. Plomp RG, Bredero-Boelhouwer HH, Joosten KF, et al. Obstructive sleep apnoea in Treacher Collins syndrome: prevalence, severity and cause. Int J Oral Maxillofac Surg 2012;41(6):696–701.
13. Akre H, Øverland B, Åsten P, et al. Obstructive sleep apnea in Treacher Collins syndrome. Eur Arch Otorhinolaryngol 2012;269(1):331–7.
14. Posnick JC, al-Qattan MM, Moffat SM, et al. Cranio-orbito-zygomatic measurements from standard CT scans in unoperated Treacher Collins syndrome patients: comparison with normal controls. Cleft Palate Craniofac J 1995;32(1):20–4.
15. Wong KR, Pfaff MJ, Chang CC, et al. A range of malar and masseteric hypoplasia exists in Treacher Collins syndrome. J Plast Reconstr Aesthet Surg 2013;66(1):43–6.
16. Travieso R, Chang CC, Terner JS, et al. A range of condylar hypoplasia exists in Treacher Collins syndrome. J Oral Maxillofac Surg 2013;71(2): 393–7.

17. Shprintzen RJ, Croft C, Berkman MD, et al. Pharyngeal hypoplasia in treacher collins syndrome. Arch Otolaryngol 1979;105(3):127–31.

18. Ma X, Forte AJ, Persing JA, et al. Reduced three-dimensional airway volume is a function of skeletal dysmorphology in Treacher Collins syndrome. Plast Reconstr Surg 2015;135(2):382e–92e.

19. Plomp RG, van Lieshout MJ, Joosten KF, et al. Treacher collins syndrome: a systematic review of evidence-based treatment and recommendations. Plast Reconstr Surg 2016;137(1):191–204.

20. Ma X, Forte AJ, Berlin NL, et al. Reduced three-dimensional nasal airway volume in treacher collins syndrome and its association with craniofacial morphology. Plast Reconstr Surg 2015;135(5):885e–94e.

21. Cobb AR, Green B, Gill D, et al. The surgical management of Treacher Collins syndrome. Br J Oral Maxillofac Surg 2014;52(7):581–9.

22. Ali-Khan S, Runyan C, Nardini G, et al. Treacher collins syndrome and tracheostomy: decannulation using mandibular distraction osteogenesis. Ann Plast Surg 2018;81(3):305–10.

23. Kobus K, Wójcicki P. Surgical treatment of treacher collins syndrome. Ann Plast Surg 2006;56(5):549–54.

24. Baas EM, Horsthuis RBG, de Lange J. Subjective alveolar nerve function after bilateral sagittal split osteotomy or distraction osteogenesis of mandible. J Oral Maxillofac Surg 2012;70(4):910–8.

25. Scolozzi P, Link DW II, Schendel SA. Computer simulation of curvilinear mandibular distraction: accuracy and predictability. Plast Reconstr Surg 2007;120(7):1975–80.

26. Resnick CM. Virtual surgical planning for mandibular distraction in infants with robin sequence. Plast Reconstr Surg Glob Open 2017;5(6):e1379.

27. Chang EI, Jenkins MP, Patel SA, et al. Long-term operative outcomes of preoperative computed tomography–guided virtual surgical planning for osteocutaneous free flap mandible reconstruction. Plast Reconstr Surg 2016;137(2):619–23.

28. Miller JJ, Kahn D, Lorenz HP, et al. Infant mandibular distraction with an internal curvilinear device. J Craniofac Surg 2007;18(6):1403–7.

29. Tessier P, Tulasne JF. Stability in correction of hypertelorbitism and Treacher Collins syndromes. Clin Plast Surg 1989;16(1):195–204.

30. Miloro M. Mandibular distraction osteogenesis for pediatric airway management. J Oral Maxillofac Surg 2010;68(7):1512–23.

31. Heller JB, Gabbay JS, Kwan D, et al. Genioplasty distraction osteogenesis and hyoid advancement for correction of upper airway obstruction in patients with Treacher Collins and Nager syndromes. Plast Reconstr Surg 2006;117(7):2389–98.

32. Zellner E, Steinbacher DM. Pediatric plastic and reconstructive surgery. In: Distraction Osteogenesis. Stuggart: Thieme; 2018. p. 99–111.

33. Denny AD, Talisman R, Hanson PR, et al. Mandibular distraction osteogenesis in very young patients to correct airway obstruction. Plast Reconstr Surg 2001;108(2):302–11.

34. Cohen SR, Simms C, Burstein FD. Mandibular distraction osteogenesis in the treatment of upper airway obstruction in children with craniofacial deformities. Plast Reconstr Surg 1998;101(2):312–8.

35. Miller JJ, Schendel SA. Invited discussion: surgical treatment of treacher collins syndrome. Ann Plast Surg 2006;56(5):555–6.

36. Kaban LB, Seldin EB, Kikinis R, et al. Clinical application of curvilinear distraction osteogenesis for correction of mandibular deformities. J Oral Maxillofac Surg 2009;67(5):996–1008.

37. Moss ML, Salentijn L. The logarithmic growth of the human mandible. Acta Anatomica 1970;77(3):341–60.

38. Schendel SA. Curvilinear distraction. J Oral Maxillofac Surg 2009;67(12):2696–7 [author reply: 2697–8].

39. Ricketts RM. The biologic significance of the divine proportion and Fibonacci series. Am J Orthod 1982;81(5):351–70.

40. Ritter L, Yeshwant K, Seldin EB, et al. Range of curvilinear distraction devices required for treatment of mandibular deformities. J Oral Maxillofac Surg 2006;64(2):259–64.

41. Handler MZ, Alabi O, Miller J. Curvilinear mandibular distraction in a patient with mandibulofacial dysostosis associated with Diamond-Blackfan anemia. J Craniofac Surg 2009;20(5):1417–9.

42. Flores RL. Neonatal mandibular distraction osteogenesis. Semin Plast Surg 2014;28(4):199–206.

43. Morris R, Beckett J, Steinbacher DM. Simultaneous costochondral ramus-condyle reconstruction and mandibular distraction for hemifacial microsomia. J Oral Maxillofac Surg 2012;70(10):e541–6.

44. Murage KP, Costa MA, Friel MT, et al. Complications associated with neonatal mandibular distraction osteogenesis in the treatment of Robin sequence. J Craniofac Surg 2014;25(2):383–7.

45. Aizenbud D, Hazan-Molina H, Thimmappa B, et al. Curvilinear mandibular distraction results and long-term stability effects in a group of 40 patients. Plast Reconstr Surg 2010;125(6):1771–80.

46. Hopper RA, Kapadia H, Susarla S, et al. Counterclockwise craniofacial distraction osteogenesis for tracheostomy-dependent children with treacher collins syndrome. Plast Reconstr Surg 2018;142(2):447–57.

47. Steinbacher DM. Discussion: counterclockwise craniofacial distraction osteogenesis for tracheostomy-dependent children with treacher collins syndrome. Plast Reconstr Surg 2018;142(2):458–62.

48. Pereira AR, Neves P, Rosa J, et al. Curvilinear segmental mandibular reconstruction utilizing distraction osteogenesis and early open callus

manipulation. Plast Reconstr Surg Glob Open 2017;
5(1):e1229.

49. Zhou L, Shang H, Feng Z, et al. Segmental curvilinear distraction osteogenesis. Med Hypotheses 2012;79(4):427–9.

50. Zhou L, Liu G, Han Z, et al. Grain size effect on wear resistance of a nanostructured AISI52100 steel. Scripta Materialia 2008;58(6):445–8.

51. Obwegeser HL. Variations of a standard approach for correction of the bird-face deformity. J Cranio Maxillofac Surg 1988;16(6):247–65.

52. da Silva Freitas R, Tolazzi AR, Alonso N, et al. Evaluation of molar teeth and buds in patients submitted to mandible distraction: long-term results. Plast Reconstr Surg 2008;121(4):1335–42.

53. Bresnick S, Walker J, Clarke-Sheehan N, et al. Increased fistula risk following palatoplasty in Treacher Collins syndrome. Cleft Palate Craniofac J 2003;40(3):280–3.

54. Posnick JC, Ruiz RL. Treacher Collins syndrome: current evaluation, treatment, and future directions. Cleft Palate Craniofac J 2000;37(5):434.

55. Taylor JA. Bilateral orbitozygomatic reconstruction with tissue-engineered bone. J Craniofac Surg 2010;21(5):1612–4.

56. Bauer BS. Reconstruction of microtia. Plast Reconstr Surg 2009;124(1 Suppl):14e–26e.

57. Marsella P, Scorpecci A, Pacifico C, et al. Bone-anchored hearing aid (Baha) in patients with Treacher Collins syndrome: tips and pitfalls. Int J Pediatr Otorhinolaryngol 2011;75(10):1308–12.

58. Coleman SR. Facial augmentation with structural fat grafting. Clin Plast Surg 2006;33(4):567–77.

59. Wake MJC. Craniofacial anomalies: growth and development from a surgical perspective. Ann R Coll Surg Engl 1997;79(3):238–9.

Counterclockwise Craniofacial Distraction Osteogenesis

Richard A. Hopper, MD, MS[a,b],*, Howard D. Wang, MD[a,b],
Ezgi Mercan, PhD[a], Hitesh Kapadia, PhD[a,b,c]

KEYWORDS

- Treacher Collins syndrome • Craniofacial microsomia • Hemifacial microsomia
- Midface hypoplasia • Distraction osteogenesis • Midface distraction • Mandibular distraction
- Upper airway obstruction

KEY POINTS

- The skeletal deformity of Treacher Collins syndrome and some cases of bilateral craniofacial microsomia are characterized by a high occlusal plane in addition to mandibular and midface hypoplasia.
- This bimaxillary rotational deformity results in upper airway narrowing of the oropharynx and nasopharynx and can result in tracheostomy dependence.
- Counterclockwise craniofacial distraction osteogenesis (C3DO) increases the airway volume at both the nasopharyngeal and oropharyngeal levels through rotation of the entire subcranial skeleton.
- In cases without an adequate condylar to skull base relationship, such as in Pruzansky types IIB and III mandibular deformities, a staged approach with enucleation of the second molar follicles and temporomandibular joint reconstruction with costochondral graft is required before C3DO.
- C3DO can result in successful decannulation of tracheostomy-dependent patients with a rotational deformity, when previous attempts of single jaw surgery or choanal atresia surgery have been unsuccessful.

BACKGROUND

Treacher Collins syndrome is an autosomal dominant condition characterized by abnormal development of craniofacial structures derived from the first and second branchial arches.[1] Clinical features can include hypoplastic zygomas, micrognathia, microtia, conductive hearing loss, coloboma of the eyelids, down-slanting palpebral fissures, and cleft palate. Severe presentation is characterized by hypoplasia and clockwise rotation of the maxillomandibular complex, contributing to upper airway obstruction and tracheostomy dependence.[2,3] The prevalence of obstructive sleep apnea in Treacher Collins syndrome patients has been reported to range from 25% to 91%, with a significant subset requiring tracheostomy.[4–7] In the most severe cases, patients remain tracheostomy-dependent despite multiple surgical interventions, including isolated lengthening of mandible through distraction osteogenesis.[8]

Three-dimensional airway analysis of Treacher Collins syndrome has revealed reduced airway volume at multiple levels, including the nasal and retroglossal region. Furthermore, the degree of maxillomandibular hypoplasia and clockwise rotation both contribute to the reduced airway

[a] The Craniofacial Center, Seattle Children's Hospital, 4800 Sand Point Way Northeast, Seattle, WA 98105, USA;
[b] Division of Plastic Surgery, Department of Surgery, University of Washington; [c] Department of Orthodontics, School of Dentistry, University of Washington
* Corresponding author. Division of Craniofacial and Plastic Surgery, Seattle Children's Hospital, 4800 Sand Point Way Northeast, Seattle, WA 98105.
E-mail address: richard.hopper@seattlechildrens.org

Clin Plastic Surg 48 (2021) 445–454
https://doi.org/10.1016/j.cps.2021.02.006
0094-1298/21/Published by Elsevier Inc.

volume.[9,10] The importance of counterclockwise rotation to treat obstructive airway disease is well recognized.[11,12] Tessier proposed the integral procedure in 1985 to correct the rotational deformity in Treacher Collins syndrome using a combination of Le Fort II and mandibular osteotomies.[13] This operation was limited, however, by the need for extensive bone grafting, high rates of relapse, and challenge with overcoming the restrictive soft tissue envelope.[14]

The counterclockwise craniofacial distraction osteogenesis (C3DO) shares some similarities to the integral procedure described by Tessier but leverages the gradual stretching of the surrounding soft tissue envelope characterized by distraction osteogenesis. C3DO combines subcranial and bilateral mandibular distraction around a nasofrontal pivot point to achieve counterclockwise rotation of the maxillomandibular complex and expansion of the entire upper airway.[15] The goal of the operation is to achieve decannulation in tracheostomy-dependent children. Early results of this operation in tracheostomy-dependent children with Treacher Collins syndrome have demonstrated a large magnitude of palatal rotation and a high success rate of decannulation.

INDICATIONS

The primary indication for C3DO is severe airway obstruction with tracheostomy dependence in the setting of maxillomandibular deficiency and a high occlusal plane (**Fig. 1**). Many patients who undergo this operation have had unsuccessful attempts to remove the tracheostomy tube using other procedures, including isolated mandibular distraction, and often are dependent on gastrostomy tube for feeding. In addition to Treacher Collins syndrome, severe presentations of other conditions, such as craniofacial microsomia and acrofacial dysostosis, also have benefited from this operation.

All patients require computed tomography (CT) imaging to assess the bony and soft tissue anatomy and undergo a formal airway evaluation by a pediatric otolaryngologist to characterize the airway anatomy and levels of obstruction. A combination of restricted nasopharyngeal volume, small choana, oropharyngeal obstruction from retroglossia, and a high palatal plane indicates the patient would benefit from rotational advancement of the maxillomandibular complex. CT-based virtual surgical planning (VSP) is used to plan the osteotomy and traction pin placements, and a craniofacial orthodontist fabricates an occlusal splint with traction posts to coordinate final jaw positioning. At the authors' center, the C3DO

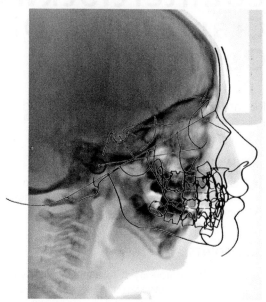

Fig. 1. Lateral cephalogram tracing of a tracheostomy-dependent patient with Treacher Collins syndrome who would be a candidate for the C3DO procedure for airway improvement with overlayed Bolton normal tracing. The deformity is characterized by a subcranial clockwise rotation deformity with a high occlusal plane. This has caused compression of the nasopharyngeal and oropharyngeal airway cavities.

operation is not performed before the age of 7, and the surgery preferably is performed closer to the age of 10. This timing optimizes bone stability, allows eruption of permanent molars and central incisors for splint stability, and from the authors' experience provides airway improvement that lasts until the final orthognathic treatment at maturity.

A staged approach is required in patients with abnormal temporomandibular joints, such as Kaban-Pruzansky type IIB and type III mandibles. The first stage is enucleation of second molar follicles that is in the line of the eventual mandible osteotomy, along with iliac crest corticocancellous grafting to augment the posterior mandible and facilitate enucleation site healing. The second stage takes place approximately 9 months later to place bilateral costochondral grafts to establish a centric relation. The subcranial rotational surgery then is planned as a third stage approximately 9 months to 12 months after the second stage. Depending on the patient's mandibular anatomy, the first 2 stages may be combined if there is adequate bone stock for fixation of the costochondral graft and planning of the final mandible osteotomy.

SURGICAL TECHNIQUE
Stage 1: Enucleation of Mandible Second Molar Follicles and Iliac Crest Bone Grafting

- Enucleation of tooth follicles is performed through an external approach using the Risdon incisions that are used for subsequent stages.
- Subperiosteal dissection then is performed along the inferior border of the mandibular body and up to the apex of the mandibular ramus remnant.
- A piezoelectric saw is used to create a bony window over the dental follicle to allow enucleation.
- The extraction site is burred to create a recipient bed for bone grafting, with care taken to avoid damage to the inferior alveolar nerve that typically is in close proximity.
- Both cancellous bone graft and a piece of medial cortical bone are harvested from the iliac crest.
- The cancellous bone graft is used to pack the extraction site, and the cortical graft is used to augment the posterior mandible and secured with a lag screw.
- All incisions are closed, and the extraction site is allowed to heal for approximately 9 months before the next stage.

Stage 2: Temporomandibular Joint Reconstruction with Costochondral Graft

- The authors use VSP and stereotactic navigation guidance to ensure accurate placement of costochondral grafts relative to the skull base.
- The Risdon incisions are reopened to expose the inferior border of the hypoplastic mandible.
- VSP cutting guides are used to shave off the prominence of the mandibular angle to allow for better apposition of the costochondral grafts to the mandible.
- VSP positioning guides are used to identify the desired angle of graft placement, and blunt finger dissection is used to create a pocket toward the skull base just lateral to the pterygoid plates.
- Stereotactic navigation then is used within the pocket to confirm the landing point of the graft on the skull base.
- A third or fourth costochondral graft is harvested with a length determined by VSP planning and 5 mm of cartilage cap with intact perichondrium.

- The VSP occlusal splint is used to establish the desired maxillomandibular relationship. Minor closure of an anterior open bite is possible if there is sufficient mandible mobility.
- Positioning guides are used to insert the rib graft in the appropriate orientation (**Fig. 2**), and stereotactic navigation can be used again to confirm the placement of the graft.
- Once the location has been confirmed, the rib graft is fixated with titanium plates and screws.
- The positioning guide then is removed, and the incisions are closed.
- Orthodontic bone anchors are secured anteriorly between the central incisors for placement of elastics postoperatively.
- The patient is maintained on a soft diet for a few weeks, and the C3DO surgery can be performed 9 months later.

Stage 3: Counterclockwise Craniofacial Distraction Osteogenesis

- A Le Fort II or Le Fort III osteotomy is performed, based on the degree of hypoplasia of the zygomas, through a coronal incision and subgaleal dissection.
- The anterior edge of the temporalis origin is released but the remaining muscle is left in place to prevent atrophy.
- Exposure of the nasofrontal region, lateral orbital rim, anterior part of the zygomatic arch, and the medial and lateral orbital walls is performed.
- Next, the nasofrontal osteotomy is performed with a piezoelectric saw, and a 5-mm wedge of bone is removed to create the hinge for rotation.
- The piezoelectric saw is used to continue along the medial orbital wall behind the medial canthus bilaterally.
- An osteotome is used to complete the medial orbital wall osteotomy down to the floor.
- A reciprocating saw then is used to release the zygomatic arch at its junction with the zygomatic body and cut from the inferior orbital fissure through the junction of the lateral and inferior orbital rims.
- Next, an osteotome is inserted into the inferior orbital fissure and directed medially to complete the orbital floor osteotomy toward the previously made medial wall osteotomy.
- An osteotome is placed in the suborbital edge of the inferior orbital fissure and directed inferiorly along the posterior wall of the maxillary sinus, finishing with a pterygomaxillary

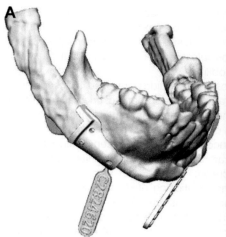
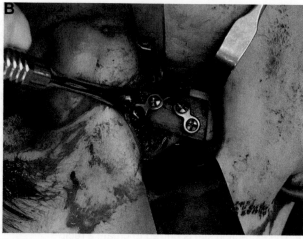

Fig. 2. (*A*) VSP for accurate positioning of costochondral grafts in a patient with severe mandibular hypoplasia. (*B*) Positioning of the graft with the use of the custom guide through a Risdon incision. Establishment of a temporomandibular relationship with costochondral grafts is performed in selected patients 9 months to 12 months before the C3DO procedure.

osteotomy. If needed, an intraoral mucosal access can be used to complete the pterygomaxillary disjunction.

- Due to the severe clockwise rotation deformity of the maxilla, this osteotomy needs to be immediately below the skull base to avoid damage to the maxillary molar follicles.
- The septal disjunction then is performed with an osteotome through the nasofrontal region, aiming toward the posterior nasal spine.
- Down-fracturing then is performed with gentle manual pressure and the midface is fully mobilized with Rowe-Kiley forceps.
- Steel wires (28 gauge) or 3-0 polydioxanone sutures are placed through bone holes at the nasofrontal osteotomy site to create a hinge for the rotational movement.
- Prior to closure of the scalp incision, lateral canthopexies should be performed if future zygomatic reconstruction is not required.
- Once the scalp is closed, the preexisting Risdon incisions are used to access the mandible.
- VSP can be helpful to avoid injury to the mandibular tooth follicles and the inferior alveolar nerve. Additionally, it can help to achieve precise positioning of the transfacial pins to allow for parallel placement of the external mandibular distractors.
- Preplanned cutting/positioning guides are adapted to the mandible and secured in place.
- The positioning guides are used to drill the predicted holes bilaterally for the transfacial pins

- The planned inverted-L osteotomies positioned behind the lingula are started with a piezoelectric saw, but the inferior cortex is left intact to maintain mandibular stability during pin insertion.
- The cutting guides are removed.
- Next, 2 pairs of 0.078-in transfacial pins are passed through the predrilled holes on 1 ramus and behind the tonsillar pillar into the pharynx. A Frazier suction tip then is passed through the contralateral ramal holes into the pharynx to receive the tips of the pins. The Frazier tip acts as a guiding device; with withdrawal of the Frazier suction, the pins are guided out the contralateral holes.
- The mandibular osteotomies then are completed, and the patient is placed into the custom acrylic occlusal splint with extraoral traction posts from an embedded facebow. Suspension wires from the piriform rim and lateral maxillary buttress secure the splint.
- Maxillomandibular fixation is achieved using circummandibular and suspension wires from the piriform aperture and the lateral buttress.
- Multivector mandibular external distraction devices are attached to the transfacial pins.
- A halo external midface distraction device is secured using cranial pins.
- The activation posts are secured with 24-gauge wires to the traction posts on the splint and the vector is set at 45o upwards (**Fig. 3**A)
- The patient is kept sedated and monitored in the intensive care unit for 48 hours after surgery.

A
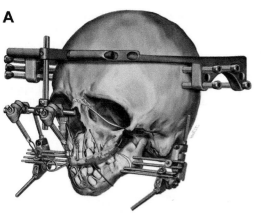

B
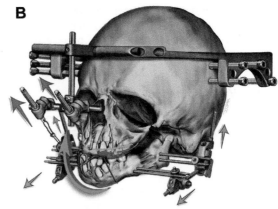

Fig. 3. Artistic rendering before (*A*) and after (*B*) the bimaxillary subcranial rotation movement achieved with the C3DO procedure. The rotation is based on a wire or suture hinge at the nasofrontal osteotomy, with a wedge of bone removed to avoid impingement. Arrows indicate the direction of distraction. Orange: active distraction at the occlusal splint; Blue: passive distraction at the mandibular osteotomies; Green: overall direction of the maxillomandibular complex. See text for technical details. (*Illustrations by* Joseph Chovan, Cincinnati, OH.)

- After a 5-day latency period, the activation period is initiated by turning the midface distraction device until there is tension on the splint wires. This ensures the traction force is on the midface device to avoid compression of the temporomandibular joints.
- The midface device exerts the rotational pull at 1 mm/d using the nasofrontal wire as a hinge.
- The mandibular distractors are activated at the same rate as the midface device to maintain proximity of the mandibular condyles with the skull base.
- Weekly serial lateral cephalograms monitor the progress of distraction.
- Once the pogonion is in vertical line with the nasofrontal junction, the midface distraction arm angle is increased to as vertical as possible to maximize end rotation.
- The endpoint of activation is a normalized palatal plane, which requires an average rotation of 25° (see **Fig. 3**B).
- After 5 days of consolidation, the patient is taken back to the operating room to release the maxillomandibular fixation and allow for independent mandibular and maxilla movement during the consolidation phase. Elastic traction is maintained using the bone anchors.

Removal of Distraction Devices and Zygomatic Reconstruction

- After a 12-week consolidation period, the patient is taken back to the operating room for removal of distractors.
- Simultaneous zygoma reconstruction with cranial bone graft can be accomplished with

the assistance of VSP in conditions such as Treacher Collins syndrome.
- Custom guides identify the ideal curvature on the parietal bone donor site to harvest bilateral full-thickness calvarial bone grafts for bilateral zygoma reconstruction with titanium fixation.
- The cranial defects then are reconstructed with split calvarial bone graft from the remaining bone and fixated with resorbable plates.

CLINICAL OUTCOMES
Clinical Series

The authors have performed C3DO on 15 patients, with an age range from 3 years to 19 years and an average age of 8 years. Six had a diagnosis of Treacher Collins syndrome, 5 bilateral craniofacial microsomia, and 1 each of Nager syndrome, auriculocondylar syndrome, Miller syndrome, and radiation-induced hypoplasia. All received this treatment for obstructive airway disease in the presence of a clockwise rotation deformity.

Cephalometric Changes

Follow-up lateral cephalograms of the authors' initial series of 5 patients obtained between 5 months and 9 months after device removal demonstrated a relapse in the palatal plane of 5°, sella-nasion-A point angle (SNA) of 2°, and mandibular advancement of 7 mm.[15] These proportional changes are consistent with those described by smaller rotational movements from Le Fort I traditional orthognathic surgery.[16,17] To anticipate this relapse, the authors' current cephalometric goals are to demonstrate average palatal plane rotation of 20° to 25°, sella-nasion-B point angle increase of 15° to 20°, and SNB increase of 20° to 25°. Preliminary analysis of patients with longer follow-up after C3DO has shown stability of the palate plane rotation but with progressive bimaxillary retrusion from lack of growth and early relapse (**Fig. 4**).

Airway Volume Changes

The authors have measured airway volume using preoperative and postconsolidation CT scans. By addressing both the maxilla and the mandible with a counterclockwise rotation, the upper airway volume is increased at the nasal, nasopharyngeal, and oropharyngeal levels (**Fig. 5**). Preliminary analysis also demonstrates a significantly larger increase in the total upper airway volume compared with mandibular distraction alone (Hopper R, MD, unpublished data, 2019).

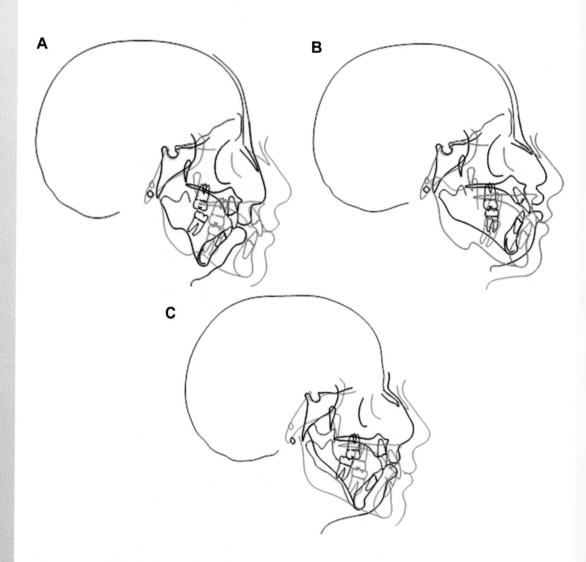

Fig. 4. Lateral cephalogram tracings (*black*) of a patient with Treacher Collins syndrome with age-matched Bolton normal superimpositions (*green*). (*A*) Before C3DO, the clockwise deformity is evident compared with age-matched normal with bimaxillary retrusion greater in the mandible than the maxilla and a high palate angle (22°). (*B*) After the C3DO procedure, the palate angle has been normalized to 8° and the maxilla and mandible approached normal position. (*C*) Five years later, there has been some reduction of bimaxillary advancement relative to the older age-matched Bolton normal, partially from lack of postsurgical growth and part from relapse. The palate plane correction has remained stable (8°). The authors anticipate this patient, as with other C3DO cases, will benefit from Le Fort I and mandible advancement but without the need of further rotational correction.

A

B

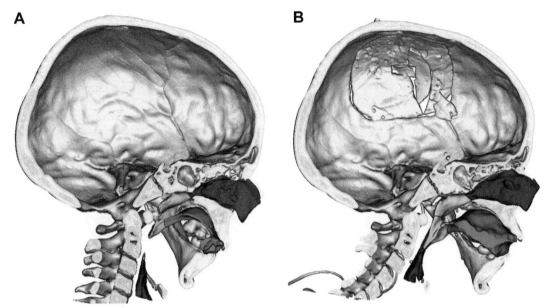

Fig. 5. Preoperative (*A*) and postoperative (*B*) renderings of the changes in the upper airway spaces achieved through the C3DO procedure. The greatest increase is in the nasopharynx, followed by the oropharynx.

Sleep Endoscopy and Polysomnography Changes

Comparing preoperative and postoperative sleep endoscopy studies, in the authors' initial series, the tongue base airspace improved from Chan-Parikh classification[18] grade 3 (complete obstruction) to grade 1 (0%–50% obstruction), and the Cormack-Lehane grading[19] of direct laryngoscopy view improved from grade 3 (epiglottis only) to grade 1 (normal—anterior commissure visible) (**Fig. 6**). Polysomnography studies performed a minimum of 3 months after C3DO with the tracheostomy capped showed near normalization of the apnea-hypopnea index, with an average of 5.5.[15]

Decannulation

Of the 11 previously tracheostomized patients with at least 1-year follow-up, 9 (82%) have remained

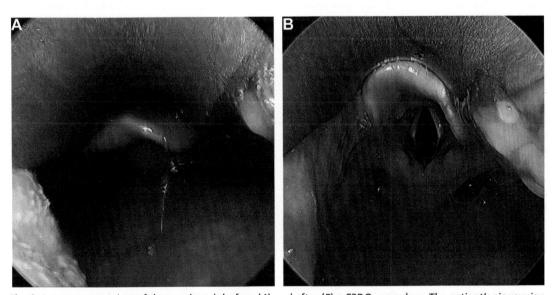

Fig. 6. Laryngoscope view of the vocal cords before (*A*) and after (*B*) a C3DO procedure. The patient's airway visualization has decreased from a Cormack-Lehane[19] grade 3 (epiglottis only, airway at risk) to a grade 1 (normal).

decannulated after the C3DO operation despite being tracheostomy-dependent since a young age and having undergone multiple previous airway surgeries, including mandibular distraction osteogenesis and choanal atresia surgery. One adolescent patient with Nager syndrome and one 3-year-old Treacher Collins patient failed decannulation. They both had successful subcranial rotation of the bony skeleton and improved airway space, but soft tissue prolapse was noted on endoscopy and further soft tissue airway surgeries are planned.

Complications

There have been no serious complications after C3DO and no prolonged morbidity or mortality. There has been no evidence of nonunion or lack of generate formation after the distraction. One patient who had porous polyethylene malar implants with repeated periorbital infections required removal of the implants. One patient with Treacher Collins syndrome and previous cleft palate repair and 1 with radiation-induced hypoplasia developed severe velopharyngeal insufficiency, presumably secondary to the palate rotation and increased nasopharyngeal space.

DISCUSSION

Patients with Treacher Collins syndrome and severe upper airway obstruction often require tracheostomy. Isolated repeated mandibular distraction traditionally has been performed in an attempt to avoid the need for tracheostomy or achieve decannulation.[20,21] Although mandibular distraction may increase the oropharyngeal airway by addressing the sagittal deficiency of the mandible, it does not adequately address the complete upper airway obstruction that has been described.[8,9] The C3DO procedure produces a counterclockwise rotation of the entire maxillomandibular complex with the pivot point at the nasofrontal hinge and uses the power of distraction osteogenesis to achieve the rotational movement envisioned by Tessier more than 3 decades ago.[13] This novel technique addresses both the sagittal deficiency and the high occlusal plane characteristic of patients with Treacher Collins syndrome and other conditions. At the conclusion of distraction, the greatest magnitude of advancement occurs at the pogonion by rotation at the nasion, resulting in a large increase in the nasopharyngeal and oropharyngeal airway volumes.

The challenges of treating severe airway obstruction in Treacher Collins syndrome patients are well recognized. One of the larger series of Treacher Collins syndrome patients treated with primary bilateral mandibular distraction reported the rate of successful decannulation to be 4 of 19 (21%).[21] Biskup and colleagues[22] reported on a retrospective study of 25 patients with Treacher Collins syndrome–related airway obstruction treated with either isolated mandibular distraction or combined maxillary and mandibular linear distraction. The decannulation rate in this study was 7 of 18 (39%). The authors' early experience has demonstrated C3DO to be an effective technique to achieve stable decannulation of patients with Treacher Collins syndrome and severe airway obstruction. The authors have performed C3DO on 7 patients with Treacher Collins syndrome who were tracheostomy-dependent despite having undergone multiple previous airway surgeries. Six of these were decannulated after C3DO and remain decannulated on last follow-up, for a success rate of 86%, which is greater than in previous reported series.

Craniofacial microsomia is another condition with rotational deformity and airway obstruction that can be amenable to treatment with C3DO. In a multicentered study of 755 patients with craniofacial microsomia, obstructive sleep apnea was identified in 17.6% and tracheostomy was required in 4.6% of patients, with a higher incidence in those with more severe phenotypes (Pruzansky type IIB/III mandibles) or bilaterally affected individuals.[23] The authors have performed C3DO on 3 consecutive tracheotomized patients with bilateral craniofacial microsomia and have achieved successful stable decannulation in all.

Nonfunctional esthetic benefits of C3DO include a shortening of the vertical length of the upper face, improved malar prominence, and shortening of nasal dorsal length with increased tip projection (**Fig. 7**). The authors anticipate that all patients will require definitive traditional orthognathic surgery at skeletal maturity to correct any residual malocclusion and further advance the maxillomandibular complex. The authors have observed that the rotation correction of C3DO is stable; therefore, the final orthognathic surgery is limited to linear advancement, avoiding the challenges of rotational correction at maturity (see **Fig. 4**).[24,25]

In comparison to the procedure integral described by Tessier, C3DO harnesses the stability of counterclockwise rotation achieved by the use of distraction osteogenesis to achieve a degree of simultaneous maxillomandibular rotation that has not been reported previously. The authors' early results have shown that the movement is relatively stable, and none of the decannulated patients has needed repeat tracheostomy.

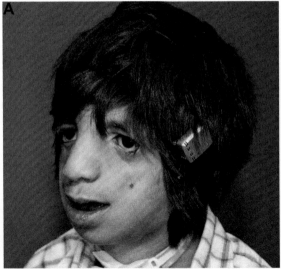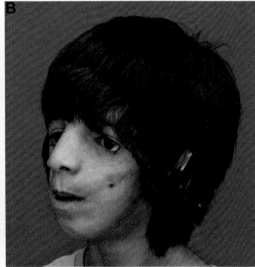

Fig. 7. Oblique view changes before (*A*) and 2 years after (*B*) C3DO in a patient with Treacher Collins syndrome. At the time of device removal, the patient underwent bilateral zygomatic reconstruction with full-thickness cranial grafts. The subcranial rotation movement achieved shortening of the upper midface height with increased nasal tip and chin projection.

SUMMARY

The authors' early experience with C3DO has yielded a high success rate of decannulation in patients with Treacher Collins syndrome and craniofacial microsomia. For patients who are tracheostomy-dependent and have a clockwise rotational deformity of the subcranial facial skeleton, C3DO has become the authors' operation of choice over mandibular distraction at a recommended age of 7 years or older.

CLINICS CARE POINTS

- During the activation phase, ensure the majority of the force exerted to achieve the subcranial rotation is on the midface pull rather than from mandibular distraction to minimize pressure on the condyles or costochondral grafts.

- Start with a 45o upward midface distraction vector until the pogonion is directly under the nasion and then verticalize the activation arms as much as possible to complete the rotation.

- Counsel patients with previous cleft palate repair on the risk of velopharyngeal insufficiency from palate rotation and increased nasopharyngeal space.

DISCLOSURE

Dr R.A. Hopper is the inventor on a patent licensed to KLS Martin LP. No other financial interest to disclose.

REFERENCES

1. Positional cloning of a gene involved in the pathogenesis of treacher collins syndrome. The treacher collins syndrome Collaborative Group. Nat Genet 1996;12:130–6.
2. Chong DK, Murray DJ, Britto JA, et al. A cephalometric analysis of maxillary and mandibular parameters in Treacher Collins syndrome. Plast Reconstr Surg 2008;121:77e–84e.
3. Kapadia H, Shetye PR, Grayson BH, et al. Cephalometric assessment of craniofacial morphology in patients with treacher Collins syndrome. J Craniofac Surg 2013;24:1141–5.
4. Akre H, Overland B, Asten P, et al. Obstructive sleep apnea in Treacher Collins syndrome. Eur Arch Otorhinolaryngol 2012;269:331–7.
5. Plomp RG, Bredero-Boelhouwer HH, Joosten KF, et al. Obstructive sleep apnoea in Treacher Collins syndrome: prevalence, severity and cause. Int J Oral Maxillofac Surg 2012;41:696–701.
6. Sher AE, Shprintzen RJ, Thorpy MJ. Endoscopic observations of obstructive sleep apnea in children with anomalous upper airways: predictive and therapeutic value. Int J Pediatr Otorhinolaryngol 1986;11:135–46.

7. Vallino-Napoli LD. A profile of the features and speech in patients with mandibulofacial dysostosis. Cleft Palate Craniofac J 2002;39:623–34.

8. Sorin A, McCarthy JG, Bernstein JM. Predicting decannulation outcomes after distraction osteogenesis for syndromic micrognathia. Laryngoscope 2004; 114:1815–21.

9. Ma X, Forte AJ, Berlin NL, et al. Reduced three-dimensional nasal airway volume in treacher collins syndrome and its association with craniofacial morphology. Plast Reconstr Surg 2015;135: 885e–94e.

10. Ma X, Forte AJ, Persing JA, et al. Reduced three-dimensional airway volume is a function of skeletal dysmorphology in Treacher Collins syndrome. Plast Reconstr Surg 2015;135:382e–92e.

11. Goncalves JR, Gomes LC, Vianna AP, et al. Airway space changes after maxillomandibular counterclockwise rotation and mandibular advancement with TMJ Concepts(R) total joint prostheses: three-dimensional assessment. Int J Oral Maxillofac Surg 2013;42:1014–22.

12. Rubio-Bueno P, Landete P, Ardanza B, et al. Maxillomandibular advancement as the initial treatment of obstructive sleep apnoea: is the mandibular occlusal plane the key? Int J Oral Maxillofac Surg 2017;46:1363–71.

13. Tulasne JF, Tessier PL. Results of the Tessier integral procedure for correction of Treacher Collins syndrome. Cleft Palate J 1986;23(Suppl 1):40–9.

14. Tessier P, Tulasne JF. Stability in correction of hypertelorbitism and Treacher Collins syndromes. Clin Plast Surg 1989;16:195–204.

15. Hopper RA, Kapadia H, Susarla S, et al. Counterclockwise craniofacial distraction osteogenesis for tracheostomy-dependent children with treacher collins syndrome. Plast Reconstr Surg 2018;142: 447–57.

16. Goncalves JR, Cassano DS, Wolford LM, et al. Post-surgical stability of counterclockwise maxillomandibular advancement surgery: affect of articular disc repositioning. J Oral Maxillofac Surg 2008;66: 724–38.

17. Reyneke JP, Bryant RS, Suuronen R, et al. Postoperative skeletal stability following clockwise and counter-clockwise rotation of the maxillomandibular complex compared to conventional orthognathic treatment. Br J Oral Maxillofac Surg 2007;45:56–64.

18. Chan DK, Liming BJ, Horn DL, et al. A new scoring system for upper airway pediatric sleep endoscopy. JAMA Otolaryngol Head Neck Surg 2014;140: 595–602.

19. Cormack RS, Lehane JR, Adams AP, et al. Laryngoscopy grades and percentage glottic opening. Anaesthesia 2000;55:184.

20. Plomp RG, van Lieshout MJ, Joosten KF, et al. Treacher collins syndrome: a systematic review of evidence-based treatment and recommendations. Plast Reconstr Surg 2016;137:191–204.

21. Ali-Khan S, Runyan C, Nardini G, et al. Treacher collins syndrome and tracheostomy: decannulation using mandibular distraction osteogenesis. Ann Plast Surg 2018;81:305–10.

22. Biskup NI, Pan BS, Elhadi-Babiker H, et al. Decannulation and airway outcomes with maxillomandibular distraction in treacher collins and Nager syndrome. J Craniofac Surg 2018;29:692–7.

23. Caron C, Pluijmers BI, Maas B, et al. Obstructive sleep apnoea in craniofacial microsomia: analysis of 755 patients. Int J Oral Maxillofac Surg 2017;46: 1330–7.

24. Birgfeld C, Heike C. Craniofacial microsomia. Clin Plast Surg 2019;46:207–21.

25. Nguyen PD, Caro MC, Smith DM, et al. Long-term orthognathic surgical outcomes in Treacher Collins patients. J Plast Reconstr Aesthet Surg 2016;69: 402–8.

Craniosynostosis
Posterior Cranial Vault Remodeling

Laura S. Humphries, MD[a], Jordan W. Swanson, MD, MSc[b], Scott P. Bartlett, MD[b], Jesse A. Taylor, MD[b],*

KEYWORDS

- Craniofacial distraction osteogenesis • Posterior cranial vault distraction osteogenesis
- Syndromic craniosynostosis • Nonsyndromic craniosynostosis • Intracranial expansion
- Cranial vault remodeling

KEY POINTS

- Posterior cranial vault distraction osteogenesis is a powerful, reliable, low-morbidity method for intracranial expansion, particularly useful in treating turribrachycephaly seen in syndromic craniosynostosis.
- Application of posterior cranial vault distraction osteogenesis as a first step in intracranial expansion in syndromic craniosynostosis achieves larger intracranial volume gains than other methods.
- Posterior cranial vault distraction osteogenesis preserves the frontal cranium for future frontofacial procedures, which may be negated or delayed owing to compensatory posterior cranial vault distraction osteogenesis-related cranial remodeling.
- Complications associated with posterior cranial vault distraction osteogenesis include cerebrospinal fluid leak, infection, and device failure.

INTRODUCTION

Craniosynostosis (CS) is the premature fusion of the cranial sutures that often occurs in infancy or early childhood. Its presence may result in cephalocranial disproportion, or constricted intracranial space that limits the growth and development of a child's brain. Expansion of the intracranial space is the primary goal of surgical intervention for CS. Cranial expansion aims to correct cranial dysmorphology and to optimize neurocognitive development by ensuring adequate cerebral space both globally and regionally, including the relief or prevention of elevated intracranial pressure (ICP).

CS comes in a variety of presentations. CS may affect one major cranial suture as in single-suture CS (metopic, sagittal, unicoronal, or unilambdoid), or may affect multiple sutures, as in multisuture CS. By convention, "pancraniosynostosis" refers to patients with CS involving more than 3 major cranial sutures.[1,2] Minor suture CS may be isolated or occur in combination with major suture fusion.[3] The degree of cranial dysmorphology associated with minor suture fusion may vary,[4,5] and the impact of its presence on ICP is unknown.[3]

Patients with CS may or may not be associated with a known syndrome, of which the most common are Crouzon, Apert, Pfeiffer, Sathre Chotzen, and Muenke syndromes (**Fig. 1**).[6] Patients with syndromic craniosynostoses have high rates of multisuture CS[6] manifesting in turribrachycephaly, elevated ICP, hydrocephalus and/or cerebral tonsillar herniation (ie, Chiari malformation).[7,8] These syndromes have genetic underpinnings, namely involving mutations of the FGFR1, FGFR2, FGFR3, and TWIST 1 genes, with autosomal-dominant inheritance patterns (see **Fig. 1**).

The methods of intracranial expansion have evolved over time, but the principal goals of

[a] Division of Plastic and Reconstructive Surgery, University of Mississippi Medical Center, Children's of Mississippi Hospital, 2500 N. State Street, Jackson, MS 39216, USA; [b] Division of Plastic and Reconstructive Surgery, The Children's Hospital of Philadelphia, 3401 Civic Center Boulevard, Philadelphia, PA 19104, USA
* Corresponding author.
E-mail address: jataylor@gmail.com
Twitter: @ls_humphries (L.S.H.)

Clin Plastic Surg 48 (2021) 455–471
https://doi.org/10.1016/j.cps.2021.03.001
0094-1298/21/© 2021 Elsevier Inc. All rights reserved.

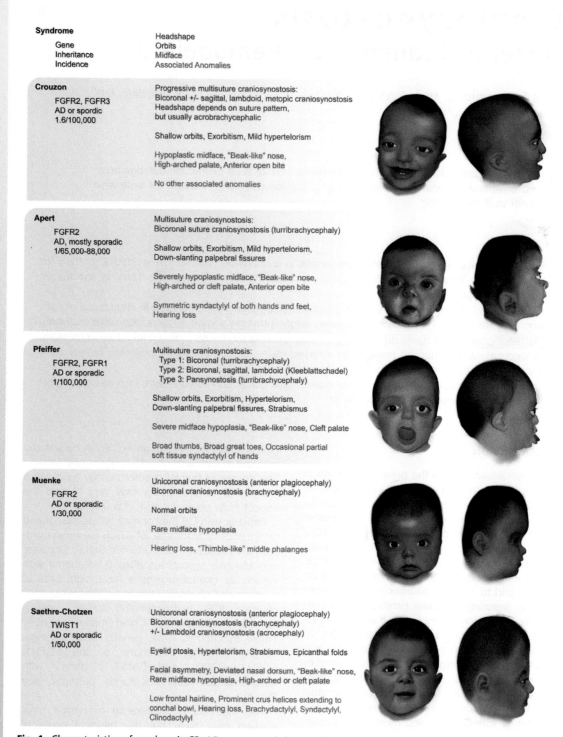

Syndrome Gene Inheritance Incidence	Headshape Orbits Midface Associated Anomalies
Crouzon FGFR2, FGFR3 AD or spordic 1.6/100,000	Progressive multisuture craniosynostosis: Bicoronal +/- sagittal, lambdoid, metopic craniosynostosis Headshape depends on suture pattern, but usually acrobrachycephalic Shallow orbits, Exorbitism, Mild hypertelorism Hypoplastic midface, "Beak-like" nose, High-arched palate, Anterior open bite No other associated anomalies
Apert FGFR2 AD, mostly sporadic 1/65,000-88,000	Multisuture craniosynostosis: Bicoronal suture craniosynostosis (turribrachycephaly) Shallow orbits, Exorbitism, Mild hypertelorism, Down-slanting palpebral fissures Severely hypoplastic midface, "Beak-like" nose, High-arched or cleft palate, Anterior open bite Symmetric syndactylyl of both hands and feet, Hearing loss
Pfeiffer FGFR2, FGFR1 AD or sporadic 1/100,000	Multisuture craniosynostosis: Type 1: Bicoronal (turribrachycephaly) Type 2: Bicoronal, sagittal, lambdoid (Kleeblattschadel) Type 3: Pansynostosis (turribrachycephaly) Shallow orbits, Exorbitism, Hypertelorism, Down-slanting palpebral fissures, Strabismus Severe midface hypoplasia, "Beak-like" nose, Cleft palate Broad thumbs, Broad great toes, Occasional partial soft tissue syndactylyl of hands
Muenke FGFR2 AD or sporadic 1/30,000	Unicoronal craniosynostosis (anterior plagiocephaly) Bicoronal craniosynostosis (brachycephaly) Normal orbits Rare midface hypoplasia Hearing loss, "Thimble-like" middle phalanges
Saethre-Chotzen TWIST1 AD or sporadic 1/50,000	Unicoronal craniosynostosis (anterior plagiocephaly) Bicoronal craniosynostosis (brachycephaly) +/- Lambdoid craniosynostosis (acrocephaly) Eyelid ptosis, Hypertelorism, Strabismus, Epicanthal folds Facial asymmetry, Deviated nasal dorsum, "Beak-like" nose, Rare midface hypoplasia, High-arched or cleft palate Low frontal hairline, Prominent crus helices extending to conchal bowl, Hearing loss, Brachydactylyl, Syndactylyl, Clinodactylyl

Fig. 1. Characteristics of syndromic CS. AD, autosomal dominant.

expanding intracranial space for a growing brain and correcting cranial dysmorphology have remained the same. In the early years of craniofacial surgery, surgeons focused on expanding the anterior cranial vault alone (bilateral frontal orbital advancement and remodeling [BFOAR])[8,9] or in conjunction with midface advancement (monobloc) to address concurrent midface hypoplasia.[8,10–13]

However, publications in the 1990s and thereafter demonstrated that open anterior cranial vault reconstruction early in life in the syndromic population is associated with high reoperation rates[4] for elevated ICP and recurrent cranial dysmorphology.[12] As a result, attention has shifted from anterior to posterior cranial vault expansion as an initial approach to treat syndromic CS[4] for patients without indications for a monobloc, such as severe exorbitism and obstructive sleep apnea.[14,15] Additionally, studies have shown that posterior cranial vault remodeling achieved greater intracranial volumetric expansion than that achieved by frontal surgery.[16] However, posterior vault remodeling could be technically challenging owing to large bridging veins, a thinned out cranium, limited soft tissue stretch, and the potential for relapse.[3–5] However, specific relapse rates and the need for repeat procedures owing to recurrent cranial deformity are not reported in the literature. Additionally, there are no craniometric studies to date investigating the degree of linear and volumetric expansion that is achieved with conventional open posterior vault reconstruction.

The question then became: how do we expand the posterior cranial vault to yield the maximum amount of intracranial volume while minimizing the risks and challenges associated with posterior vault reconstruction? This development set the stage for posterior cranial vault expansion with distraction osteogenesis. The history, approach, advantages, disadvantages, techniques and overall outcomes of posterior cranial vault distraction osteogenesis (PVDO) is the focus of the remainder of this article.

HISTORY OF POSTERIOR CRANIAL VAULT DISTRACTION OSTEOGENESIS

Distraction osteogenesis is the process by which gradual separation of bone segments at an osteotomy site results in new bone formation and bone lengthening. Bony healing of distraction mimics that of intramembranous ossification, with direct formation of bone rather than forming through a cartilaginous intermediate.[4] A long history of distraction osteogenesis precedes its application in the context of cranial vault expansion. The roots of distraction osteogenesis originate in orthopedic literature, whereby femur[17] and tibia[10] lengthening were described in the early 20th century. The technique was not adopted immediately owing to high morbidity, but Debastiani[18] and Ilizarov[19,20] popularized it in the latter half of the 20th century. Through intense clinical and histologic study, Ilizarov refined the concepts, principles and techniques of distraction; he published on the importance of appropriate bony fixation, refined distraction protocols, and described histology of distraction-related healing.[19,20]

Multiple animal studies validated the application of distraction the setting of the human facial skeleton.[21–24] One early study applied distraction to a frontal craniotomy in a white rabbit.[25] The results demonstrated advancement of the osteotomized segment compared with the sham and control groups. Histologically, they demonstrated callous bone deposition within the gap between the transport segment and the stable cranial bone segment.[25]

McCarthy and colleagues[26] were the first to publish applying distraction osteogenesis to the craniofacial skeleton in a clinical case description of mandibular distraction osteogenesis. Soon thereafter, distraction was applied to other aspects of the facial skeleton with success, including the cranial vault.[27–31] Early works of distraction in the cranial vault described transverse bilateral temporal distraction for sagittal craniosynostsis,[32,33] unilateral frontal distraction for unicoronal CS,[34] and bifrontal cranial distraction for patients with syndromic CS.[32,33,35–37] This approach in the syndromic population aligned with the philosophy of the time: treat the frontofacial area first. Studies demonstrated clinical success with this approach: faster operative times, lower blood loss rates, and greater intracranial volume gain for frontal cranial distraction compared with conventional cranial vault remodeling (mean 20.9% vs 10.7%).[38]

This moment in craniofacial history was critical: there was a shift toward posterior cranial vault expansion as a first step in treating syndromic CS and a search for maximizing intracranial expansion while minimizing relapse. In this moment, White and colleagues[39] described the initial series of posterior cranial vault distraction in 6 patients with Apert or Crouzon syndromes and multisuture CS with concern for elevated ICP. Patients were a mean age of 1.4 years and underwent PVDO and with median distraction distance of 24 mm (range, 18–30 mm). All patients had successful decreases in elevated ICP as determined by radiographs or fundoscopy.[39] Over the course of the next decade, PVDO has emerged as a powerful tool for cranial expansion, particularly in the syndromic and multisuture CS populations. Since 2009, we have adopted PVDO as our preferred initial cranial vault expansion technique in syndromic patients owing to its low complication rates,[40] low morbidity,[7] large volumetric expansion,[13,14] improvement in both frontal[41] and occipital morphologies,[42] the ability to resolve a Chiari malformation in some instances,[16] and the ability to delay frontal surgery.[15]

POSTERIOR CRANIAL VAULT DISTRACTION OSTEOGENESIS APPROACH AND TIMING

PVDO aims to gradually enlarge cranial volume through the movement of an osteotomized, vascularized posterior cranial segment. This gradual expansion improves abnormal cranial morphology, improves cerebral blood flow and cerebrospinal fluid flow, and aims to prevent or alleviate existing elevated ICP.[8] **Table 1** details the advantages and disadvantages of PVDO.

PVDO has been incorporated into a treatment algorithm for patients with syndromic CS at the Children's Hospital of Philadelphia, based on superior outcomes identified early in the use of PVDO at our institution[8,15] (**Fig. 2**). Given the multiorgan system effects of syndromic CS, it is important to frequently assess for and treat airway obstruction (nasopharyngeal or oropharyngeal), ocular protection (exorbitism with corneal exposure), and cerebral perfusion (severe cranial restriction).[15] Decompressive craniectomy or ventriculoperitoneal (VP) shunts should be considered for elevated ICP at an age of less than 3 months. If indicated, patients undergo tarsorrhaphy and/or tracheostomy before PVDO. PVDO is generally completed at 3 to 9 months of age, depending on severity of cephalocranial disproportion and ICP status. Then, patients are allowed to grow.

We anticipate that the progression of related deformities may need additional surgical treatment and are guided by a philosophy of optimizing function and minimizing the number of surgical procedures when planning additional interventions. Deformities may involve different anatomic levels alone or in combination: intracranial pathology (recurrent or persistently elevated ICP), cranial dysmorphology (frontal bone retrusion, turribrachycephaly), orbit (exorbitism, hypertelorism), nasal length (short), midface hypoplasia (central vs lateral), orthodontic or dental (abnormal maxillary dental arc, anterior open bite, high-arched palate), and obstructive sleep apnea. Patients may require a midface-only versus cranial vault-only expansion or both. The procedures may occur simultaneously (ie, monobloc) or in a staged fashion (see **Fig. 2**).[8,15] Following this treatment algorithm, we identified common syndrome-specific management patterns for interventions after PVDO as an initial intervention (**Fig. 3**).[15] Similar approaches have been supported by a number of studies, with the emphasis on early cranial expansion within the first year of life to optimize cognitive outcomes.[43–50]

POSTERIOR CRANIAL VAULT DISTRACTION OSTEOGENESIS TECHNIQUE
Distractor Type and Number

We generally use parallel, bitemporal, semiburied, self-ratcheting distractors for PVDO. The number

Table 1
PVDO advantages and disadvantages

Advantages	Disadvantages

Theoretic[8]
  Vascularized osteotomy
  Gradual expansion of soft tissue envelope
  Facilitation of new bone creation
	Prolonged treatment time[3–5]

Technical[3]
  Shorter operative times than conventional surgery
  No need for bone grafts
	Large bridging posterior veins[6] compared with frontal surgery
	Thinned out calvarium[6]
	Relying on parental compliance for advancement
	Need for operation to remove devices

Application and outcomes
  Favorable perioperative morbidity profile[7,8]
  Reliability of use in various populations (syndromic CS, nonsyndromic CS, early infancy, older patients)[8,9]
  Greater cranial volume gain over alternative methods[8,10–13]
  Alleviate elevated ICP in infants who are not old enough to have a conventional CVR[4]
  Aesthetic improvement in turribrachycephaly[12]
  Decrease reoperation rates in syndromic CS for elevated ICP[4] or frontal dysmorphology[14,15]
  Decreased incidence of post-PVDO Chiari malformation rates[16]
	Semiburied device risk for infection, poor aesthetics[3–5]
	Inability to simultaneously reshape gross contour abnormalities (flattened hypoplastic areas or compensatory bulges)[4]

Abbreviations: CVR, cranial vault remodeling; PVDO, posterior vault distraction osteogenesis.

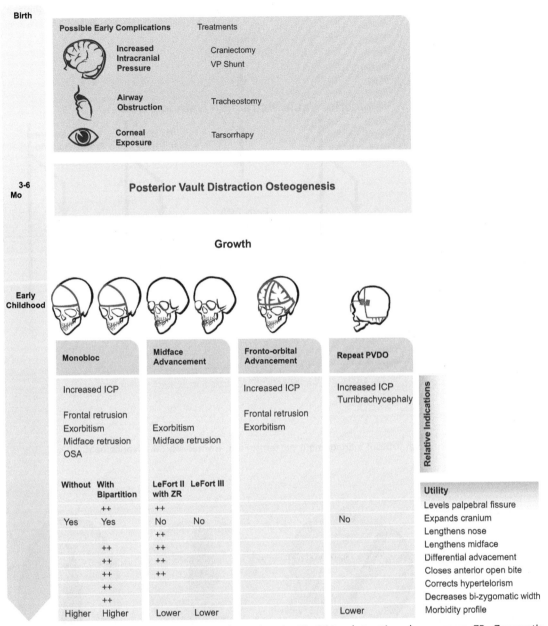

Fig. 2. Treatment algorithm of patients with syndromic CS. OSA, obstructive sleep apnea; ZR, Zygomatic Repositioning.

of distractors varies between institutions. Early in its adoption, 3 to 4 distractors were used for PVDO.[36,39,51,52] However, using 2 distractors has the following advantages[3]: (1) it offers sufficient control over the distraction vector while minimizing the chance of bone segment collision in the setting of multiple nonparallel vectors; (2) the lower device burden simplifies distraction regimen for parents and lowers the chance for device malfunction;

and (3) using fewer devices saves intraoperative time and is less expensive.

Distraction Vector and Technique for Application

To achieve PVDO, distractors may be applied in an anterior–posterior direction, transverse direction, or a combination of the two. In patients with severe

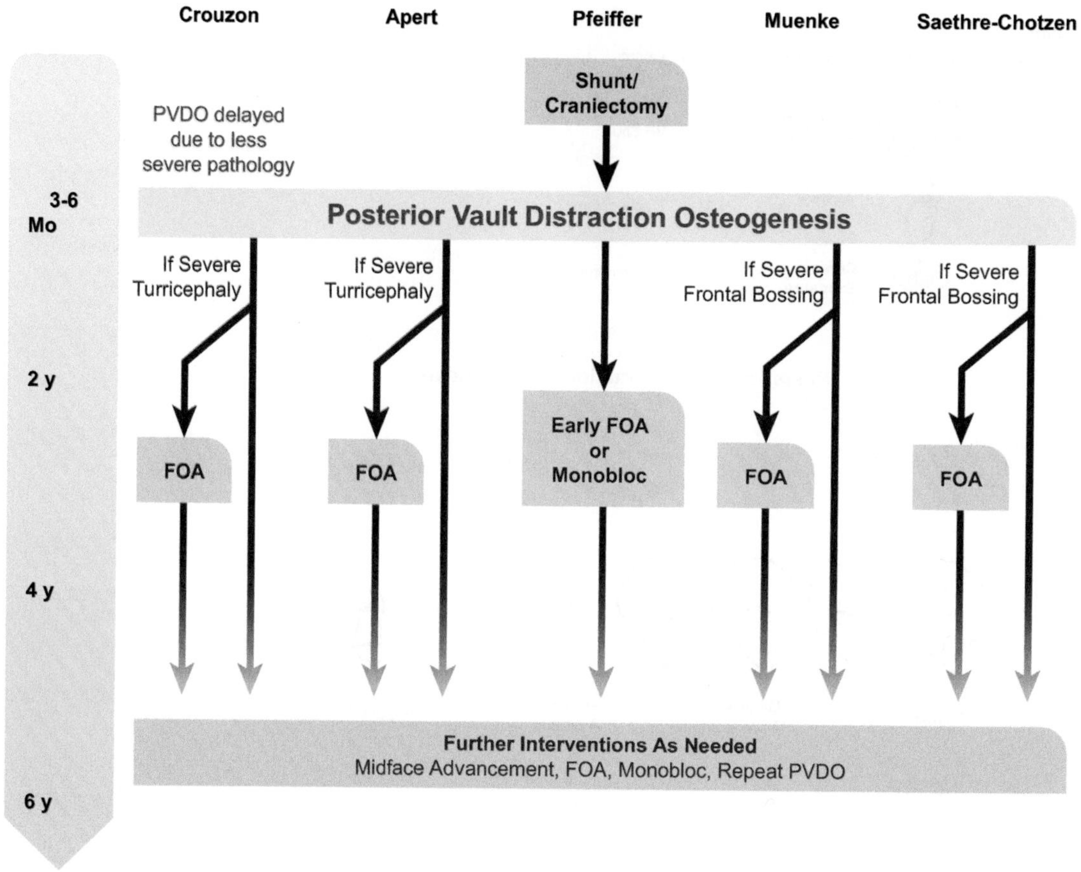

Crouzon	Apert	Pfeiffer	Muenke	Saethre-Chotzen

Shunt/ Craniectomy

PVDO delayed due to less severe pathology

3-6 Mo

Posterior Vault Distraction Osteogenesis

If Severe Turricephaly | If Severe Turricephaly | | If Severe Frontal Bossing | If Severe Frontal Bossing

2 y

FOA | FOA | **Early FOA or Monobloc** | FOA | FOA

4 y

Further Interventions As Needed
Midface Advancement, FOA, Monobloc, Repeat PVDO

6 y

Fig. 3. Syndrome-specific craniofacial management patterns. FOA, frontal orbital advancement.

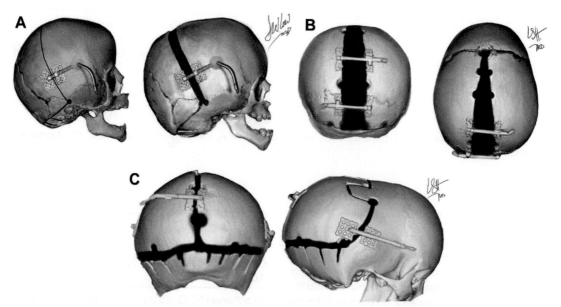

Fig. 4. Surgical technique for PVDO. (*A*) Univector distraction in the posterior–inferior direction. (*B*) Univector distraction in the transverse direction, (*C*) Multivector distraction in the posterior and transverse directions.

turribrachycephaly, we use posterior distraction, with a slight inferior vector to lower the cranial height.[3] Details The df our operative sequence are as follows (**Fig. 4**).

- Patient position: Prone.
- Approach:
  - Bicoronal stealth incision, subgaleal dissection.
  - Careful cautery of venous channels.
- Craniotomy:
  - Coronally oriented craniotomy in the mid-parietal region; low transverse osteotomy across occipital bones in the region of the torcula.
  - Limited dural dissection.
  - In older patients, high parietal "tongue-in-groove" osteotomies may be used to maximize bone-to-bone contact and the minimize contiguity of cranial defects.
- Steps are taken to improve cranial morphology after distraction, specifically preventing (1) step-off between the transport and stable cranial segments and (2) excursion across an open lambdoid suture.
  - Low occipital barrel stave osteotomies with greenstick out-fracture: barrel staves help to mitigate the step-off.
  - Barrel stave lagging: The barrel staves may be lagged to the transport segment with sutures to further smooth the bony transition throughout expansion.
  - Lambdoid suture plating: Open lambdoid sutures may be rigidly fixated with resorbable plates and screws to prevent excursion across the open suture. This maneuver allows for the parietal and occipital bones to transport in concert, although plating the lambdoid sutures may have deleterious effects on occipital growth.
- Device placement: Two distraction devices are placed in a parasagittal, colinear position with either a directly posterior or posterior-inferior vector. Four to 6 blunt, non–self-tapping screws are used to fixate each footplate to the bone. Additionally, the dura directly underlying the baseplates is fully dissected and protected while screws are placed to minimize risk of a durotomy. Gelfoam may be placed between the skull and the dura beneath footplates to limit potential contact between screws and dura.
- Distractor arms exit anteriorly through the incision or a separate stab incision through the scalp. This orientation directs the push force on the posterior bone flap, and patients are less likely to lay on the distractor arms.[3] Flexible or hinged activation arms can be used to minimize the rigidity of distractor arms and risk of hardware fracture. Remotely detachable activating arms can be removed at the completion of activation for the duration of consolidation.
- Drains: Drains are used at the discretion of the surgeon, with postoperative removal in 2 to 3 days.
- Dressing: A sterile, soft headwrap is placed and removed on postoperative day 2.

Variations in Technique

One can apply asymmetric transverse posterior distraction in cases of cephalocranial disproportion with minimal or scaphocephalic dysmorphology.[53] In this technique, posterior cranial osteotomies are performed described elsewhere in this article, with the addition of a sagittally oriented midline osteotomy of the cranial segments. The distractors are placed perpendicular to the midline osteotomy posteriorly, and a hinge is placed at the junction of the coronal sutures and frontal bone. The transverse-directed expansion increases posterior cranial volume, and normalizes scaphocephalic head shape.[53] One can also apply a combination of posterior and transverse expansion in cases where the cranial vault requires both sagittal and coronal expansion, as necessary.

Postoperative Management

Postoperatively, patients recover in the intensive care unit for close hemodynamic and neurologic monitoring. We start active distraction after a latency of 3 to 5 days. Active distraction occurs at a rate of 0.5 mm twice daily or 1 mm once daily until the desired length of distraction is achieved.[3,17] In the early PVDO experience, the mean active phase lasted 28.5 days (range, 21–42 days), and achieved a mean advancement of 23 mm (range, 19–32 mm).[3] We removed distractors after a mean 77-day consolidation period (range, 42–100 days). We monitor progress of advancement and evaluate for hardware failure with weekly or biweekly 2-view anteroposterior and lateral plain radiographs during active distraction.[3] An accelerated cranial distraction timeline has been reported with apparent success, using a latency of 2 days, activation of 1 mm twice daily, and a 4-week consolidation period.[54]

CLINICAL CASES

We provide clinical examples with corresponding figures of anterior-posterior, transverse, and combined anterior–posterior and transverse PVDO.

Posterior Cranial Vault Distraction Osteogenesis

A 6-month old baby girl with Apert syndrome and bicoronal CS who underwent PVDO in a posterior-inferior vector to achieve intracranial expansion and address her turribrachycephaly (**Fig. 5**). The total distraction distance was 35 mm. Before PVDO, she had a gastrostomy tube placed to assist with nutrition and nasal dilation for choanal stenosis.

Transverse Cranial Vault Distraction Osteogenesis

A 3-year-old girl who presented for a workup for headaches was found to have papilledema on fundoscopy and sagittal CS on a computed tomography scan (**Fig. 6**). Given the normocephalic head shape, intracranial expansion was achieved with a transverse posterior cranial distraction of 30 mm. Her headaches resolved after PVDO.

Posterior and Transverse Cranial Vault Distraction Osteogenesis

A 9-year-old boy with a diagnosis of pseudotumor cerebri and minor suture CS presented with symptoms of headaches, obtundation, confusion, possible seizures, and evidence of elevated ICP on lumbar puncture (30 mm Hg) and

fundoscopy (papilledema) (**Fig. 7**). The patient's mother wanted to avoid the placement of VP shunt; thus, cranial distraction was performed to maximally expand the intracranial space. The patient's head shape was relatively normocephalic; thus, PVDO was performed in a combined posterior and transverse vector. He achieved 30 mm of posterior expansion and 24 mm transverse expansion. After expansion, his sleep habits, mood, headaches, and school performance improved significantly.

POSTERIOR CRANIAL VAULT DISTRACTION OSTEOGENESIS OUTCOMES

We categorize studies of PVDO outcomes into 3 types: perioperative outcomes, craniometric outcomes, and clinical outcomes.

Perioperative Outcomes

A few studies have looked at the safety and perioperative morbidity profile of PVDO.[3,7] In the early days of applying PVDO, the Children's Hospital of Philadelphia described similar safety and morbidity profiles as conventional cranial vault remodeling, with regard to mean total surgery time, intensive care unit length of stay, overall hospital length of stay, estimated blood loss, total blood donor exposures, and intraoperative or

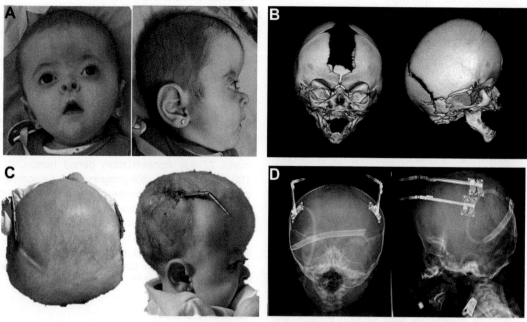

Fig. 5. Posterior PVDO for syndromic CS. (*A*) Preoperative photographs demonstrating turribrachycephaly. (*B*) Preoperative 3D computed tomography scan demonstrating bicoronal CS. (*C*) Postoperative photographs in consolidation. (*D*) Postoperative plain skull radiographs before distraction demonstrating parasagittal placement of distractors in posterior–inferior vector.

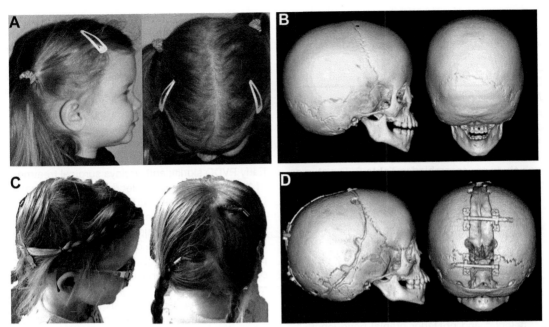

Fig. 6. Transverse PVDO for normocephalic sagittal CS. (*A*) Preoperative photographs demonstrating normal head shape. (*B*) Preoperative 3D computed tomography scan demonstrating sagittal CS. (*C*) Postoperative photographs in consolidation. (*D*) Postoperative 3D computed tomography scan demonstrating transverse posterior cranial expansion.

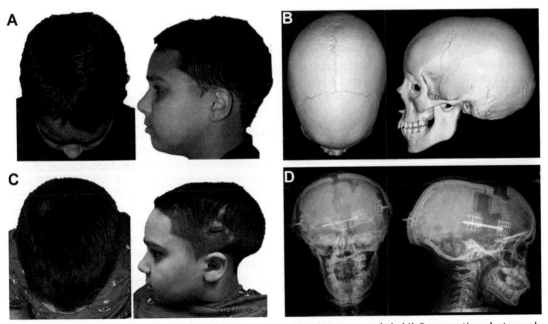

Fig. 7. Posterior and transverse PVDO for normocephalic pseudotumor cerebri. (*A*) Preoperative photographs demonstrating normal head shape. (*B*) Preoperative 3D computed tomography scan demonstrating minor suture CS. (*C*) Postoperative photographs in consolidation. (*D*) Postoperative plain skull radiographs demonstrating transverse and posterior cranial expansion.

postoperative complications.[7] There are no more recent studies comparing perioperative PVDO outcomes with conventional PVR outcomes.

Craniometric Outcomes

Many studies have evaluated different craniometric outcomes that result from PVDO. These studies focus on volume changes, posterior cranial base and vault morphology, and anterior cranial base and vault morphology changes. The details of each study are assembled in **Table 2**. The studies cumulatively support the following conclusions.

- PVDO increases intracranial volume by approximately 20% to 25%,[10,11,13,14,17,41,42,55–57] which is more than other methods of intracranial expansion, including free floating posterior bone flap,[10] lambdoid springs,[10] and bifronto-orbital procedures.[11,13,14]
- PVDO increases the posterior cranial vault height[14] and posterior cranial base length,[42] and provides a greater relative increase in the posterior fossa volume than entire intracranial volume.[57]
- PVDO increases the total surface area of the foramen magnum.[42,57]
- PVDO improves frontal vault dimensions, resulting from the decrease in the frontal bossing angle,[39,41,58] basofrontal angle,[14] and supraorbital retrusion.[41]
- Although anecdotally PVDO improves the turricephalic head shape, no craniometric studies directly investigate this clinical observation. Only 1 study found that, although posterior cranial vault height significantly increased after PVDO, the anterior and middle cranial heights did not on short follow-up.[14] The conclusion from this finding was that PVDO, at least with short-term follow-up, does not lead to worsening of turricephaly in the syndromic CS population. By redirecting brain growth posteriorly through PVDO, we hypothesize that brain growth is no longer primarily directed in a superior direction, thus improving turricephaly. PVDO also improves the ratio of anteroposterior skull length to height, thereby decreasing the appearance of turricephaly.

Clinical Outcomes

Improvement of elevated intracranial pressure
Completion of PVDO results in an improvement or resolution of elevated ICP.[39,59] Outcomes used to determine resolution (eg, fundoscopy), however, have a low sensitivity (11%–40%) compared with the gold standard direct ICP measurements.[60–62]

Optical coherence tomography was recently validated for detecting elevated ICP in patients with CS, with greater specificity (89%).[63] Optical coherence tomography shows promise to more accurately track elevated ICP-related changes in the retina in this population.

Rates of and perioperative outcomes of bilateral frontal orbital advancement and remodeling after posterior cranial vault distraction osteogenesis
Early PVDO significantly delays surgical treatment of the anterior cranium, decreases the number of BFOAR procedures required in the first 5 years of life (0.6 vs 1.15 per patient; $P = .023$), and may result in fewer major craniofacial procedures in the first 5 years of life compared with syndromic patients treated without early PVDO.[15] A subset of patients, however, require BFOAR after PVDO to treat frontal bossing and supraorbital retrusion. Patients who undergo BFOAR may have slightly longer operative and anesthesia times, and a greater technical difficulty with incision closure (59% vs 19%; odds ratio, 8.6; $P = .038$) than primary BFOAR patients of similar demographics.[64] Thus, if indicated, BFOAR can be performed safely in patients with previous PVDO.

New-onset craniosynostosis after posterior cranial vault distraction osteogenesis
Patients may develop new-onset CS after PVDO.[65] In 1 series, 89.5% of patients with patent lambdoid sutures and 41.2% of patients with patent sagittal sutures before PVDO developed new-onset suture fusion after PVDO. The cases were detected radiographically on routine post-PVDO imaging and the long-term implications are unknown, but to date in our experience with these patients we have not observed any untoward effects of this radiographic finding.

Effect of posterior cranial vault distraction osteogenesis on tonsillar herniation (Chiari malformation) and ventriculoperitoneal shunts
Patients with some forms of syndromic CS have relatively high rates of Chiari malformation[66] and hydrocephalus.[67–70] PVDO results in a decreased incidence of developing Chiari malformation compared with patients who underwent posterior vault reconstruction (2.0% vs 17.4%; $P = .033$).[16] Two patients in a single series had improvement in Chiari malformation after PVDO, but none after open vault surgery.[16] However, there was no significant difference in new-onset hydrocephalus requiring shunt placement between groups after either intervention (4.1% vs 4.3%; $P = .999$) and no patients had an improvement in shunt-dependent hydrocephalus. Thus, the increase in

Table 2
Craniometric outcomes of PVDO

Study	Patients/ Groups	Intracranial Volume Expansion	Posterior Craniometrics	Anterior Craniometrics	Conclusion
Serlo et al,[17] 2011	PVDO (10)	↑20.2% (10.2%–28.5%)			Volume predictions: PVDO ↑ICV Formula for volume gained per mm distraction: Vc = (pi)* r^2*h/2, r = AP distance distracted
Nowinski et al,[10] 2012	Free floating posterior bone flap (2)	↑13% and 24%			PVDO has significant opportunity for intracranial expansion
	Lambdoid springs (2)	↑18% and 25%			
	PVDO (2)	↑22% and 29%			
Choi et al,[11] 2012	PVDO simulations	20 mm advancement: ↑23.9%			Computer simulated PVDO demonstrates 35% greater ICV increase than BFOAR
	BFOAR simulations	↑17.7%			
Goldstein et al,[14] 2013	PVDO (11)	↑21% (7.5%–50%) overall, $P<.001$ ↑28% (10.8%–66%) for age <1 y, $P = .01$	Posterior cranial ht: ↑ 12.2% (0%–35%) overall, $P = .002$ ↑ 19.5% (9.2%–29%) for age <1y, $P = .02$	Anterior cranial ht: no ⊿ Middle cranial ht: no ⊿ Basofrontal angle: ↓3.9% (0%–12%), $P = .003$	PVDO may reduce tendency of worsening turribrachycephaly PVDO may improve frontal morphology by decreasing frontal bossing
Derderian et al,[13] 2015	PVDO (15)	↑274 cm³ (142 cm³ corrected for growth)			PVDO has significantly more intracranial volume expansion than BFOAR
	BFOAR (15)	↑144 cm³ (66 cm³ corrected for growth) uncorrected			Volume gain

(continued on next page)

Table 2
(continued)

Study	Patients/ Groups	Intracranial Volume Expansion	Posterior Craniometrics	Anterior Craniometrics	Conclusion
		intergroup difference, $P = .009$; corrected $P = .0017$			per mm was similar, but trending toward greater gains for PVDO
Samra et al,[58] 2015	Apert patients PVDO (7)			Frontal bossing angle: ↓7.6%	PVDO results in frontal morphologic changes that may delay or defer BFOAR
Shimizu et al,[17] 2016	PVDO (7)	↑21% (13%–34%)			Estimated mean 6.31 mm³ of volume gain per mm of distraction
Salokorpi et al,[56] 2017	PVDO (31)	↑17.4% (14.5%– 23.2%) by 3D photos ↑20.8% (19.3%– 21.9%) by 2D cephalograms			Able to calculate ICV from 3D photographs, and 2D cephalograms
terMaaten et al,[41] 2018	PVDO (12)	↑249 cm³ overall, $P<.001$ (205 cm³ corrected for growth) ↑380 cm³, $P<.001$ for age <1 y (302 cm³ corrected for growth) ↑302 cm³ for age <1 y was sig more than 122 cm³ for age >1 y ($P = .01$) ↑23% overall; 45.5% for age <1 y; 10.5% age >1 y		Supraorbital retrusion: ↓ 5.44→4.45 mm ($P<.001$), held true for patients without previous BFOAR Basofrontal angle: ↓2.92°, $P = .003$ overall ↓3.33° age <1 y vs ↓2.58° age >1 y, $P = .0079$ ↓2.85° for previous BFOAR, $P = .0097$ ↓3.09° for no previous BFOAR,	PVDO ↓ frontal retrusion and frontal bossing in syndromic CS with turribra-chycephaly

(continued on next page)

Table 2
(continued)

Study	Patients/ Groups	Intracranial Volume Expansion	Posterior Craniometrics	Anterior Craniometrics	Conclusion
				$P = .0164$ Anterior cranial ht: no Δ Anterofrontal angle: no Δ	
Bauder et al,[57] 2015	PVDO (10)	Total ICV ↑299 cm³, $P = .0069$	Posterior fossa:total ICV: ↑9.5% ($P = .0051$) FM: ↑0.22 cm ($P = .074$) and 0.18 cm ($P = .0284$) dimensions, with ↑0.72 cm² TSA, $P = .028$		PVDO results in relative ↑in posterior fossa volume to net ICV TSA of foramen magnum expands with PVDO
Mazzaferro et al,[42] 2019	PVDO (12)		Cranial base distances N-TS: ↑1.9 mm, $P = .015$ N-pFM: ↑3.4 mm, $P = .010$ N-OP: ↑9.1, $P = .003$ pFM-OP: ↑4.3 mm N-TS, N-pFM, FM width measurements ↑ more for age <1 y vs >1 y Posterior Vault Inflection Angle: ↑5.4°, $P = .0414$ Foramen magnum FM TSA: ↑52.1 mm² ($P = .002$), FM length: ↑0.9 mm ($P = .05$) FM width: ↑0.6 mm ($P = .05$)		PVDO ↑ Δ in length of the posterior cranial base PVDO ↑ Δ size of the foramen magnum Posterior cranial vault changes in order of most to least were N-OP > FM-OP > N-FM > N-TS: thus, there is an expansion at the anterior cranial base *and* posterior cranial base Posterior vault inflection angle ↑ indicates posterior cranial base was flattened

Abbreviations: 2D, 2-dimensional; 3D, 3-dimensional; AP, anteroposterior; BFOAR, bifrontal orbital advancement reconstruction; FM, foramen magnum; ht, height; ICV, intracranial volume; N, nasion; OP, occipital protuberance; pFM, opisthion; PVDO, posterior vault distraction osteogenesis; TS, tuberculum sellae; TSA, total surface area.

posterior fossa volume and foramen magnum dimensions may contribute to preventing development of Chiari malformation, but PVDO is unlikely to affect intracranial hydrodynamics.

Posterior cranial vault distraction osteogenesis in nonsyndromic and older patients

Although much of the literature on PVDO has been published in the context of younger syndromic CS patients, its effectiveness has also been studied in older patients. Patients with syndromic multisuture CS undergoing PVDO were compared. The older cohort was mean 9.2 years and the younger cohort was a mean of 0.7 year old.[71] Intraoperatively, the older cohort had less weight-based blood loss (mean 58.6 mL/kg vs 7.0 mL/kg, $P = .0092$) and weight-based transfusion (mean 70.1 mL/kg vs 21.1 mL/kg; $P = .0023$) than the younger patients. The groups did not differ in regard to length of stay, distracted distance, time in consolidation, or length of follow-up. Thus, PVDO is safe and effective in older patients with complex multisuture CS.

PVDO may be applied to nonsyndromic patients with complex CS. In 1 series, nonsyndromic patients were older (4.04 vs 2.55 years; $P = .046$), had a higher rate of signs of raised ICP (68.4% vs 25.0%), and a lower rate of bicoronal CS (15.8% vs 45.5%; $P = .044$).[9] There were no differences in perioperative complications or total cranial distraction length. All nonsyndromic patients with evidence of elevated ICP preoperatively had resolution after PVDO at 22 months of follow-up. Thus, in contrast with syndromic patients where PVDO is often applied early to prevent the development of elevated ICP, PVDO is often applied in nonsyndromic patients to treat existing ICP elevation.

Complications of posterior cranial vault distraction osteogenesis

Despite its many advantages, PVDO has the potential for complications.[7,40] Multiple series describe the specific complications, which are summarized by a comprehensive literature review by Greives and colleagues (**Table 3**).[40] In this review, they

Table 3
Complications and their considerations after PVDO

Complication Type	Incidence	Considerations
CSF leak/ dural injury[14,40]	9.8% (8/86)[40]	Use blunt, non–self-drilling screws to prevent small dural tears May insert Gelfoam endocranially under distractor to protect dura from overlying screws If there is a dural tear, it may need pericranial graft for repair ↑ latency phase to allow for dural injury healing Lumbar drain or extraventricular drain for persistent CSF leak
Wound infections/device exposure[40]	6.9% (6/86)[40]	Usual treatment with local wound care and oral antibiotics If frank purulence in distractor pocket and systemic signs/symptoms then may need for operative debridement with or without hardware removal with or without rigid fixation to maintain distracted distance
Device failure[40]	5.8% (5/86)[40]	Example: footplate disengagement from bone,[3] failure/breakage[73] Pins fail to thread properly, screws and plates lift off the bone, distal pins break off during the distraction phase[40]
Dural sinus bleeding[40]	2.3% (2/86)[40]	Hold firm, constant pressure over site of bleeding with large piece of un-=cut gelfoam as the initial step Manage with neurosurgical assistance
External trauma to distractor[40]	2.3% (2/86)[40]	Examples: breakage of distractor arm, breakage of extension arm[3]
VP shunt complication[72]	35.7% (5/14 patients with shunts)[72]	External component of semiburied distractor may contribute to increased incidence of VP shunt related complications in this group. Counsel parents of risks, discuss alternatives to PVDO

Abbreviations: CSF, cerebrospinal fluid; PVDO, posterior vault distraction osteogenesis.

reported a mean 30% overall complication rate (range, 12.5%–100%). There were no reported deaths or long-term morbidities. Complications in order of frequency include cerebrospinal fluid leak, wound infection, device exposure, device failure, dural sinus bleeding, and external trauma to the distractor. To prevent these complications, care must be taken to ensure careful dural dissection off the cranial bone at the site of craniotomy, protection of the dura when placing self-tapping screws into the distractor plates, and expedient management of postoperative signs of infection.

A subsequent study explored VP shunt complications in 14 patients with VP shunts who underwent PVDO compared with 8 patients with shunts who underwent posterior vault reconstruction.[72] Shunt complications were significantly greater in the PVDO group (5/14) than in the PVR group (0/8) (P = .0093). Specific complications in this group included prolonged cerebrospinal fluid leak (n = 2), shunt malfunction (n = 4), shunt infection (n = 4), wound infection (n = 3), wound dehiscence (n = 1), and hospital readmissions (n = 17). Although the specific factors that contribute to higher complication rates in patients with VP shunts are not elucidated, shunt exposure during and after PVDO may contribute to shunt-related complications warranting additional caution.

SUMMARY

PVDO is a powerful surgical tool that increases intracranial volume for patients with syndromic CS, thereby treating and/or preventing elevated ICP and addressing cranial dysmorphology. Its application has safely been expanded to include older and nonsyndromic children with complex craniosynostoses. PVDO increases volume in the pos terior vault, but it also decreases forehead bossing and improves supraorbital retrusion, thereby positively impacting frontal cranial morphology. This effect delays or negates the need for BFOAR in select syndromic patients before the age of 5 years. Furthermore, PVDO results in a lower incidence of Chiari malformations in the syndromic population compared with open cranial vault reconstruction. When diligent care in the technique is executed, complications may be limited.

CLINICS CARE POINTS

- PVDO is safe and effective in patients with syndromic CS, nonsyndromic CS patients, and older children.

- PVDO may occur in a strict posterior–inferior vector, or a transverse component may be considered in patients with normocephalic or dolicocephalic complex CS.

- Barrel stave osteotomies and lagging of the transport segment to the barrel staves may assist in expanding the posterior fossa and prevent a palpable and visible occipital step-off.

- Dural protection during the parieto-occipital craniotomy and during distractor fixation will help prevent complications related to cerebrospinal fluid leak, which can be exacerbated during active distraction.

ACKNOWLEDGMENTS

The authors would like to acknowledge Dr David W. Low and Dr Christopher Kalmar for their creativity and contributions to this article. The authors would like to thank Chris Kalmar, MD, for his thoughtful contribution to this article.

DISCLOSURE

The authors have nothing to disclose.

REFERENCES

1. Chumas PD, Cinalli G, Arnaud E, et al. Classification of previously unclassified cases of craniosynostosis. J Neurosurg 1997;86(2):177–81.
2. Blount JP, Louis RG Jr, Tubbs RS, et al. Pansynostosis: a review. Childs Nerv Syst 2007;23(10):1103–9.
3. Steinbacher DM, Skirpan J, Puchała J, et al. Expansion of the posterior cranial vault using distraction osteogenesis. Plast Reconstr Surg 2011;127(2):792–801.
4. Derderian CA, Bartlett SP. Open cranial vault remodeling. J Craniofac Surg 2012;23(1):229–34.
5. Mitchell BT, Swanson JW, Taylor JA. A new, single-stage, distraction-mediated, cranial vault expansion technique for the multisuture deformity. J Craniofac Surg 2015;26(6):1923–5.
6. Fearon JA, Rhodes J. Pfeiffer syndrome: a treatment evaluation. Plast Reconstr Surg 2009;123(5):1560–9.
7. Taylor JA, Derderian CA, Bartlett SP, et al. Perioperative morbidity in posterior cranial vault expansion. Plast Reconstr Surg 2012;129(4):674e–80e.
8. Taylor JA, Bartlett SP. What's new in syndromic craniosynostosis surgery? Plast Reconstr Surg 2017;140(1):82e–93e.
9. Zhang RS, Wes AM, Naran S, et al. Posterior vault distraction osteogenesis in nonsyndromic patients: an evaluation of indications and safety. J Craniofac Surg 2018;29(3):566–71.

10. Nowinski D, Di Rocco F, Renier D, et al. Posterior cranial vault expansion in the treatment of craniosynostosis. Comparison of current techniques. Childs Nerv Syst 2012;28(9):1537–44.

11. Choi M, Flores RL, Havlik RJ. Volumetric analysis of anterior versus posterior cranial vault expansion in patients with syndromic craniosynostosis. J Craniofac Surg 2012;23(2):455–8.

12. Goldstein JA, Paliga JT, Bailey RL, et al. Posterior vault distraction with midface distraction without osteotomy as a first stage for syndromic craniosynostosis. J Craniofac Surg 2013;24(4):1263–7.

13. Derderian CA, Wink JD, McGrath JL, et al. Volumetric changes in cranial vault expansion. Plast Reconstr Surg 2015;135(6):1665–72.

14. Goldstein JA, Paliga JT, Wink JD, et al. A craniometric analysis of posterior cranial vault distraction osteogenesis. Plast Reconstr Surg 2013;131(6):1367–75.

15. Swanson JW, Samra F, Bauder A, et al. An algorithm for managing syndromic craniosynostosis using posterior vault distraction osteogenesis. Plast Reconstr Surg 2016;137(5):829e–41e.

16. Lin LO, Zhang RS, Hoppe IC, et al. Onset and resolution of Chiari malformations and hydrocephalus in syndromic craniosynostosis following posterior vault distraction. Plast Reconstr Surg 2019;144(4):932–40.

17. Serlo WS, Ylikontiola LP, Lähdesluoma N, et al. Posterior cranial vault distraction osteogenesis in craniosynostosis: estimated increases in intracranial volume. Childs Nerv Syst 2011;27(4):627–33.

18. De Bastiani G, Aldegheri R, Renzi-Brivio L, Trivella G. Limb lengthening by callus distraction (callotasis). J Pediatr Orthop 1987;7(2):129–34.

19. Ilizarov GA. The tension-stress effect on the genesis and growth of tissues. Part I. The influence of stability of fixation and soft-tissue preservation. Clin Orthop Relat Res 1989;(238):249–81.

20. Ilizarov GA. The tension-stress effect on the genesis and growth of tissues: part II. The influence of the rate and frequency of distraction. Clin Orthop Relat Res 1989;(239):263–85.

21. Snyder CC, Levine GA, Swanson HM, et al. Mandibular lengthening by gradual distraction. Preliminary report. Plast Reconstr Surg 1973;51(5):506–8.

22. Michieli S, Miotti B. Lengthening of mandibular body by gradual surgical-orthodontic distraction. J Oral Surg 1977;35(3):187–92.

23. Karp NS, Thorne CH, McCarthy JG, et al. Bone lengthening in the craniofacial skeleton. Ann Plast Surg 1990;24(3):231–7.

24. Karp NS, McCarthy JG, Schreiber JS, et al. Membranous bone lengthening: a serial histological study. Ann Plast Surg 1992;29(1):2–7.

25. Barone CM, Ferder M, Jimenez DF, et al. Distraction of the frontal bone outside the cranial plane: a rabbit model. J Craniofac Surg 1993;4(3):177–81.

26. McCarthy JG, Schreiber J, Karp N, et al. Lengthening the human mandible by gradual distraction. Plast Reconstr Surg 1992;89(1):1–8 [discussion: 9–10].

27. Cohen SR, Rutrick RE, Burstein FD. Distraction osteogenesis of the human craniofacial skeleton: initial experience with new distraction system. J Craniofac Surg 1995;6(5):368–74.

28. Polley JW, Figueroa AA, Charbel FT, et al. Monobloc craniomaxillofacial distraction osteogenesis in a newborn with severe craniofacial synostosis: a preliminary report. J Craniofac Surg 1995;6(5):421–3.

29. Polley JW, Figueroa AA. Distraction osteogenesis: its application in severe mandibular deformities in hemifacial microsomia. J Craniofac Surg 1997;8(5):422–30.

30. Cohen SR. Craniofacial distraction with a modular internal distraction system: evolution of design and surgical techniques. Plast Reconstr Surg 1999;103(6):1592–607.

31. Cohen SR, Boydston W, Hudgins R, et al. Monobloc and facial bipartition distraction with internal devices. J Craniofac Surg 1999;10(3):244–51.

32. Sugawara Y, Hirabayashi S, Sakurai A, et al. Gradual cranial vault expansion for the treatment of craniofacial synostosis: a preliminary report. Ann Plast Surg 1998;40(5):554–65.

33. Yonehara Y, Hirabayashi S, Sugawara Y, et al. Complications associated with gradual cranial vault distraction osteogenesis for the treatment of craniofacial synostosis. J Craniofac Surg 2003;14(4):526–8.

34. Kobayashi S, Honda T, Saitoh A, et al. Unilateral coronal synostosis treated by internal forehead distraction. J Craniofac Surg 1999;10(6):467–71 [discussion: 472].

35. Hirabayashi S, Sugawara Y, Sakurai A, et al. Frontoorbital advancement by gradual distraction. Technical note. J Neurosurg 1998;89(6):1058–61.

36. Nonaka Y, Oi S, Miyawaki T, et al. Indication for and surgical outcomes of the distraction method in various types of craniosynostosis. Childs Nerv Syst 2003;1(1):1.

37. Akai T, Iizuka H, Kawakami S. Treatment of craniosynostosis by distraction osteogenesis. Pediatr Neurosurg 2006;42(5):288–92.

38. Kim S-W, Shim K-W, Plesnila N, et al. Distraction vs remodeling surgery for craniosynostosis. Childs Nerv Syst 2006;23(2):201–6.

39. White N, Evans M, Dover MS, et al. Posterior calvarial vault expansion using distraction osteogenesis. Childs Nerv Syst 2009;25(2):231–6.

40. Greives MR, Ware BW, Tian AG, et al. Complications in posterior cranial vault distraction. Ann Plast Surg 2016;76(2):211–5.

41. Maaten ter NS, Mazzaferro DM, Wes AM, et al. A craniometric analysis of frontal cranial morphology following posterior vault distraction. J Craniofac Surg 2018;1–5. https://doi.org/10.1097/SCS.0000000000004473.

42. Mazzaferro DM, Maaten ter NS, Wes AM, et al. A craniometric analysis of the posterior cranial

base after posterior vault distraction. J Craniofac Surg 2019;30(6):1692–5.

43. Renier D, Lajeunie E, Arnaud E, et al. Management of craniosynostoses. Childs Nerv Syst 2000;16(10–11):645–58.

44. Arnaud E, Meneses P, Lajeunie E, et al. Postoperative mental and morphological outcome for nonsyndromic brachycephaly. Plast Reconstr Surg 2002;110(1):6–12 [discussion: 13].

45. Mathijssen IMJ, Arnaud E. Benchmarking for craniosynostosis. J Craniofac Surg 2007;18(2):436–42.

46. Arnaud E, Marchac D, Renier D. Reduction of morbidity of the frontofacial monobloc advancement in children by the use of internal distraction. Plast Reconstr Surg 2007;120(4):1009–26.

47. Honnebier MB, Cabiling DS, Hetlinger M, et al. The natural history of patients treated for FGFR3-associated (Muenke-type) craniosynostosis. Plast Reconstr Surg 2008;121(3):919–31.

48. Fitzgerald O'Connor EJ, Marucci DD, Jeelani NO, et al. Ocular advancement in monobloc distraction. Plast Reconstr Surg 2009;123(5):1570–7.

49. de Jong T, Bannink N, Bredero-Boelhouwer HH, et al. Long-term functional outcome in 167 patients with syndromic craniosynostosis; defining a syndrome-specific risk profile. J Plast Reconstr Aesthet Surg 2010;63(10):1635–41.

50. Mathijssen IMJ. Guideline for care of patients with the diagnoses of craniosynostosis: working group on craniosynostosis. J Craniofac Surg 2015;26(6):1735–807.

51. Anderson PJ, Tan E, David DJ. Simultaneous multiple vector distraction for craniosynostosis syndromes. Br J Plast Surg 2005;58(5):626–31.

52. Komuro Y, Hashizume K, Koizumi T, et al. Cranial expansion with distraction osteogenesis for multiple-suture synostosis in school-aged children. J Craniofac Surg 2009;20(2):457–60.

53. Lao WW, Denny AD. Internal distraction osteogenesis to correct symptomatic cephalocranial disproportion. Plast Reconstr Surg 2010;126(5):1677–88.

54. Nowinski D, Saiepour D, Leikola J, et al. Posterior cranial vault expansion performed with rapid distraction and time-reduced consolidation in infants with syndromic craniosynostosis. Childs Nerv Syst 2011;27(11):1999–2003.

55. Shimizu A, Komuro Y, Shimoji K, et al. Quantitative analysis of change in intracranial volume after posterior cranial vault distraction. J Craniofac Surg 2016;27(5):1135–8.

56. Salokorpi N, Vuollo V, Sinikumpu J-J, et al. Increases in cranial volume with posterior cranial vault distraction in 31 consecutive cases. Neurosurgery 2017;81(5):803–11.

57. Bauder AR, Wink JD, Swanson JW, et al. An analysis of posterior vault distraction and its effects on the posterior fossa and cranial base. Plast Reconstr Surg 2015;136(4S):52–3.

58. Samra F, Swanson JW, Mitchell B, et al. Posterior vault distraction osteogenesis conveys anterior benefit in apert syndrome. Plast Reconstr Surg 2015;136(4S):51.

59. Spruijt B, Rijken BFM, Ottelander den BK, et al. First vault expansion in apert and Crouzon-Pfeiffer syndromes: front or back? Plast Reconstr Surg 2016;137(1):112e–21e.

60. Rangwala LM, Liu GT. Pediatric idiopathic intracranial hypertension. Surv Ophthalmol 2007;52(6):597–617.

61. Nazir S, O'Brien M, Qureshi NH, et al. Sensitivity of papilledema as a sign of shunt failure in children. J AAPOS 2009;13(1):63–6.

62. Xu W, Gerety P, Aleman T, et al. Noninvasive methods of detecting increased intracranial pressure. Childs Nerv Syst 2016;32(8):1371–86.

63. Swanson JW, Aleman TS, Xu W, et al. Evaluation of optical coherence tomography to detect elevated intracranial pressure in children. JAMA Ophthalmol 2017;135(4):320–9.

64. Zhang RS, Lin LO, Hoppe IC, et al. Perioperative outcomes of secondary frontal orbital advancement after posterior vault distraction osteogenesis. J Craniofac Surg 2019;30(2):503–7.

65. Tahiri Y, Paliga JT, Bartlett SP, et al. New-onset craniosynostosis after posterior vault distraction osteogenesis. J Craniofac Surg 2015;26(1):176–9.

66. Rijken BFM, Lequin MH, de Rooi JJ, et al. Foramen magnum size and involvement of its intraoccipital synchondroses in Crouzon syndrome. Plast Reconstr Surg 2013;132(6):993e–1000e.

67. Collmann H, Sörensen N, Krauß J. Hydrocephalus in craniosynostosis: a review. Childs Nerv Syst 2005;21(10):902–12.

68. Cinalli G, Sainte-Rose C, Kollar EM, et al. Hydrocephalus and craniosynostosis. J Neurosurg 1998;88(2):209–14.

69. Cinalli G, Chumas P, Arnaud E, et al. Occipital remodeling and suboccipital decompression in severe craniosynostosis associated with tonsillar herniation. Neurosurgery 1998;42(1):66–71 [discussion: 71–3].

70. Copeland AE, Hoffman CE, Open VTSG. Clinical significance of venous anomalies in syndromic craniosynostosis. Plast Reconstr Surg Glob Open 2018. https://doi.org/10.1097/GOX.0000000000001613.

71. Li J, Gerety PA, Xu W, et al. A perioperative risk comparison of posterior vault distraction osteogenesis in an older pediatric population. J Craniofac Surg 2016;27(5):1165–9.

72. Azzolini A, Magoon K, Yang R, et al. Ventricular shunt complications in patients undergoing posterior vault distraction osteogenesis. Childs Nerv Syst 2020;36(5):1009–16.

73. Lee JA, Park DH, Yoon SH, et al. Distractor breakage in cranial distraction osteogenesis for children with craniosynostosis. Pediatr Neurosurg 2008;44(3):216–20.

Craniosynostosis
Le Fort III Distraction Osteogenesis

Paul A. Mittermiller, MD[a], Roberto L. Flores, MD[b],*, David A. Staffenberg, MD[a]

KEYWORDS

- Le Fort III distraction osteogenesis • Midface hypoplasia • Midface distraction • Internal distraction
- External distraction

KEY POINTS

- Le Fort III distraction is used to improve the airway and midface appearance at the level of the infraorbital rims.
- Device selection (external or internal) is critical for technical success and patient satisfaction.
- A multidisciplinary craniofacial team is critical for evaluating and treating patients with craniofacial anomalies.
- The surgeon-orthodontist relationship is important preoperatively and postoperatively to control and adjust the Le Fort III distraction vector.

INTRODUCTION

In 1950, Sir Harold Gillies published a Le Fort III pattern osteotomy.[1] This procedure was performed in a 14-year-old patient to improve the appearance of her midface. She had midface retrusion, including the maxillary dental arch, infraorbital rims, and zygomas. After the osteotomies, advancement of the midface was performed and held in place with intermaxillary wiring. After 2 weeks, the intermaxillary wires were removed and the patient was transitioned to a metal cap splint that was attached to the teeth and secured to a plaster head cap. After 5 weeks, this device was removed. There is some disagreement regarding the success of the procedure, but in his original paper, Gillies himself stated the patient developed relapse of the advancement.[1–4]

Paul Tessier is credited for designing the Le Fort III osteotomy technique used today, and demonstrating stability in midface advancement.[4] The results of his initial 14 cases were first reported at the 1967 Fourth International Congress of Plastic and Reconstructive Surgery in Rome and he subsequently published his techniques in 1971.[4,5]

Tessier modified Gillies' approach by using a coronal incision and moving the medial orbital osteotomy from along the anterior lacrimal crest to behind the posterior lacrimal crest, preserving the medial canthus and lacrimal apparatus within the Le Fort III segment.[5] In addition, bone grafts were used to maintain the advancement and a traction system was implemented to prevent relapse.[3,4]

The concept of distraction osteogenesis was first developed in the 1950s by G. A. Ilizarov.[6] Compressive forces were supposed to be applied on a patient who had developed hypertrophic nonunion. The compression device was turned in the wrong direction and applied distraction instead of compression forces. He subsequently observed findings on a radiograph of the site, which he believed was the result of osteogenesis.

The technique of distraction osteogenesis was first applied to the human craniofacial skeleton by Joseph McCarthy and colleagues[7] and reported in 1992. This procedure was undertaken to lengthen the human mandible in a child with craniofacial microsomia.[7] The possibility of applying distraction osteogenesis to the midface

[a] Hansjörg Wyss Department of Plastic Surgery, NYU Langone Health, 222 East 41st Street, 22nd floor, New York, NY, 10017, USA; [b] Hansjörg Wyss Department of Plastic Surgery, Cleft and Craniofacial Surgery, NYU Langone Health, 222 East 41st Street, 22nd floor, New York, NY, 10017, USA
* Corresponding author.
E-mail address: Roberto.Flores@nyulangone.org

Clin Plastic Surg 48 (2021) 473–485
https://doi.org/10.1016/j.cps.2021.03.003

was suggested in laboratory work by Staffenberg and McCarthy presented at the International Society of Craniofacial Surgeons in Oaxaca, Mexico, in 1993, and published in 1995.[8,9] The first midface distraction performed on a human was subsequently performed in 1993 by Muhlbauer in Germany and presented in 1995. In 1996, Chin and Toth[10] published a series of patients who underwent internal distraction, including 1 patient who underwent Le Fort III advancement.[11]

Since the original Le Fort III distraction, surgeons and device manufacturers have continued to modify their devices and techniques. Both internal and external distractors have had multiple iterations in design, and some internal devices have been modified to include absorbable components.[12] The first external distraction device was used on the midface in 1997 by Polley and Figueroa[13] after performing a Le Fort I osteotomy. The use of the external distractor subsequently expanded for use in patients following Le Fort III osteotomies.[13]

INDICATIONS
Indications for Le Fort III Advancement

The indications for a Le Fort III advancement include shallow orbits with exorbitism, airway obstruction owing to midface retrusion, and class III malocclusion.[14,15] Although absolute and relative indications have been published previously, it is notable that the severity of many indications are subject to interpretation and can be temporized by less invasive interventions.[14] For example, a clear definition of severe exorbitism has not been codified and most cases of exorbitism can be temporized or conservatively managed by a tarsorrhaphy and eye lubrication. Sleep studies can quantify the severity of airway obstruction, but the sleep study values for which midface distraction is indicated have not been defined. Furthermore, continuous positive airway pressure and adenoidectomy can also be used as temporizing measures. If supraorbital retrusion is present with signs of increased intracranial pressure, monobloc advancement with or without distraction can be considered.

Conventional Versus Distraction Le Fort III Advancement

The indication for distraction osteogenesis versus traditional Le Fort III advancement with bone grafts is determined by the age of the patient and the degree of advancement required. A traditional Le Fort III advancement is ideal for patients who have completed facial growth and require smaller advancements (<10–12 mm).[16,17] Advantages include completion of surgery in a single operation, greater control of the final position of the midface, and better restoration of occlusion.[18] In an adult patient, a Le Fort I osteotomy may be required at the time of the Le Fort III or as a second surgery, to restore functional occlusion. The midface should be positioned to correct exorbitism and restore convexity to the midface as the priority, rather than to optimize occlusion. The midface is most frequently advanced forward along the Frankfurt horizontal so the inferior orbital rim is properly positioned in regard to the globe (orbitale advanced to the cornea). The remaining malocclusion is corrected with a Le Fort I, which can be altered as needed in 3 dimensions without distorting the midface, orbits, or nose. The authors prefer to undertake this procedure as a combined operation with an occlusal wafer and class III elastics offering postoperative stability to the advancement. The disadvantages include longer operative times, need for bone graft, and increased blood loss compared with a midface distraction.[17]

The growing face presents different priorities for care. Restoration of occlusion is not the surgical goal of surgery, because the patient will require further midface growth. Therefore, overcorrection of the anterior position of the maxilla and orbitale are the end points of distraction. The patient should be placed in an anterior crossbite with a moderate degree of enophthalmos. This degree of overcompensation is a matter of clinical judgment; however, it should be noted that maxillary growth is typically limited after pterygoid separation. Therefore, the older the patient is at the time of the procedure, the less likely it is that the patient will require a second distraction. Conversely, patients who undergo midface distraction at an early age (≤5 years of age) are more likely to require a second midface distraction before skeletal maturity and, therefore, a greater degree of overcompensation is required. Of course, patients who require an early midface surgery typically have a more severe expression of the condition; however, the limits of anterior facial growth after midface distraction should be kept in mind regarding the timing of surgery and the extent of midface advancement. Overcorrection can be difficult for the patient and family members because, although the distraction process will bring their facial appearance to normal, overcorrection will continue to advance the patient's midface to an improved but perhaps also abnormal appearance.[19] However, our experience indicates that overcorrection is very well-tolerated and accepted with appropriate preoperative consultation. We believe that early midface distraction is reserved for patients with severe anatomic airway obstruction who will require a tracheostomy or who are tracheostomy dependent. Patients should not have a significant secondary airway anomaly precluding successful airway restoration by midface distraction. Performing conventional Le Fort III advancement in a child is rarely, if ever, indicated. A large degree of midface advancement is more difficult using conventional techniques. Additionally, if a secondary Le Fort III is required, the retained rigid fixation hardware can complicate the procedure.[20]

A Le Fort III distraction can advance the midface to a greater degree than a conventional Le Fort III advancement.[17,20] This procedure is ideal when performed in a growing child in whom an overcorrection of the advancement is required to compensate for future facial growth. A Le Fort III distraction can simplify any subsequent midface advancement, because there are no indwelling rigid internal fixation plates[18]; however, a repeat osteotomy of a previously distracted bony site may have other challenges. There may be areas of fibrous union or nonunion in specific sites of osteogenesis creating difficulty in bony separation or subsequent bone generation. When compared with the conventional Le Fort III advancement, a Le Fort III distraction has been shown to have shorter operative time, less blood loss, and a decreased length of hospital stay.[17] It has also been reported to have lower costs than conventional Le Fort III advancements.[21]

Age Considerations for Surgical Distraction

The age at which midface distraction should be performed is a topic of active debate. As stated elsewhere in this article, in patients with severe airway obstruction or exorbitism, early correction can be justified to correct these functional impairments.[22] If the deformity is less severe, delaying surgical intervention until a later age (8–11 years) can provide benefits, such as limiting the possibility of requiring a repeat Le Fort III advancement owing to relapse or initial incomplete advancement.[22,23] Additionally, awaiting the eruption of the 6-year molars can decrease complications associated with the pterygomaxillary disjunction.

One concern about performing Le Fort III osteotomies in a growing child is the potential risk of midfacial growth impairment. Multiple studies have demonstrated that, after Le Fort III osteotomies in patients with craniofacial dysostoses, there is continued vertical growth with minimal anterior growth of the midface.[19,23–25] However, patients with craniofacial dysostosis have been shown to exhibit impaired forward growth of the maxilla, even without an operation.[16,26] Therefore, it is not entirely known how much of the impairment of midfacial growth seen after Le Fort III osteotomies is due to the underlying pathology versus the surgery itself. There are no known studies evaluating the effect on midfacial growth of Le Fort III osteotomies in patients without craniofacial pathology.[16] Considering what is known about the phases of pediatric midface growth and the lack of anterior growth maxillary growth after distraction, parents and surgeons should be aware of the increased risk of recurrence of the facial dysmorphology as the child grows and the potential need for repeat midface surgery before facial maturity in children who undergo midface distraction before the age of 7 years.

There are additional considerations when considering early distraction. Children younger than 3 years of age tend to have thinner skulls, leading to the potential for poor retention of the calvarial pins with the use of external distractors.[16] Furthermore, performing midface distraction on patients younger than 3 years of age can be difficult owing to poor patient cooperation.[14] For these reasons, when early Le Fort III is indicated, internal distraction osteogenesis devices may be favored.

If elective midface distraction is being considered in an adolescent patient with no immediate need for intervention (eg, corneal exposure, airway obstruction), one should consider delaying the procedure until skeletal maturity.[14] This practice prevents the need to estimate the degree of advancement required. When performed at skeletal maturity, the Le Fort III segment can be brought into its ideal position. Delaying surgery until skeletal maturity should be weighed against the psychological benefits obtained from performing the surgery earlier. This information should be included in discussion of timing with the patient and family.[27]

PREOPERATIVE WORKUP AND PLANNING
Physical Examination

One should evaluate the periorbital region to assess the degree of exorbitism, the position of the supraorbital and infraorbital rims, the degree of scleral show, and the amount of lower eyelid support. Extraocular motility should be assessed, and a baseline ophthalmologist evaluation is recommended. Patients with syndromic craniosynostosis should already be followed routinely by an ophthalmologist. The mouth should be evaluated, assessing the occlusion, degree of maxillary arch constriction, degree of dental compensation, dental crowding, condition of the teeth, and orientation of the occlusal plane. The condition of the teeth is critical if an external distraction device is used because they serve as an anchor for the device. The skull should be palpated to assess for any cranial defects.

Dental and Orthodontic Assessments

The patient should be evaluated by a dentist and orthodontist before the operation to assess the condition of the teeth.[14] They should be evaluated for dental decay and treated accordingly.

If an external distractor is chosen for the operation, the patient should undergo fabrication of a dental splint. The considerations for choosing an external versus internal distractor are included elsewhere in this article.

Ophthalmology Assessment

Referral to an ophthalmologist is critical for diagnosing the presence of papilledema, strabismus, anisometropia, astigmatism, and ametropia.[14] In particular, the ophthalmologist should be asked to evaluate for evidence of corneal exposure.

Respiratory Evaluation

Patients with craniofacial dysostosis commonly have airway obstructions at the level of the nasopharynx.[28] One must be aware of other potential areas of obstruction, because this can occur at multiple levels in syndromic patients. For example, patients with Pfeiffer syndrome more commonly have tracheal stenosis and bronchial abnormalities, making a midface advancement only partially effective for improving the patient's airway.[28] Therefore, the workup should include nasoendoscopy and a sleep study for at-risk patients.[14] Nasoendoscopy will identify a second location of anatomic airway obstruction that can preclude successful restoration of airflow by midface distraction. This assessment is recommended for patients with Pfeiffer syndrome. A sleep study will quantify the severity of airway obstruction and identify the presence of central sleep apnea. This type of assessment with provide an objective assessment of airflow and can be useful in determining the indication and timing of midface advancement. Patients with a Chiari malformation may exhibit a degree of central sleep apnea that will not improve with midface advancement. If a sleep study is obtained preoperatively, a postoperative evaluation should also be performed to assess for changes in airflow.

General Health and Specialist Evaluation

The general health of the patient should be considered before the operation. These considerations include having had regular visits with the child's pediatrician or specialists for optimization of medical problems including cardiac, neurologic, genetic, ophthalmologic, and respiratory anomalies.[14]

Photographs

Standardized medical photography is useful for the planning, documentation, and assessment of results.[14] Standard photographs should include frontal, three-quarters, profile, submental vertex, bird's eye, occlusal, and oculomotor photographs. If 3-dimensional photography is available, it should be considered.

Imaging

A computed tomography (CT) scan is helpful for operative planning, especially when previous surgery has been performed. The scan is useful for evaluating the morphology of the facial skeleton, the quality and quantity of bone, and the dimensions of the airway and orbits. If the procedure is a repeat advancement, CT imaging is critical for determining the quality of bone and for confirming the presence and location of any existing hardware. The quality of bone can help determine the appropriate placement of the distraction devices and may impact the decision to use external versus internal devices. A critical absence of bone from resorption after prior procedures may indicate bone grafting before or after advancement. It is also important to rule out nasofrontal and nasopharyngeal encephaloceles.

Cephalograms can be obtained preoperatively and subsequently repeated postoperatively to determine the degree of translation and rotation of the Le Fort III segment during device activation. On occasion, the patient's age or behavioral factors may make reliable cephalograms impossible, whereas CT scans may be performed with anesthesia.

Panoramic radiographs are useful for evaluating the patient's dentition and are generally not needed for preoperative evaluation. This information is readily available on CT images.

Choice of External Versus Internal Distraction

No single device is ideal in every situation, and each has its own advantages. Internal distractors are rapidly applied, less visibly conspicuous, and have less of a psychological impact on the patient and family.[22] The devices are lower profile and, therefore, have a decreased risk for accidental trauma.[14] Being inconspicuous and less vulnerable to trauma make them ideal for patients who would otherwise be unlikely to tolerate an external distractor (those patients with attention deficit hyperactivity disorder, behavioral challenges, and gait disturbance). Because the internal devices are activated posteriorly, it is easy for 1 parent to hold the child facing them on their lap while the other parent activates the devices. Some practitioners perceive that the primary disadvantage of internal distractors is that, once placed, these devices are limited to a single vector for distraction.[14] One should keep in mind that the single vector for advancement of the midface is along the Frankfurt horizontal, although 1 side may be advanced further than the other if that is indeed indicated. The occlusal correction is addressed by the Le Fort I at a later date. These internal devices have been used effectively in patients as young as 3 years and even younger in patients who undergo very early monobloc distraction. Rotation of the Le Fort III segment can occur during the distraction, resulting in more movement of the zygomaticomaxillary complex than at the level of the occlusal plane.[29] If manipulation of the device is required or if malfunction occurs, the device needs to be surgically adjusted under anesthesia,[14] although this tends to occur more frequently with external devices. If the patient has thin bone, the device is at a greater risk for dislodgement and distraction failure.[16] The internal devices are very well-tolerated once distraction is completed and the activation arms are removed. Removal of the devices may be more difficult if there is significant growth of bone over the plates.[16] Removal of the devices is done through the lower part of the coronal scars on an outpatient basis.

External devices have the advantage of being more stable than internal distractors owing to the broad points of fixation to the craniofacial skeleton.[14] If the distraction vector needs to be adjusted, the adjustment can be performed postoperatively in a cooperative patient without surgical intervention.[14,23] Removal of the external device is relatively simple and can be performed without surgical exposure.[29] If the patient has poor or absent dentition, the application of a dental splint may not be possible, but distraction can still be performed with the use of skeletal anchors or osseointegrated implants.[29] A disadvantage of the external devices is that they are large and physically imposing.[14] This factor can impact the patient and family psychologically. Because the device is larger, it is also at a greater risk of accidental trauma and dislodgement. There have also been reports of accidental and gradual intracranial pin migration.[30] This risk is greater in young children (<3 years of age) in whom the cranial bone may still be thin and in patients with complex craniosynostosis in whom previous cranial surgery has rendered the skull thin. Some surgeons have advocated for the placement of a titanium mesh if thin areas of bone are encountered on CT scan or at the time of surgery. If transcutaneous wires attached to fixation screws are used, this practice has the potential to result in unsightly scarring.[30]

Virtual Surgical Planning and Image-Guided Systems

Virtual surgical planning has been reported and can be helpful for visualizing the planned movements.[31–33] However, the benefit of these systems in the background of the added costs are still pending. Image-guided systems have also been used in an attempt to more safely perform the Le Fort III osteotomies, claiming particular benefit for the nasofrontal and pterygomaxillary osteotomies, which are commonly performed in a blind fashion and can result in significant morbidity with incorrect trajectories.[34,35] Although these systems can be of potential use for the novice surgeon, these systems should not be required in experienced hands.

OPERATIVE TECHNIQUES
Preoperative Setup

The patient is intubated with an orotracheal tube and the globes are protected using corneal shields with or without lid sutures to prevent corneal injury during the operation. Because corneal shields alone may be easily dislodged during the surgery, the surgeon must constantly reassess the ocular protection during the surgery. Packed red blood cells should be available and in the room. Tranexamic acid may be used to help decrease blood loss.[36] A low blood pressure should be maintained during pterygomaxillary disjunction and the nasofrontal separation.

Exposure for Osteotomies

A coronal incision is designed and infiltrated with weight-based local anesthetic with epinephrine. Frequently, the scar from prior cranial vault surgery is reopened and may be revised later upon closure. The scalp flap is elevated anteriorly in the subperiosteal plane to the orbits. The lateral orbital rim and anterior aspect of the zygomatic arch is exposed. When conventional Le Fort III is performed, the majority of the arch is exposed. Subperiosteal degloving of the orbits is completed.

The lateral orbital exposure should include identification of the lateral aspect of the inferior orbital fissure. In syndromic patients with severe midface retrusion, this structure may be quite narrow. The inferior orbital fissure marks the boundary between the skull base and the facial skeleton at the lateral orbit. Medial orbital dissection must allow for the identification of the posterior lacrimal crest and the anterior ethmoid artery. Again, in syndromic patients, the distance between these important landmarks is diminished and the anterior ethmoid should be preserved carefully. The anterior ethmoid artery marks the junction of the skull base and the facial skeleton in the medial orbit.

The anterior aspect of the temporalis muscle is dissected from the posterior aspect of the lateral orbital rim and the anterior zygomatic arch. The pterygomaxillary suture is exposed by inserting a periosteal elevator behind the zygomatic body and dissecting inferiorly along the lateral wall of the lateral maxilla until the pterygomaxillary suture is reached. It is important to maintain a subperiosteal plan to prevent injury to the internal maxillary artery during ostetomy.[37] In cases where there is severe midface retrusion, making complete pterygomaxillary separation from above challenging, a Kawamoto osteotome can be used to complete a transoral osteotomy typically performed during a Le Fort I.

Exposure for Internal Distraction

If an internal distractor is used, the anterior footplate is positioned at the junction between the arch and the lateral orbital rim. The temporal muscle is taken down and split vertically above the helix of the ear to allow the temporal (skull base) footplate to be secured.

Osteotomies

Detailed descriptions of all osteotomies performed in the Le Fort III procedure and many cardinal craniofacial procedures are available through a freely accessibly surgical simulator CIVApro. This can be accessed through the website, www.myface.org/civa or through the smartphone app (CIVApro) available for the iPhone and Android.

Internal Distractor Placement

If internal distractors are used, they are placed through the coronal incision. Multiple internal distractor designs have been used for Le Fort III distraction, with the primary difference being the lateral projection, size, and location of the footplates. The anterior footplate is commonly placed at the junction of the zygoma and lateral orbital rim.[38,39] The posterior footplate can be attached to the temporal bone immediately above the root of the helix, which is typically thicker bone.[38,39] This placement allows the two to be placed parallel to each other and the Frankfurt horizontal (**Fig. 1**). The temporalis muscle may be draped

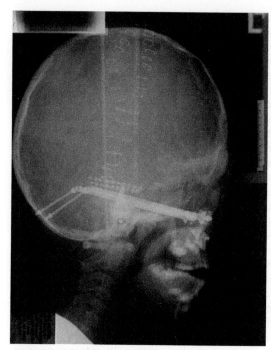

Fig. 1. Lateral cephalogram demonstrating placement of internal distractors. (Patient of DAS).

over the distractor or split so the distractor can lie along the deep temporal fascia (**Fig. 2**).

External Distractor Placement

The external distractor is applied after closure of the incisions. A halo frame is positioned on the skull with the horizontal component lying roughly 2 cm above the supraorbital rim and with the vertical rod in the facial midline.[14] There are a variety of techniques to secure the Le Fort III segment to the distractor frame. One method is to use a rigid occlusal splint alone that is connected to the central rod.[14] The occlusal splint can also be suspended by wires to outriggers attached to the central rod. It is important to prestretch the wires to avoid the possibility of premature consolidation from stretching during distraction. Fixation posts can also be secured to the nasomaxillary buttress or zygoma to provide additional points of fixation.[17,38]

Vector Choice

The ideal vector for distraction depends on the individual patient. Anterior translation of the segment is the primary goal. If the patient has a presurgical anterior open bite, the advancement can be performed with a clockwise rotation.[40] If improved midface or dorsal nasal lengthening is desired, the vector is angled downward from the

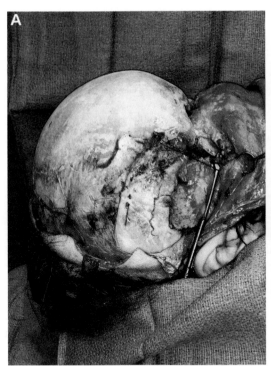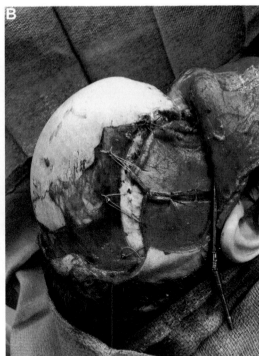

Fig. 2. Placement of internal distractors before temporalis resuspension (*A*) and after temporalis resuspension (*B*). (Patient of DAS).

Frankfort horizontal plane.[23] Care should be taken with a downward vector, because this will increase orbital volume faster than a horizontal distraction, possibly limiting the advancement at the orbital level if enophthalmos occurs sooner than expected.[19] In these cases, a Le Fort II distraction with simultaneous zygomatic repositioning, described elsewhere in this issue of Clinics in Plastic Surgery, may be considered.

It has been shown that, when using an external distractor with wired attachments, the Le Fort III segment has a tendency to rotate in a counterclockwise direction with the posterior nasal spine moving inferiorly.[41] Serial cephalograms will detect this clockwise rotation of the Le Fort III segment during activation, providing the opportunity for correction before the start of consolidation.

With an external distractor and wired attachments to the midface, obtaining midface advancement with minimal rotation can be obtained with a net force vector applied to a point roughly 54% of the distance between the maxillary occlusal plane and the mobilized nasion.[40] With a direction of pull roughly parallel to the maxillary occlusal plane. The midface tends to rotate in a counterclockwise direction when the vector is moved closer to the

occlusal plane and tends to rotate in a clockwise rotation when moved closer to the nasion.

Additional methods for attempting to control the midface have been reported. The cat's cradle technique involves circumferentially wiring the maxilla and wired attachment to the external device.[42] A separate group has reported fabrication of custom zygomatic fixation plates that are then attached to the external device through parallel connecting pins.[43] Alternatively, a dental splint is rigidly attached to the external device (**Fig. 3**).[41] With this technique, a dental splint is prefabricated and at the time of surgery is cemented to the maxillary arch with dental cement. The splint can be reinforced posteriorly with steel wires passing around the zygoma and anteriorly with a wire passed from the anterior nasal spine to the dental splint. This can be useful when the patient has only deciduous teeth present. The splint is then rigidly attached to the vertical rod of the external distraction device. With this technique, there is no need for additional zygomatic fixation posts and the associated transcutaneous wiring.[41] This form of dental fixation effectively counteracts the masseteric forces and prevents counterclockwise rotation of the Le Fort segment.[41] This is our

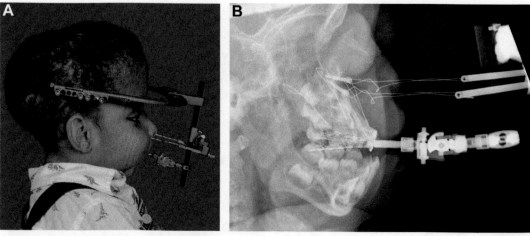

Fig. 3. External distraction device with rigidly attached dental splint. This is shown in the photograph (*A*) and lateral cephalogram (*B*). (Patient of RLF).

preferred method of Le Fort III distraction when an external device is used.

POSTOPERATIVE PERIOD

The postoperative latency period is 5 to 7 days, after which activation commences at a rate of 1 mm per day, split into twice daily 0.5 mm advancements.[14,44] The end point for distraction depends on the age of the patient. In a growing child, distraction is performed to a point of overcorrection.[14] The exact degree of overcorrection is not well-defined. It has been suggested that the average midface grows slightly more than 1.0 cm between 8 years of age and skeletal maturity.[23] This number can be used to guide the degree of overcorrection. It is important to place the infraorbital rims into their desired location with less importance placed on the occlusion, because this can be corrected with a Le Fort I after skeletal maturity has been reached. Although we do not typically perform Le Fort III distraction on the skeletally mature patient, the end point in this patient population would be correction of enophthalmos and orthotopic malar position. A concurrent Le Fort I may be required in these cases. Lateral cephalograms can be performed during the activation period to help guide the degree of distraction.[14] After the activation period, the bone is allowed to consolidate for 2 months to prevent relapse.[41,44] Other institutions implement a consolidation period as short as 4 weeks.[45]

COMPLICATIONS

Complications involved with Le Fort III distractions include zygomaticomaxillary complex fractures, cerebrospinal fluid leakage from dural tears, infection, corneal exposure, damage to maxillary tooth buds, asymmetric advancement, and incomplete advancement.[14,16,46,47] Major morbidities that have been reported with Le Fort III osteotomies include blindness and death, although these complications should be exceedingly rare in experienced hands.[48] Complications may occur with bony healing, resulting in premature consolidation or nonunion.

Complications related to distraction with internal devices include dislodging of the device and misplacing screws into the maxillary tooth buds.[16] One should note that these devices were designed with anterior footplates that wrap around the anterior aspect of the maxilla. Current designs mitigate this risk by only resting against the lateral orbital rim and can be retained with a single optional screw. A major concern with the use of internal devices is fracturing the zygomaticomaxillary buttress, either during the Le Fort osteotomy or as a result of distraction.[29,39] This process can result in distraction of the zygoma, while leaving the maxilla behind. For this reason, the use of internal distractors demands absolute precision with the osteotomies, preserving all of the buttresses. If the lateral orbital osteotomy did not travel properly through the inferior orbital fissure, there is a weakening along the zygomaticomaxillary buttress. As mentioned elsewhere in this article, once the osteotomy is complete, the Le Fort III must be carefully interrogated to test for any sign of instability. If a fracture is identified, it should be fixated accordingly.

Complications related to distraction with an external device include pin loosening, frame migration, frame dislodgement, and intracranial migration of the halo fixation pins.[46,49]

LONG-TERM RESULTS

The advancement obtained through Le Fort III distraction in preadolescent patients has been shown to be stable for up to 10 years after the operation.[50] It is important to note the distinction between surgical relapse and phenotypic relapse. If the midface is not overcorrected at the time of the original operation, the patient may redevelop the appearance of midface recession. This phenotypic relapse is most often due to continued mandibular growth with a stable maxillary position.[50] It is unlikely to be due to surgical relapse, or actual posterior movement of the maxilla.[50] Therefore, to account for continued normal mandibular growth with minimal anterior maxillary growth during teenage years, overcorrection at the time of distraction is critical for obtaining appropriate maxillomandibular positioning at the time of skeletal maturity.[18,50] See **Figs. 4** and **5** for results obtained with Le Fort III distraction using internal distractors.

The airway improvement results from increasing the volume of the nasopharyngeal and velopharyngeal airspaces.[28] Although Le Fort III distraction can be effective in improving airway obstruction in patients with severe midface retrusion, there can be evidence of recurrence of the airway obstruction owing to increase in physiologic needs as the patient grows.[23,28] Furthermore, not all patients may benefit from Le Fort III distraction alone, suggesting another anatomic or physiologic cause of airflow disfunction.[16]

SECONDARY PROCEDURES

The need for a second Le Fort III distraction has been associated with greater degree of preoperative midface hypoplasia, advancement at a younger age (7.1 years vs 9.5 years), and failure to overcorrect the midface position at the original operation.[23]

If there continues to be upper airway obstruction after Le Fort III distraction and the midface is located in an appropriate position, the patient should be evaluated for tonsillectomy or adenoidectomy if they were not performed preoperatively.[14]

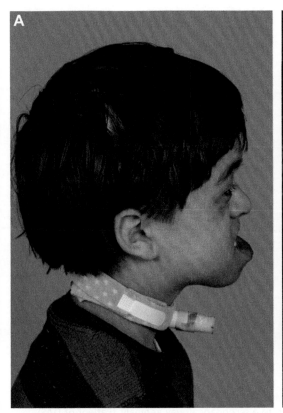 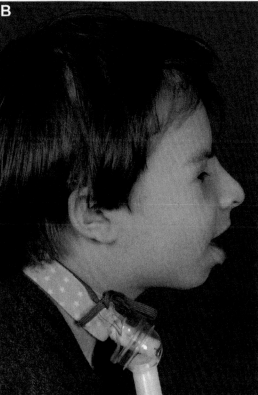

Fig. 4. Patient before and after internal distraction. Note overcorrection of midface position. (Patient of DAS).

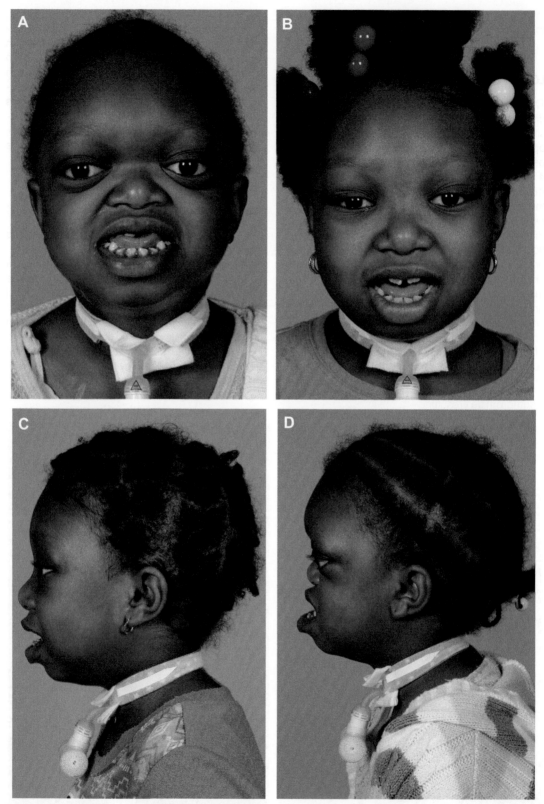

Fig. 5. Patient before (*A*, *C*) and after (*B*, *D*) internal distraction. Tracheostomy was managed by an outside otolaryngologist and remained in place postoperatively owing to a secondary airway anomaly. (Patient of DAS).

Complete endoscopic airway assessment, if not already completed, should be performed.

A goal of the Le Fort III distraction is to bring the infraorbital rims and zygomas into optimal relationships. This does not always result in optimal occlusal relationships. If that is the case, orthognathic surgery may be required at the time of skeletal maturity.[14]

Periorbital and facial fat injection has been increasingly used to refine the appearance of patient affected with craniofacial anomalies.[51] Bone substitutes can be used to fill voids and contour deformities of the cranium and temporal areas.[52]

SUMMARY

Le Fort III distraction improves midfacial hypoplasia associated with craniofacial dysostosis and can result in stable, large advancements of the midface, resulting in improvements in facial convexity, globe protection, occlusion and airflow. It can be performed using internal and external distraction devices based on the preference of the surgeon and patients. The ideal age of distraction is yet to be determined and should be based on the severity of the deformity and functional compromise resulting from midface retrusion. When performed in the growing child, distraction should result in overcorrection because the maxilla will have minimal to no anterior growth, whereas the remainder of the face grows until skeletal maturity. If necessary, a Le Fort III with or without a Le Fort I procedure can be performed at skeletal maturity.

CLINICS CARE POINTS

- Le Fort III distraction is advantageous over conventional Le Fort III advancement when a large movement is required in a growing patient.

- Overcorrection is important in the growing child.

- Le Fort III distraction performed at a later age will be less likely to require a secondary distraction or midface advancement.

- Posterior descent of the midface can be avoided with an occlusal splint.

- The patient may require subsequent operations despite a technically successful Le Fort III advancement.

DISCLOSURE

The authors have nothing to disclose.

REFERENCES

1. Gillies H, Harrison SH. Operative correction by osteotomy of recessed malar maxillary compound in a case of oxycephaly. Br J Plast Surg 1950;3(2): 123–7.
2. Waterhouse N. The history of craniofacial surgery. Facial Plast Surg 1993;9(2):143–50.
3. Wolfe SA. A man from Héric. In: Wolfe SA, editor. The life and work of Paul Tessier, MD, Father of craniofacial surgery, Vol. I. San Bernardino (CA): lulu.com; 2012. p. 236–8.
4. Ghali MG, Srinivasan VM, Jea A, et al. Craniosynostosis surgery: the legacy of Paul Tessier. Neurosurg Focus 2014;36(4):E17.
5. Tessier P. The definitive plastic surgical treatment of the severe facial deformities of craniofacial dysostosis. Crouzon's and Apert's diseases. Plast Reconstr Surg 1971;48(5):419–42.
6. Illizarov S. The Ilizarov method: history and scope. In: Rozbruch SR, Ilizarov S, editors. Limb lengthening and reconstruction surgery. New York: Informa healthcare; 2007. p. 1–18.
7. McCarthy JG, Schreiber J, Karp N, et al. Lengthening the human mandible by gradual distraction. Plast Reconstr Surg 1992;89(1):1–8 [discussion 9-10].
8. Staffenberg DA, Wood RJ, McCarthy JG, et al. Midface distraction advancement in the canine without osteotomies. Ann Plast Surg 1995;34(5):512–7.
9. Staffenberg DA, Wood RJ, Grayson BH, et al. Midface advancement in the canine without osteotomies. Fifth biannual congress of the international society of craniofacial surgery. Mexico: Oaxaca; 1993.
10. Cohen SR, Rutrick RE, Burstein FD. Distraction osteogenesis of the human craniofacial skeleton: initial experience with new distraction system. J Craniofac Surg 1995;6(5):368–74.
11. Chin M, Toth BA. Distraction osteogenesis in maxillofacial surgery using internal devices: review of five cases. J Oral Maxillofac Surg 1996;54(1):45–53 [discussion 54].
12. Cohen SR, Holmes RE. Internal Le Fort III distraction with biodegradable devices. J Craniofac Surg 2001; 12(3):264–72.
13. Polley JW, Figueroa AA. Management of severe maxillary deficiency in childhood and adolescence through distraction osteogenesis with an external, adjustable, rigid distraction device. J Craniofac Surg 1997;8(3):181–5 [discussion 186].
14. McCarthy JG, Flores RL. Craniofacial distraction. In: McCarthy JG, editor. Craniofacial distraction. New York: Springer; 2017. p. 321–36.

15. Tahiri Y, Taylor J. An update on midface advancement using Le Fort II and III distraction osteogenesis. Semin Plast Surg 2014;28(4):184–92.

16. Fearon JA. Halo distraction of the Le Fort III in syndromic craniosynostosis: a long-term assessment. Plast Reconstr Surg 2005;115(6):1524–36.

17. Shetye PR, Davidson EH, Sorkin M, et al. Evaluation of three surgical techniques for advancement of the midface in growing children with syndromic craniosynostosis. Plast Reconstr Surg 2010;126(3):982–94.

18. Shetye PR, Kapadia H, Grayson BH, et al. A 10-year study of skeletal stability and growth of the midface following Le Fort III advancement in syndromic craniosynostosis. Plast Reconstr Surg 2010;126(3):973–81.

19. Shetye PR, Boutros S, Grayson BH, et al. Midterm follow-up of midface distraction for syndromic craniosynostosis: a clinical and cephalometric study. Plast Reconstr Surg 2007;120(6):1621–32.

20. Caterson EJ, Shetye PR, Grayson BH, et al. Surgical management of patients with a history of early Le Fort III advancement after they have attained skeletal maturity. Plast Reconstr Surg 2013;132(4):592e–601e.

21. Mosa AJ, Zellner E, Ho ES, et al. Le Fort III in syndromic craniosynostosis: cost comparison of distraction osteogenesis versus single-stage internal fixation techniques. Plast Surg (Oakv) 2019;27(2):125–9.

22. Nout E, Cesteleyn LL, van der Wal KG, et al. Advancement of the midface, from conventional Le Fort III osteotomy to Le Fort III distraction: review of the literature. Int J Oral Maxillofac Surg 2008;37(9):781–9.

23. Patel N, Fearon JA. Treatment of the syndromic midface: a long-term assessment at skeletal maturity. Plast Reconstr Surg 2015;135(4):731e–42e.

24. McCarthy JG, La Trenta GS, Breitbart AS, et al. The Le Fort III advancement osteotomy in the child under 7 years of age. Plast Reconstr Surg 1990;86(4):633–46 [discussion 647-639].

25. Coccaro PJ, McCarthy JG, Epstein FJ, et al. Early and late surgery in craniofacial dysostosis: a longitudinal cephalometric study. Am J Orthod 1980;77(4):421–36.

26. Kreiborg S. Craniofacial growth in plagiocephaly and Crouzon syndrome. Scand J Plast Reconstr Surg 1981;15(3):187–97.

27. Bachmayer DI, Ross RB, Munro IR. Maxillary growth following LeFort III advancement surgery in Crouzon, Apert, and Pfeiffer syndromes. Am J Orthod Dentofacial Orthop 1986;90(5):420–30.

28. Flores RL, Shetye PR, Zeitler D, et al. Airway changes following Le Fort III distraction osteogenesis for syndromic craniosynostosis: a clinical and cephalometric study. Plast Reconstr Surg 2009;124(2):590–601.

29. Gosain AK, Santoro TD, Havlik RJ, et al. Midface distraction following Le Fort III and monobloc osteotomies: problems and solutions. Plast Reconstr Surg 2002;109(6):1797–808.

30. Meling TR, Hogevold HE, Due-Tonnessen BJ, et al. Midface distraction osteogenesis: internal vs. external devices. Int J Oral Maxillofac Surg 2011;40(2):139–45.

31. Gateno J, Teichgraeber JF, Xia JJ. Three-dimensional surgical planning for maxillary and midface distraction osteogenesis. J Craniofac Surg 2003;14(6):833–9.

32. Steinbacher DM. Three-Dimensional analysis and surgical planning in craniomaxillofacial surgery. J Oral Maxillofac Surg 2015;73(12 Suppl):S40–56.

33. Hopper RA, Kapadia H, Susarla SM. Surgical-orthodontic considerations in subcranial and frontofacial distraction. Oral Maxillofacial Surg Clin N Am 2020;32(2):309–20.

34. Karian LS, Phillips BZ, Morrison CS, et al. Technology to minimize the morbidity of Le Fort III osteotomies. Plast Reconstr Surg 2012;130(1):210e–2e.

35. Wood JS, Purzycki A, Thompson J, et al. The use of Brainlab navigation in Le Fort III osteotomy. J Craniofac Surg 2015;26(3):616–9.

36. Raposo-Amaral CE, Denadai R, Pereira-Filho JC, et al. Serious complications after Le Fort III distraction osteogenesis in syndromic craniosynostosis: evolution of preventive and Therapeutic strategies. J Craniofac Surg 2018;29(6):1397–401.

37. Flores RL. App for Iphone and Andriod. BioDigital Inc. Available at https://www.myface.org/civa/.

38. Robertson KJ, Mendez BM, Bruce WJ, et al. Le Fort III distraction with internal vs external distractors: a cephalometric analysis. Cleft Palate Craniofac J 2018;55(5):721–7.

39. Satoh K, Mitsukawa N, Tosa Y, et al. Le Fort III midfacial distraction using an internal distraction device for syndromic craniosynostosis: device selection, problems, indications, and a proposal for use of a parallel bar for device-setting. J Craniofac Surg 2006;17(6):1050–8.

40. Shetye PR, Giannoutsos E, Grayson BH, et al. Le Fort III distraction: part I. Controlling position and vectors of the midface segment. Plast Reconstr Surg 2009;124(3):871–8.

41. Shetye PR, Grayson BH, McCarthy JG. Le Fort III distraction: controlling position and path of the osteotomized midface segment on a rigid platform. J Craniofac Surg 2010;21(4):1118–21.

42. Havlik RJ, Seelinger MJ, Fashemo DV, et al. "Cat's cradle" midfacial fixation in distraction osteogenesis after Le Fort III osteotomy. J Craniofac Surg 2004;15(6):946–52.

43. Klammert U, Bohm H, Schweitzer T, et al. Multi-directional Le Fort III midfacial distraction using an individual prefabricated device. J Craniomaxillofac Surg 2009;37(4):210–5.

44. Hopper RA, Aspinall C, Heike C, et al. What the patients and parents do not tell you-recollections from families following external LeFort III midface distraction. Plast Surg Nurs 2009;29(2):78–85 [quiz 86-77].

45. Fearon JA. Discussion. Computed tomographic analysis of temporal maxillary stability and pterygomaxillary generate formation following pediatric Le Fort III distraction advancement. Plast Reconstr Surg 2010;126(5):1675–6.

46. Saltaji H, Altalibi M, Major MP, et al. Le Fort III distraction osteogenesis versus conventional Le Fort III osteotomy in correction of syndromic midfacial hypoplasia: a systematic review. J Oral Maxillofac Surg 2014;72(5):959–72.

47. Santiago PE, Grayson BH, Degen M, et al. The effect of an early Le Fort III surgery on permanent molar eruption. Plast Reconstr Surg 2005;115(2):423–7.

48. Czerwinski M, Hopper RA, Gruss J, et al. Major morbidity and mortality rates in craniofacial surgery: an analysis of 8101 major procedures. Plast Reconstr Surg 2010;126(1):181–6.

49. Goldstein JA, Paliga JT, Taylor JA, et al. Complications in 54 frontofacial distraction procedures in patients with syndromic craniosynostosis. J Craniofac Surg 2015;26(1):124–8.

50. Gibson TL, Grayson BH, McCarthy JG, et al. Maxillomandibular and occlusal relationships in preadolescent patients with syndromic craniosynostosis treated by LeFort III distraction osteogenesis: 10-year surgical and phenotypic stability. Am J Orthod Dentofacial Orthop 2019;156(6):779–90.

51. Denadai R, Raposo-Amaral CA, Raposo-Amaral CE. Fat grafting in managing craniofacial deformities. Plast Reconstr Surg 2019;143(5):1447–55.

52. Vu DD, Tiwana PS. Le Fort III and Le Fort II osteotomies. Atlas Oral Maxillofac Surg Clin North Am 2016; 24(1):15–25.

Le Fort II Distraction with Simultaneous Zygomatic Repositioning

Richard A. Hopper, MD, MS[a,b,]*, Howard D. Wang, MD[a,b],
Ezgi Mercan, PhD[a]

KEYWORDS

- Midface hypoplasia • Syndromic craniosynostosis • Le Fort II • Zygomatic repositioning • Le Fort III
- Distraction osteogenesis • Apert syndrome • Achondroplasia

KEY POINTS

- Apert midface hypoplasia is characterized by central nasomaxillary deficiency that is more severe than the degree of hypoplasia present at the lateral orbitomalar region.
- Le Fort II distraction with zygomatic repositioning allows for differential advancement of the central and lateral components of the midface to correct the relative central deficiency for Apert midface hypoplasia and other similar conditions.
- Early outcomes of Le Fort II distraction with zygomatic repositioning demonstrate normalization of facial ratios in patients with Apert syndrome, significant increases in the nasopharyngeal airway volume, and comparable complication profile to Le Fort III distraction.

BACKGROUND

Severe midface hypoplasia is commonly associated with syndromic craniosynostosis and can lead to several functional problems including exorbitism, airway obstruction, and malocclusion.[1] Subcranial Le Fort III distraction osteogenesis has become the standard treatment for correction of severe midface hypoplasia.[2–6] However, surgical movement of the entire midface may not adequately address all forms of midface hypoplasia. In a subset of patients, the degree of hypoplasia varies between the central nasomaxillary region and the lateral orbitozygomatic region. For example, the midface of patients with Apert syndrome is characterized by the presence of a central concavity in the setting of a retrusive midface. This is caused by a severe deficiency in the sagittal and vertical dimension of the central midface relative to the lateral midface.[7] Unlike the midface hypoplasia associated with Crouzon syndrome, the Apert facial dysmorphology has been described as an abnormal face in an abnormal position.[8]

The en bloc midface advancement achieved through Le Fort III distraction corrects exorbitism and malar hypoplasia through sagittal advancement of the inferior orbital rims and the body of the zygomas. The extent of sagittal advancement in the central nasomaxillary region with the Le Fort III operation is limited by the risk of causing enophthalmos, and vertical lengthening is limited by the risk of creating excessive orbital height. Therefore, the relative central midface vertical and axial deficiency remains undercorrected in patients with Apert syndrome after a Le Fort III operation because of these limitations imposed by the adjacent zygomas. Le Fort II distraction with simultaneous zygomatic repositioning (LF2ZR) was designed with the goal of differential and unrestricted movement of the central midface relative to the lateral zygomas, thus achieving not only

[a] The Craniofacial Center, Seattle Children's Hospital, 4800 Sand Point Way Northeast, Seattle, WA 98105, USA;
[b] Division of Plastic Surgery, Department of Surgery, University of Washington, Seattle, WA, USA
* Corresponding author. Division of Craniofacial and Plastic Surgery, Seattle Children's Hospital, 4800 Sand Point Way Northeast, Seattle, WA 98105.
E-mail address: richard.hopper@seattlechildrens.org

Clin Plastic Surg 48 (2021) 487–496
https://doi.org/10.1016/j.cps.2021.02.007
0094-1298/21/Published by Elsevier Inc.

advancement of the existing hypoplastic facial structures but also normalization of the facial ratios.[8,9]

LF2ZR involves a single surgery that first repositions and fixates the Le Fort III osteotomy to optimize lateral malar position, followed by osteotomy at the Le Fort II level to allow unrestricted movement of the central nasomaxillary region through distraction osteogenesis (**Fig. 1**). The smaller advancement and elevation of the zygoma segments correct exorbitism and malar hypoplasia, whereas the subsequent greater advancement and vertical lengthening of the Le Fort II osteotomy corrects the biconcave deformity of the syndromic midface without affecting globe position because of the support from the fixated zygomas. The LF2ZR operation was first described for the correction of the characteristic central midface deficiency associated with Apert syndrome, but the indications for LF2ZR also include other conditions where a differential magnitude of hypoplasia exists between the central and lateral midface.[10,11]

INDICATIONS
Apert and Pfeiffer Syndromes

Patients with Apert, Pfeiffer, and Crouzon syndromes share the phenotype of midface hypoplasia that is characterized by a concave lateral facial profile. Unlike Crouzon syndrome, Apert and Pfeiffer facial dysmorphology is also characterized by a more profound retrusion and vertical deficiency of the central nasomaxillary region compared with the lateral orbitozygomatic regions, resulting in an additional concave facial profile on worm's-eye view and frontal view.[8] These three conditions are also characterized by a down-slanting palpebral fissure. However, in Crouzon syndrome this is secondary to lateral canthal dystopia, whereas in Apert and Pfeiffer, it is caused by an elevation of the medial canthus from the central facial vertical impaction. The vertical lengthening and advancement of the central Le Fort II segment in LF2ZR not only corrects this biconcave deformity of Apert and Pfeiffer syndromes, but it also creates a desirable lengthening of the nose and downward movement of the medial canthus to improve the periorbital esthetics (**Fig. 2**).

Achondroplasia

Certain patients with achondroplasia share a similar facial dysmorphology with Apert syndrome where the central midface hypoplasia is more severe than the lateral midface, and associated obstructive sleep apnea is common.[10] Le Fort III distraction alone has been shown to be limited in treating the central hypoplasia of the face and the obstructive apnea in these patients.[2] LF2ZR has the potential for greater airway expansion by distracting the central nasomaxillary region independent of the zygoma positions. This differential movement treats the nasopharyngeal compression while avoiding enophthalmos (**Fig. 3**).[10]

Positive-Pressure Therapy Induced Midface Retrusion

Children with obstructive sleep apnea who require high-pressure nasal positive-pressure airway therapy at an early age can develop midface retrusion as a result of the effect of constant pressure on the growing facial structures.[12] The nasomaxillary region tends to be the most affected area, because the pressure of the mask is focused on this region, and can cause challenges in maintaining mask fit and air seal. In these patients, Le Fort II distraction with or without zygomatic repositioning depending on the degree of zygomatic retrusion can advance and lengthen the central midface to improve airway anatomy, facial balance, and fit of the pressure mask (**Fig. 4**).[11]

SURGICAL TECHNIQUE

A detailed description of the surgical technique of LF2ZR was previously published.[11] We recommend performing the operation on patients at age of 7 years or older, with an ideal age range of 9 to 12 years. Performing LF2ZR before 7 years of age can result in zygoma instability or resorption. Next is a summary of the operative steps (**Fig. 5**).

Le Fort III Osteotomy

- A coronal incision is used to expose the upper midface.
- Dissection is performed in the subperiosteal plane with reflection of the anterior portion of the temporalis muscle bilaterally to expose the anterior zygomatic arch laterally and nasofrontal region centrally.
- The zygomatic arch osteotomies are performed with a reciprocating saw just behind the body of the zygomas without disruption of the posterior temporalis muscle.
- Stepped osteotomies of the lateral orbital walls are made from the zygomaticofrontal suture down to the inferior orbital fissure using a piezoelectric or reciprocating saw.
- A small osteotome from the lateral orbit creates an osteotomy along the orbital floor from the inferior orbital fissure to the uncinate process behind the lacrimal fossa.

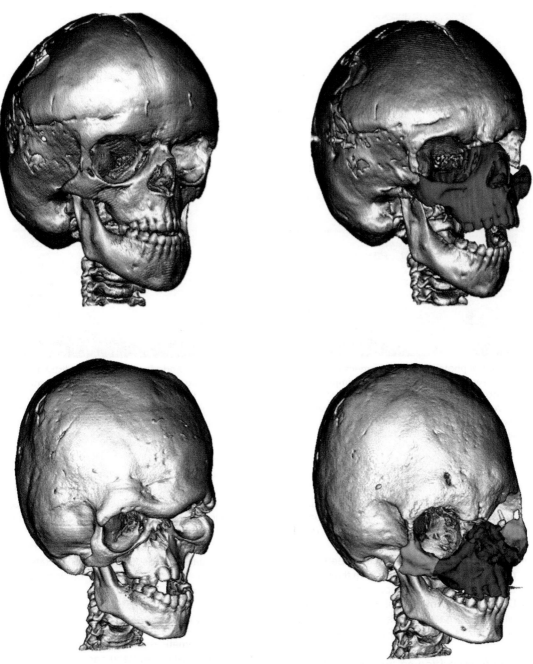

Fig. 1. Comparison of Le Fort III distraction with Le Fort II distraction with simultaneous zygomatic repositioning. Computed tomography scan of a patient with Crouzon syndrome before and after Le Fort III distraction demonstrating en bloc advancement of the midface. In contrast, computed tomography scan of a patient with Apert syndrome before and after Le Fort II distraction with simultaneous zygomatic repositioning showing segmental movement of the midface to correct the severe central retrusion.

- A piezoelectric saw is used to perform an osteotomy at the nasofrontal junction, which is carried along the medial orbital wall behind the lacrimal fossa to join the orbital floor osteotomy.

- From underneath the lateral orbit an osteotome is placed in the orbital floor osteotomy at the anterior edge of the inferior orbital fissure and used to continue the osteotomy along the posterior maxillary sinus wall,

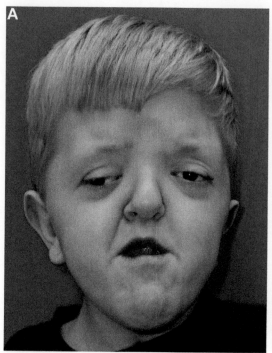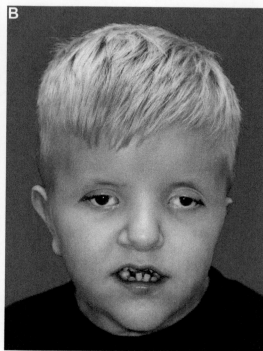

Fig. 2. Clinical photographs of a patient with Apert syndrome before (*A*) and after (*B*) Le Fort II distraction and zygomatic repositioning and forehead implant placement demonstrating the procedure's effect on frontal view appearance. The implant has achieved improved forehead contour and the repositioned zygomas have improved lower eyelid support. The inferior vector of central distraction has dropped the medial canthi to level the palpebral fissures and has lengthened the nasal dorsum and midface height. The anterior vector has effaced the deep nasolabial folds.

down to and through the pterygomaxillary junction.

- The pterygomaxillary separation is completed from this lateral coronal incision approach or from a permucosal intraoral access directly at the pterygomaxillary junction.
- A septal osteotome is used to perform the posterior septal osteotomy from the nasofrontal junction toward the posterior nasal spine.
- Down-fracture of the midface is performed with careful manual pressure, and the midface is mobilized with Rowe-Killey forceps.

Zygomatic Repositioning and Le Fort II Osteotomy

- The mobilized Le Fort III segment is tilted and advanced to place one zygoma in the desired position based on the stepped osteotomy. It is then fixated using a 1.5- to 1.7-mm titanium plate across the repositioned lateral orbital wall osteotomy.
- The typical movement of the zygoma is 5 to 8 mm anterior and 3 to 5 mm superior.
- Through an upper gingivobuccal sulcus incision, the fixated zygoma is released from the

maxilla using a piezoelectric saw lateral to the infraorbital nerve. Care is taken to preserve the zygomatic retaining ligament and periosteal attachments to avoid vascular compromise of the zygomatic segment.

- The same sequence is performed on the contralateral side to reposition, fixate, and release the contralateral orbitozygomatic complex.

Adjunctive Procedures

- The zygomatic repositioning and Le Fort II osteotomy have now been completed.
- A custom onlay forehead implant is inserted during the LF2ZR surgery to treat the forehead contour irregularities that are commonly present in Apert patients.
- In anticipation of the potential for bony step-offs that can occur after distraction of the Le Fort II segment, small wedges of bone are removed at the nasofrontal and inferior orbital osteotomy edges.
- Although the vertical distraction of the Le Fort II segment helps correct medial canthal position, lateral canthopexies should also be

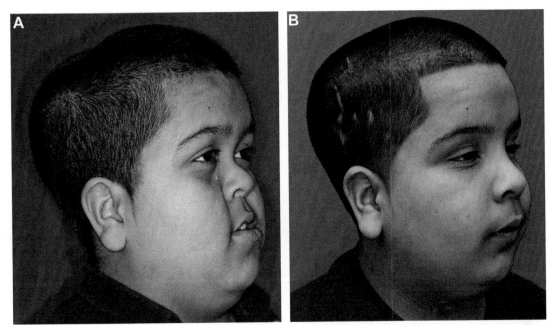

Fig. 3. Clinical photographs of a patient with achondroplasia and severe obstructive sleep apnea demonstrating changes before (*A*) and after (*B*) LF2ZR on an oblique view. Along with the improved elements seen on frontal view, the sagittal and axial biconcavity deformities of this condition are simultaneously corrected by the large Le Fort II movement relative to the zygomas. This overcorrection of the midface deficiency was followed by a sagittal split advancement of the mandible to optimize airway expansion and treat the patient's obstructive sleep apnea.

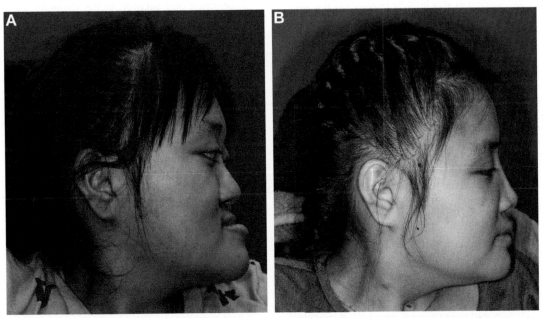

Fig. 4. Clinical photographs of a patient with neuromuscular sleep apnea and severe secondary midface retrusion from chronic positive-pressure mask treatment before (*A*) and after (*B*) Le Fort II distraction and zygomatic repositioning demonstrating changes on lateral view. The LF2ZR achieved appropriate periorbital esthetics from the repositioned zygomas and corrected the patient's anterior cross-bite deformity while creating normal facial convexity that allows improved mask fit.

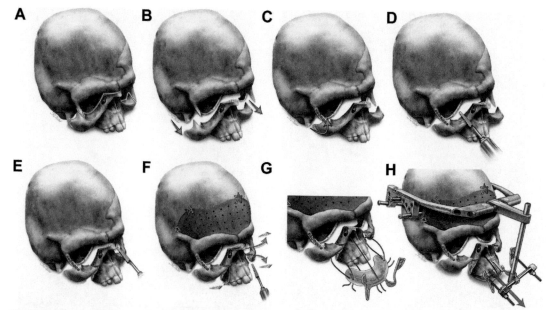

Fig. 5. Illustration of the surgical steps of Le Fort II distraction with simultaneous zygomatic repositioning. (*A, B*) Le Fort III osteotomy and mobilization through a coronal incision to achieve craniofacial separation. (*C*) Advancement and fixation of the right zygoma. (*D*) Le Fort II osteotomy through an intraoral incision. (*E*) Repositioning, fixation, and release of the left orbitozygomatic region. (*F*) Contouring of the anticipated bony prominences at the nasofrontal and zygomaticomaxillary region. A forehead onlay implant is placed to correct any contour abnormalities if indicated. (*G*) Application of a custom traction splint. (*H*) Anterior and inferior distraction of the Le Fort II segment using an external halo device. (Reprinted with permission from Hopper RA, Kapadia H, Susarla S. Le Fort II Distraction with Zygomatic Repositioning: A Technique for Differential Correction of Midface Hypoplasia. J Oral Maxillofac Surg 2018.)

performed at this time to resuspend the canthal ligament inside the superior lateral orbital wall.

- The coronal incision is then closed after thorough irrigation and resuspension of the temporalis muscle.

Le Fort II Distraction

- Through the intraoral incisions, a custom acrylic splint containing an embedded portion of a face bow with two extraoral loop extensions is secured to the maxilla using 26-gauge steel wire loops through bone holes in the piriform rim and lateral maxillary buttresses.
- The intraoral incisions are then closed, and orthodontic bone anchors are inserted at the midline of the maxilla and mandible to allow for inferior vector control with elastics during activation.
- A halo-based rigid external distraction device is secured using cranial pins with a mounted vertical midline post and transverse activation arms.
- The activation arms are set at a 30° to 45° downward vector relative to Frankfort

horizontal and secured to the maxillary traction splint extensions with 24-gauge steel wires.

Postoperative Care

- Patients are kept intubated and sedated for 2 to 3 days postoperatively in the intensive care unit until an air leak is confirmed.
- After a latency period of 3 to 5 days, distraction begins at a rate of 1 to 1.5 mm per day, with a shorter latency and faster rate used for younger patients.
- The distraction vector is decided based on the goals of augmenting the dorsal nasal length, increasing the vertical maxillary height, leveling the palpebral fissures, and correcting the maxillary occlusal plane.
- The end point of Le Fort II distraction is determined by maximizing advancement without the medial lids losing their scleral contact, and vertical lengthening that achieves a level palpebral fissure. This should bring the patient into an overjet position, demonstrating the associated mandible hypoplasia and common need for mandible advancement surgery at skeletal maturity in these patients.

- The external distraction device is removed after 6 to 8 weeks of consolidation.

CLINICAL OUTCOMES
Correction of Abnormal Facial Ratios

Patients with Apert syndrome have a relative deficiency in the facial ratios of central to lateral midface in the worm's-eye view (axial facial ratio) and the frontal view (vertical facial ratio). Our retrospective study comparing LF2ZR and Le Fort III distraction in Apert patients found that Le Fort III distraction left the abnormal facial ratio unchanged after midface advancement. In comparison, after LF2ZR surgery, the axial and vertical facial ratios of the treated Apert patients became similar to those of Crouzon patients and normal control subjects.[8] This correction was achieved through differential movements with LF2ZR in which the central midface was advanced an average of 18.0 mm and lengthened 13.5 mm compared with only 5.2 mm of advancement and 2.9 mm of lengthening for the lateral midface.[8]

In addition to correction of the abnormal facial ratio, the large magnitude and inferior vector of central midface advancement can also lead to other desirable facial changes in this patient population. Patients with Apert syndrome often have downward oriented palpebral fissures with the medial canthi positioned close to the nasofrontal junction and higher than the lateral canthi. With the medial canthi attached to the Le Fort II segment, the inferior advancement of the nasomaxillary region relative to the lateral orbital region can have a favorable effect by leveling the palpebral fissure. Other periorbital features of Apert syndrome include soft tissue bulges overlying the inferior orbital rims and prominent nasojugal folds that result from the worm's-eye concavity. These features are improved by the differential inferior and anterior movement of the medial orbit relative to the lateral orbit, which is moved superiorly. Other facial features that are improved include the short nasal dorsum, which is lengthened by the inferior distraction of the nasomaxillary complex, and the anterior open bite, which is reduced through a clockwise rotation of the palate. Thus, LF2ZR allows for correction of the abnormal facial ratios and many of the facial features that contribute to the stigmata of Apert syndrome.

Airway Changes

Severe midface hypoplasia can contribute to upper airway obstruction and is commonly associated with obstructive sleep apnea.[13] Volumetric changes to the upper airway secondary to Le Fort III distraction and LF2ZR are illustrated in **Fig. 6**. Advancement of the midface via Le Fort III distraction has been shown to increase upper airway volume, improve polysomnography study results, and lead to the resolution of obstructive sleep apnea in a subset of patients after surgery.[14–18] Previous studies have found that the greatest increase in airway volume after Le Fort III advancement occurs at the nasopharyngeal level.[15,17] Although outcomes data on airway changes after LF2ZR are limited, our center has found that improvement in sleep apnea measures and airway volume is most dependent on the magnitude of horizontal displacement of the midface, and not on the technique, palate rotation, or vertical movement.[19] Taken together, these findings emphasize the importance of fully correcting the central midface deficiency in syndromic children regardless of surgical procedure. In patients with differential central midface hypoplasia, this is not possible without a segmental procedure, such as LF2ZR.

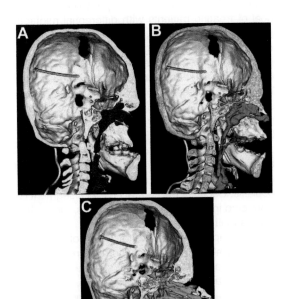

Fig. 6. Colorized airway changes on computed tomography scans of patients with Apert syndrome before midface surgery (*A*), after Le Fort III distraction advancement (*B*), and after Le Fort II and simultaneous zygomatic repositioning (*C*). Unpublished quantitative airway analysis has shown that the increase in the nasopharyngeal airway volume is more affected by the magnitude of advancement rather than the vector of distraction.

Complications

The potential complications associated with LF2ZR are similar to those of Le Fort III distraction and include hardware problems requiring adjustment in the operating room, early consolidation, relapse, adverse effects on speech, infection, bleeding, seroma, cerebral spinal fluid leak, and periorbital and ocular injuries.[14,20,21] On review of the senior author's personal experience with 67 consecutive subcranial surgeries, the overall rate of complications with LF2ZR was not greater than that with Le Fort III distraction, with the most common complication being the need to return to the operating room for adjustment of the external distraction device (unpublished data). LF2ZR does entail additional osteotomies and fixation compared with Le Fort III distraction, and in the senior author's series, the LF2ZR took 2 hours longer to complete on average.

DISCUSSION

LF2ZR is derived from a modification of the traditional Le Fort III distraction operation with the goal of treating patients with differential midface hypoplasia. Through segmental distraction of the central nasomaxillary region and repositioning of the lateral orbitozygomatic regions, the LF2ZR operation is intended for correction of the facial biconcavity present in conditions, such as Apert syndrome and achondroplasia, where the central midface retrusion is more severe compared with lateral midface hypoplasia.

The zygomatic repositioning portion of the operation improves the relationship between the orbit and the globe to correct exorbitism and malar hypoplasia. Because the central Le Fort II segment is distracted independent of the zygomas, the vector and magnitude of advancement are controlled without impacting the orbital morphology. This technique allows for not only correction of the severe central retrusion in the sagittal plane by greater magnitude of advancement, but also closure of an anterior open bite, extension of the nasal length, and improvement of the palpebral fissure orientation through a downward vector of distraction. Computed tomography scan analysis of patients with Apert syndrome who underwent LF2ZR has demonstrated significantly greater advancement and lengthening of the central midface compared with the lateral orbits, resulting in normalization of the facial ratio.[8] Smartt and colleagues[22] reported on four patients with differential midface hypoplasia from various syndromes including Apert, achondroplasia, and Goldenhar that underwent correction with LF2ZR and also found improvements in the abnormal facial ratios.

In addition to LF2ZR, other technical modifications of Le Fort III osteotomy for segmental or differential movement of the midface have also been described.[23] Denny and colleagues[24] proposed a technique for rotational advancement of the midface with an axis of rotation from the zygomaticofrontal suture to the radix to prevent contour abnormalities at the nasofrontal and zygomaticofrontal region. Our group has previously described the use of simultaneous nasal passenger grafts to achieve additional nasal augmentation and cerclage hinge control to allow for differential advancement of the midface along a gradient from one side to the other.[9]

Separating the Le Fort I segment from the Le Fort III segment has been described to allow for differential correction at the occlusal level and the orbitozygomatic level.[25–27] There has also been reports of using this technique for the treatment of midface hypoplasia associated with Apert syndrome.[28,29] In contrast to LF2ZR, the Le Fort I segmentation approach does not address the central upper midface vertical and sagittal deficiency, nor the medial canthal vertical impaction. The Apert facial dysmorphology is characterized by a short and retrusive maxilla, down-sloping palpebral slant, exorbitism, hypertelorism, prominent nasojugal groove, short nasal dorsum, and counterclockwise rotation of the occlusal plane. For Apert patients and those with similar central midface retrusion, segmentation at the Le Fort II level rather than Le Fort I level is advantageous to correct these unique facial deformities.

The group at the Great Ormand Street Hospital has proposed the use of bipartition monobloc advancement as an alternative technique for differential facial advancement.[30] This technique has the advantage of improving hypertelorism that is frequently present in Apert patients while also correcting the concave deformity on worm's-eye view. This technique, however, does require a transcranial approach and carries the associated higher risk relative to subcranial surgery.[21,31,32] In addition, it does not allow for differential vertical lengthening of the central midface or downward movement of the medial canthi. However, the bipartition monobloc approach is indicated for patients with severe hypertelorism that would not be adequately corrected by the nasal dorsal lengthening and augmentation of LF2ZR or for patients requiring simultaneous expansion of the anterior cranial fossa.

SUMMARY

Based on our center's experience, LF2ZR has a comparable safety profile to Le Fort III osteotomy but allows differential advancement of the midface to create increased facial convexity in the profile view and normalization of facial ratios on the frontal and worm's-eye view. This differential movement results in esthetically favorable periorbital and perinasal changes and improvement of an anterior open bite deformity. The unrestricted movement of the Le Fort II segment allows as much anterior advancement as is needed to treat obstructive sleep apnea. For these reasons, the LF2ZR technique has become the procedure of choice for the treatment of Apert midface hypoplasia at our center.

CLINICS CARE POINTS

- Early in his series, the senior author used transconjunctival incisions in addition to the intraoral incisions to perform the orbital rim Le Fort II osteotomies. However, lid malposition occurred in two cases likely resulting from adhesions of the anterior lamella of the eyelid to the inferior orbital rim osteotomy. The technique was modified so that the osteotomies were performed through upper gingivobuccal incisions alone, using a piezoelectric saw to allow the rim and floor cuts to be made from below through the maxillary sinus. Since this modification, we have not observed any more eyelid complications.

- Attempting to fixate both zygomas before releasing the Le Fort II segment creates strain across the midface and risk of fracture across the zygomaticomaxillary suture or displacement of the first fixated zygoma. It is important to do a sequential zygoma reposition and fixation, with release of the first zygoma before proceeding to the contralateral side.

- The choice of vector is important to achieve the desired Le Fort II movement, but too vertical a vector risks early consolidation and lack of appropriate advancement. Too horizontal a vector does not achieve the desired vertical lengthening. The senior author believes the best compromise is a 30° to 45° vector below Frankfort horizontal, but with aggressive use of bimaxillary elastics to help close any anterior open bite deformity.

DISCLOSURE

Dr R.A. Hopper is the inventor on a patent licensed to KLS Martin LP. No other financial interest to disclose.

REFERENCES

1. Taylor JA, Bartlett SP. What's new in syndromic craniosynostosis surgery? Plast Reconstr Surg 2017; 140:82e–93e.
2. Ettinger RE, Hopper RA, Sandercoe G, et al. Quantitative computed tomographic scan and polysomnographic analysis of patients with syndromic midface hypoplasia before and after Le Fort III distraction advancement. Plast Reconstr Surg 2011;127:1612–9.
3. Fearon JA. The Le Fort III osteotomy: to distract or not to distract? Plast Reconstr Surg 2001;107: 1091–103 [discussion: 1104–6].
4. Fearon JA. Midterm follow-up of midface distraction. Plast Reconstr Surg 2008;122:674–5.
5. Shetye PR, Davidson EH, Sorkin M, et al. Evaluation of three surgical techniques for advancement of the midface in growing children with syndromic craniosynostosis. Plast Reconstr Surg 2010;126: 982–94.
6. Shetye PR, Grayson BH, McCarthy JG. Le Fort III distraction: controlling position and path of the osteotomized midface segment on a rigid platform. J Craniofac Surg 2010;21:1118–21.
7. Oberoi S, Hoffman WY, Vargervik K. Craniofacial team management in Apert syndrome. Am J Orthod Dentofacial Orthop 2012;141:S82–7.
8. Hopper RA, Kapadia H, Morton T. Normalizing facial ratios in Apert syndrome patients with Le Fort II midface distraction and simultaneous zygomatic repositioning. Plast Reconstr Surg 2013;132:129–40.
9. Hopper RA, Prucz RB, Iamphongsai S. Achieving differential facial changes with Le Fort III distraction osteogenesis: the use of nasal passenger grafts, cerclage hinges, and segmental movements. Plast Reconstr Surg 2012;130:1281–8.
10. Susarla SM, Mundinger GS, Kapadia H, et al. Subcranial and orthognathic surgery for obstructive sleep apnea in achondroplasia. J Craniomaxillofac Surg 2017;45:2028–34.
11. Hopper RA, Kapadia H, Susarla SM. Le Fort II distraction with zygomatic repositioning: a technique for differential correction of midface hypoplasia. J Oral Maxillofac Surg 2018;76:2002.e1-4.
12. Roberts SD, Kapadia H, Greenlee G, et al. Midfacial and dental changes associated with nasal positive airway pressure in children with obstructive sleep apnea and craniofacial conditions. J Clin Sleep Med 2016;12:469–75.
13. Inverso G, Brustowicz KA, Katz E, et al. The prevalence of obstructive sleep apnea in symptomatic patients with syndromic craniosynostosis. Int J Oral Maxillofac Surg 2016;45:167–9.
14. Fearon JA. Halo distraction of the Le Fort III in syndromic craniosynostosis: a long-term assessment. Plast Reconstr Surg 2005;115:1524–36.

15. Flores RL, Shetye PR, Zeitler D, et al. Airway changes following Le Fort III distraction osteogenesis for syndromic craniosynostosis: a clinical and cephalometric study. Plast Reconstr Surg 2009;124:590–601.

16. Nout E, Bannink N, Koudstaal MJ, et al. Upper airway changes in syndromic craniosynostosis patients following midface or monobloc advancement: correlation between volume changes and respiratory outcome. J Craniomaxillofac Surg 2012;40:209–14.

17. Nout E, Bouw FP, Veenland JF, et al. Three-dimensional airway changes after Le Fort III advancement in syndromic craniosynostosis patients. Plast Reconstr Surg 2010;126:564–71.

18. Nelson TE, Mulliken JB, Padwa BL. Effect of midfacial distraction on the obstructed airway in patients with syndromic bilateral coronal synostosis. J Oral Maxillofac Surg 2008;66:2318–21.

19. Liu MT, Kurnik NM, Mercan E, et al. Magnitude of Horizontal Advancement is Associated with Apnea Hypopnea Index Improvement and Counter-Clockwise Maxillary Rotation After Subcranial Distraction for Syndromic Synostosis. J Oral Maxillofac Surg 2020 Dec 30.

20. Greig AV, Davidson EH, Grayson BH, et al. Complications of craniofacial midface distraction: 10-year review. Plast Reconstr Surg 2012;130:371e–2e.

21. Zhang RS, Lin LO, Hoppe IC, et al. Retrospective review of the complication profile Associated with 71 subcranial and transcranial midface distraction procedures at a single institution. Plast Reconstr Surg 2019;143:521–30.

22. Smartt JM Jr, Campbell C, Hallac R, et al. A three-dimensional study of midfacial changes following Le Fort II distraction with zygomatic repositioning in syndromic patients. J Craniofac Surg 2017;28:e728–31.

23. Hopper RA, Ettinger RE, Purnell CA, et al. Thirty years later: what has craniofacial distraction osteogenesis surgery replaced? Plast Reconstr Surg 2020;145:1073e–88e.

24. Denny AD, Kalantarian B, Hanson PR. Rotation advancement of the midface by distraction osteogenesis. Plast Reconstr Surg 2003;111:1789–99 [discussion: 1800–3].

25. Matsumoto K, Nakanishi H, Koizumi Y, et al. Segmental distraction of the midface in a patient with Crouzon syndrome. J Craniofac Surg 2002;13:273–8.

26. Brown MS, Okada H, Valiathan M, et al. 45 Years of simultaneous Le Fort III and Le Fort I osteotomies: a systematic literature review. Cleft Palate Craniofac J 2015;52:471–9.

27. Hammoudeh JA, Goel P, Wolfswinkel EM, et al. Simultaneous midface advancement and orthognathic surgery: a powerful technique for managing midface hypoplasia and malocclusion. Plast Reconstr Surg 2020;145:1067e–72e.

28. Satoh K, Mitsukawa N, Hosaka Y. Dual midfacial distraction osteogenesis: Le Fort III minus I and Le Fort I for syndromic craniosynostosis. Plast Reconstr Surg 2003;111:1019–28.

29. Takashima M, Kitai N, Murakami S, et al. Dual segmental distraction osteogenesis of the midface in a patient with Apert syndrome. Cleft Palate Craniofac J 2006;43:499–506.

30. Ponniah AJ, Witherow H, Richards R, et al. Three-dimensional image analysis of facial skeletal changes after monobloc and bipartition distraction. Plast Reconstr Surg 2008;122:225–31.

31. Fearon JA, Whitaker LA. Complications with facial advancement: a comparison between the Le Fort III and monobloc advancements. Plast Reconstr Surg 1993;91:990–5.

32. Knackstedt R, Bassiri Gharb B, Papay F, et al. Comparison of complication rate between LeFort III and monobloc advancement with or without distraction osteogenesis. J Craniofac Surg 2018;29:144–8.

Craniosynostosis
Monobloc Distraction with Internal Device and Its Variant for Infants with Severe Syndromic Craniosynostosis

Giovanna Paternoster, MD[a], Samer Elie Haber, MD[a],
Roman Hossein Khonsari, MD, PhD[a,b], Syril James, MD[a,c],
Eric Arnaud, MD[a,c],*

KEYWORDS

- Faciocraniosynostosis • Syndromic craniosynostosis • Craniofacial dysostosis
- Frontofacial monobloc advancement • Tracheostomy • Exorbitism • Sleep apnea
- Distraction osteogenesis

KEY POINTS

- Frontofacial monobloc advancement with 4 internal distractors is safe and effective before age 18 months.
- Its main indications are vision-threatening exorbitism and sleep apnea with intolerance to noninvasive ventilation.
- Overcorrection is necessary.
- Facial stability and advancement can be optimized using a transfacial pin and external traction at bedside under extended sedation.

Syndromic craniosynostosis is a complex condition commonly associated to a mutation in one of the fibroblast growth factor receptor genes.[1,2] It results in severe functional and aesthetic impairments in the craniofacial skeleton.[3–5] Surgical treatment aims to prevent further neurologic compromise and restore craniofacial dysmorphology.[6–8] Early intracranial volume expansion prevents the risks of visual and cognitive impairment due to craniocerebral disproportion and intracranial hypertension.[9–17]

The traditional strategy for syndromic craniosynostosis management is 2-stage and carries less risk for surgical morbidity than the more recent single-stage frontofacial monobloc advancement (FFMBA).[18–20] The 2-stage strategy treats the craniosynostosis first by a frontoorbital advancement before 1 year of age.[21–24] The treatment of the facial retrusion is delayed: the facial advancement (Le Fort III type) is performed at 5 to 6 years of age or even later, unless a severe breathing impairment requires an earlier surgical correction.[6–8,25–28] A secondary maxillary advancement (Le Fort I) might be necessary after 14 years of age to correct the maxillary hypoplasia caused by its congenital lack of growth, to obtain a class

[a] Unité fonctionnelle de chirurgie craniofaciale, Service de Neurochirurgie Pédiatrique, Hôpital Necker – Enfants Malades, Assistance Publique – Hôpitaux de Paris, Centre de Référence Maladies Rares CRANIOST, Filière Maladies Rares TeteCou, Université Paris Descartes, ERN Cranio, 149 rue de Sèvres, 75015, Paris, France; [b] Service de chirurgie maxillofaciale et chirurgie plastique, Hôpital Necker – Enfants Malades, Assistance Publique – Hôpitaux de Paris, Centre de Référence Maladies Rares CRANIOST, Filière Maladies Rares TeteCou, Université de Paris, Université Paris Descartes, 149 rue de Sèvres, 75015, Paris, France; [c] Clinique Marcel Sembat, Ramsay Générale de Santé, 105 boulevard Victor Hugo, 92100 Boulogne, France
* Corresponding author. 34 avenue d'Eylau, 75016 Paris.
E-mail address: drericarnaud@hotmail.com

Clin Plastic Surg 48 (2021) 497–506
https://doi.org/10.1016/j.cps.2021.02.008
0094-1298/21/© 2021 Elsevier Inc. All rights reserved.

I occlusion.[28–31] However, in this multiple-stage strategy, the facial retrusion treatment and its subsequent improvement of airways is delayed, and many teams prefer to use routine tracheostomy to address the sleep apnea syndrome.[32] Tracheostomy is considered a useful procedure, but its morbidity certainly affects the child and family quality of life.[33–38]

The simultaneous correction of the frontofacial retrusion prevents corneal desiccation resulting from exorbitism, chronic hypoxemia caused by impaired upper airway obstruction, and addresses the morphologic appearance.[39–42] MBA can correct simultaneously the frontal and the facial retrusion and increase both orbits and airways.[39,43–45] However, as a result of the necessary osteotomy of the floor of the anterior skull base, the MBA produces 2 potentially detrimental consequences: the creation of a dead space within the anterior cranial fossa and the communication between the anterior cranial fossa and the nasal cavity.[18,42,46] Consequently, infections can occur leading to reoperation and eventually to life-threatening complications such as meningitis and necrosis of the frontal bone.[18,42,46–49] The authors previously demonstrated the reduction of those risks by the use of distraction osteogenesis.[19] Thirty-years ago, the rate of infections associated with MBA was around 30% in our center, and there was an unacceptable mortality rate of 15% (Arnaud, unpublished data, 1999) in patients with a ventriculoperitoneal shunt undergoing MBA without distraction.[50]

By using FFMBA early in age and with monobloc distraction osteogenesis (MBDO) (1) the rapid growth of the brain rapidly fills the dead space and reduces the risk of infection and (2) airway obstruction associated with severe midface retrusion can be concurrently treated.[19,50] MBDO's main indications were initially restricted to vision-threatening exorbitism or severe breathing impairments in infants, in whom the benefits outweigh the risks.[46] These indications were progressively extended in our institution to include younger and less severe patients.[19,20] Although this early implementation of MBDO may be considered controversial by some, we believe that this form of early intervention will benefit appropriately indicated patients. When required, posterior skull vault expansion is chronologically performed before MBDO.[51–55] It decompresses the brain by increasing intracranial volume and can delay MBDO to a later time when the facial bones are larger and more robust.[52] However, some patients still require a very early monobloc distraction osteogenesis (VEMDO) before 18 months of age, for severe exorbitism and/or severe respiratory obstruction.

Although we and other investigators have previously presented the safety and effectiveness of VEMDO, some craniofacial surgeons worldwide remain reluctant to this procedure, because of the associated morbidity risk.[18,46–48]

We present our experience with 147 monobloc distraction procedures in infants and children with syndromic craniosynostosis operated in our unit between September 2000 and November 2018.[56,57] In a subset of our patients, who will be separately analyzed, VEMDO was performed to avoid or remove a tracheostomy. The most severely affected patients treated with VEMDO underwent surgery before 1 year of age and required a transfacial pin and external traction.[58] This surgical technique is detailed in the following section.

PATIENTS AND METHODS

Patients with syndromic craniosynostosis who underwent FFMBDO between September 2000 and November 2018 were included. Two subgroups were created based on the age at surgery: patients operated after age 18 months (group 1) and VEMDO patients who were operated before age 18 months (group 2). Charts were reviewed for demographic characteristics, tracheostomy status, polysomnographic data, fundoscopic examinations, and surgical history.

All study patients were operated by the senior author (EA) according to a standardized procedure that will be detailed later.[20,59,60] There was a slight variation in some patients of group 2 in whom 16 underwent the standard procedure and 9 had a transfacial pin inserted at the zygomatic level.

Group 1 included children older than 18 months (122 patients).

Surgical Technique

Under general anesthesia, the scalp is opened or reopened through a coronal approach. After subgaleal undermining, 2 anteriorly based paramedial frontal periosteal flaps are dissected and prepared to isolate the skull from the nasal cavities.[61] Temporal muscle flaps are also elevated to expose the lateral aspects of the orbits. The osteotomy lines are marked and a long tenon (bandeau extension) designed bilaterally behind the supraorbital bar within the flattest part of the temporal fossa. This modification will facilitate consolidation at the upper level of the orbit if limited osteogenesis occurs at other bony sites. A frontal bone craniotomy is performed for intracranial access. Subsequently, the monobloc osteotomies are completed as previously described.[19] A complete bilateral pterygomaxillary disjunction is confirmed visual through complete movement of the monobloc segment using pediatric Rowe forceps. This complete liberation of the skull base from the face is critical to avoid insufficient advancement and/or bending of the hemifaces during activation. Two internal distractors (Arnaud cranial distractors, KLS Martin, Tuttlingen, Germany) are inserted at the extremity of each bony tongue, as parallel to each other as possible. The distractors are fixed with Champy 2 mm in diameter, 3- to 5-mm long metallic screws or SonicWeld™ rivets (KLS Martin, Tuttlingen, Germany). Sealing of the anterior cranial fossa from the nasal cavities is performed by crossing the 2 pericranial flaps at the midline after transposing them across the orbital roof and suturing their anterior border to the supraorbital bar using resorbable sutures through the bone. This biological seal is reinforced by applying 1 mL of fibrin glue. The bony forehead flap is trimmed at its inferior edge by resecting 2 laterally based small triangles and fixed to the upper edge of the supraorbital bar by 4 to 6 stainless steel 3/10 mm wires; this allows for the posterior tilting of the forehead and contributed to the reduction of the future retrofrontal dead space. Two other distractors (Marchac maxillary distractors) are used at the lower aspect of the temporal fossa, with the anterior part located behind the zygomatic bone. Fixation is done with metallic Champy neuro screws (smooth tip). The distraction is started at day 3 unless a significant cerebrospinal fluid (CSF) leak is noted (**Fig. 1**).

Group 2 of 25 children aged 18 months or less underwent VEMDO (**Table 1**).

In 9 patients an additional surgical step was carried out with the insertion of a 20- to 22-mm Kirschner wire (K-wire) transfacially (zygoma to zygoma). In 6 of these patients, the transfacial pin was attached to an external pulley system providing external traction anteriorly (1–3 kg weight). The target traction weight was achieved with the head slightly lifted from the surface of the bed (**Fig. 2**). This last subgroup is detailed later in **Table 2**.

Six children aged 4 to 12 months presented with severe syndromic craniosynostosis: Crouzon syndrome (n = 2), Crouzon with Acanthosis nigricans (n = 1), and Pfeiffer syndrome (n = 3). None of the patients had been previously operated at the anterior craniofacial level. All 6 patients presented with at least one feature of severe syndromic craniosynostosis: 2 had major exorbitism, which threatened visual function, and 5 had early tracheostomy for major respiratory impairment. Indirect signs of increased intracranial pressure were evident in all 6 patients. Surgical history included a ventriculoperitoneal shunt in one patient (Pfeiffer), a posterior vault decompression

without distraction in another patient, and a foramen magnum decompression with posterior vault decompression in one patient to treat cerebellar tonsillar herniation (Chiari malformation). In the 4 patients without imminent threat to corneal scarring, initial management consisted of brain decompression using posterior release of the cranial vault. This first procedure was followed by insertion of a ventriculoperitoneal shunt. One of these 4 patients, a child with Pfeiffer syndrome presenting with a cloverleaf skull, had been previously shunted at another institution. This patient presented with a severe flatness of the posterior aspect of the skull secondary to exclusive supine positioning as well as shunt over drainage. In this case, our initial procedure was bony release of the posterior aspect of the skull with foramen magnum decompression, and the replacement of the shunt valve by a flow-regulating low-flow ventriculoperitoneal shunt (Integra®, Plainsboro Township, New Jersey, USA). All preliminary procedures are summarized in **Table 2**. These procedures were then followed by VEMDO, which was undertaken to protect the eyes in 2 out of 6 and to remove the tracheostomy in 5 out of 6 as described.

When performing VEMDO in patients younger than 1 year, the frontal processes of the malar bones are too weak and too small to withstand the translational forces generated by the lower pair of distractors. Therefore, a metallic microplate is used to reinforce the frontozygomatic junction at each side. Following this reinforcement, a transzygomatic pin (1.8- or 2.0-mm K-wire) is inserted by percutaneously drilling from one zygomatic process to the other. During this procedure, care is being taken to travel under the floor of the orbit and not puncture the globe. This step is technically challenging due to the diminutive size of the zygomatic bones secondary to the clinical condition and young patient age. The pin is cut 2 cm from the skin surface bilaterally and the ends covered by a rubber tube to protect the patient from injury. Temporal muscles are transposed anteriorly and fixed at the frontozygomatic level with the assistance of drill holes created in the bone. In 3 out of 6 patients, a third cranial distractor was transversally implanted in the region of the vertex to attempt a reduction of the associated turricephaly. Distraction is initiated intraoperatively (5 mm) to decompress the brain. The resultant coronal bony gap is filled with autologous bone dust and fibrin glue. The scalp is closed in 2 layers over a suction drain, with care taken to exteriorize the detachable activation rods of the cranial distractors. Average surgical time was 3 hours 15 minutes (ranging

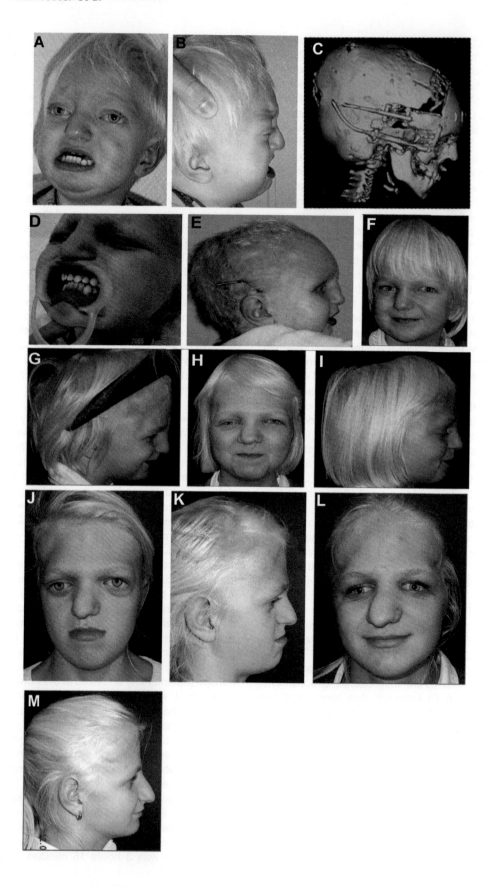

2:45–3:45). All patients were transfused intraoperatively. Patients were kept under sedation and assisted ventilation for a minimum of 48 hours: this allowed for assessment of soft tissue swelling and CSF leaks. External traction was applied the following day and under sedation. An orthopedic pulley system was attached to the free ends of the transfacial pin. The traction weight varied from 1 to 3 kg, with a clinical endpoint of the head being slightly lifted from the bed. If a CSF leak was noted in the immediate postoperative period then the traction was delayed several days. External traction is applied until the clinical endpoint is reached (approximately 1 week). The consolidation period is 5 to 6 months.

RESULTS

One hundred forty-seven patients were included. The mean age at surgery was 4.0 ± 3.0 years. Group 1 included 122 patients and group 2 included 25 patients.

In Group 1, the mean age at surgery was 57.8 ± 48.7 months and mean follow-up was 6.8 ± 4.1 years.

Mean preoperative apnea hypopnea index (AHI) was 22.7 ± 20.6 per hour. Half of the patient cohort were normalized (AHI less than 5/h), and 45% were improved but not cured after MBDO.[57] In the 6 cases in which a tracheostomy was present, 3 patients (50%) underwent decannulation after facial advancement. Variables associated with the success of decannulation included the presence or absence of secondary airway anomalies, cardiac conditions, previous ear, nose, and throat procedures, and the degree of maxillary advancement.

Exorbitism was corrected in 95% of patients, but superior results to globe position were obtained when the child was at least 3 years at the time of surgery.[62] In 75% of patients, occlusion was restored to class I or II.

In group 2, mean age at surgery was 13 ± 4 months (range 3–18 months), and mean follow-up was 8.2 ± 3.2 years (range: 1–15.25 years) (see **Table 1**). There were 13 boys and 12 girls. Eight patients (32%) had Crouzon

syndrome, 14 patients (56%) had Pfeiffer, and 3 patients (12%) had Apert syndrome. Ten patients (40%) presented with a tracheostomy. Fourteen patients (56%) had posterior cranial vault decompression, 4 patients (16%) had foramen magnum decompression, and 7 patients (28%) had a ventriculoperitoneal shunt before VEMDO.

Of the 10 patients who presented with a preintervention tracheostomy, 5 (50%) were decannulated right after VEMDO, and 3 (30%) required an additional intervention for decannulation (1 adenotonsillectomy and 2 mandibular distraction with adenotonsillectomy). Preoperative polysomnographies were available in 12 of 15 nontracheotomized patients (80%). Mean preoperative AHI was 23 ± 16 per hour. One-year and 2-year postoperative polysomnographies were available in 8 patients. One year postoperatively, mean AHI was 13.8 ± 15.3 per hour. At 2 years, mean AHI was 9.5 ± 11.7 per hour. Paired Wilcoxon signed rank test was underpowered (only 7 pairs) and did not reach statistical significance at 1 year and 2 years postoperatively ($P = .15$ and $P = .15$, respectively).

- Group 2: 19 patients underwent VEMDO according to the standard MBDO technique and 6 had a transfacial pin and application of external traction (**Table 2**). In this latter subset, the decannulation rate was 60% (3/5).

Overcorrection was performed in all patients to help limit the number of secondary procedures. The clinical endpoint of distraction in these cases is enophthalmos and (at times) exaggerated class II occlusion. We observed tooth bud damage in the area of the molars in all patients undergoing the transfacial pin procedure. Early relapse was noted in one patient who underwent facial advancement using only 2 internal distractors. Our surgical technique was modified to include 4 distractors based on these findings.

DISCUSSION

In order for a procedure to remain in the armamentarium of a craniofacial team, it must be simple

---

Fig. 1. A 16-month-old girl with Crouzon syndrome (A, B) presenting Angle class III occlusion with severe respiratory symptoms and sleep apnea. Monobloc distraction was performed using 4 internal distractors (C). Overcorrection was achieved (D, E). Two years postoperatively: overcorrection remains (age 3.5 years) (F, G). Five years postoperatively, age 6.5 years: no respiratory symptoms, regular school, normal physical activity (H, I). Ten years postoperatively (age 12 years): relapse of maxillary retrusion. Still no respiratory symptoms (J, K). Le Fort III facial advancement was performed for aesthetic correction. Age 15 years: 2 years after the Le Fort III and 14 years after the primary monobloc (L, M).

Table 1
Demographic characteristics of patients undergoing very early monobloc distraction osteogenesis (age 18 months or less)

	Frequency (%) (n = 25)	Mean ± SD
Sex		
Male	13 (52%)	
Female	12 (48%)	
Age (mo)		13.5 ± 3.9
Syndrome		
Crouzon	7 (28%)	
Pfeiffer	8 (33%)	
Apert	8 (33%)	
Crouzon with acanthosis nigricans	1 (5%)	
Tracheostomy at presentation	9 (36%)	
Tonsillectomy, turbinectomy, and/or adenoidectomy before VEMDO[a]	7 (28%)	
Foramen magnum decompression (Chiari) before VEMDO[a]	5 (20%)	
Posterior vault decompression before VEMDO[a]	14 (56%)	
Ventriculo-peritoneal shunt or endoscopic third ventriculostomy before VEMDO[a]	6 (24%)	

[a] VEMDO, very early monobloc distraction osteogenesis.

enough to be performed by a competent craniofacial surgeon and be associated with an acceptable complication rate. One of the pending questions is whether the monobloc with distraction at a very early age meets those fundamental requirements. However, by performing the MBDO in childhood (and in the absence of shunt), the rate of complications can be significantly reduced.[19] Yet the VEM carries inherent risks related to surgery, risks at an early age, and to the subsequent intensive care management, which are critical to this operation. Technically, the VEMDO is simple to perform in young patients. It is even simpler than in older children, as the bones are softer and mobilization of the bony segments simpler. However, it is not unusual to keep the children intubated under sedation for a few days until the swelling decreases.

In our entire cohort of children undergoing MBDO, improvement of respiratory impairment to normative values was obtained in only half of the cases,[39,56] although some degree of improvement was almost universally obtained. It should be noted that there is a known incidence of secondary airway anomalies in patients with syndromic craniosynostosis, which could contribute to these findings. Furthermore, associated Chiari malformation and central sleep apnea, hypotonia, difficulty swallowing, cardiac and pulmonary anomalies, choanal atresia, and hypotonia can all contribute to respiratory impairment. In the subgroup of VEM that underwent a transfacial pin, we achieved a decannulation rate of 60%. We believe that the transfacial pin can stabilize the midface and empower the surgeon to obtain a tremendous frontofacial advancement, which may be contributory to our findings. However, damage to the molars was consistently seen, and this injury has to be balanced with the potential benefit to tracheostomy removal and/or airway improvement. We have anecdotally observed that night counter positive airways pressure in childhood can aggravate facial retrusion in the long term. The preliminary removal of adenoids and tonsils was critical to obtain better results, because secondary enlargement of those structures is provoked by the inflammation generated by the inner distractors.

At an orbital level, we previously demonstrated that normalization of orbital shape and size was better obtained when the procedure was carried out after 3 to 5 years of age.[62] However, risks of globe herniation could simply be corrected at a very early age using VEMDO, and orbital morphology could be corrected, if necessary, after 10 years of age on a stable orbit. The use of microplates to reinforce the frontozygomatic suture is certainly helpful to stabilize the orbital ring during osteotomy and distraction. The very early age should not prevent the surgeon from performing the pterygomaxillary disjunction with specially designed small Rowe forceps. Again, the risks of surgery should be weighed against the benefits of this intervention, and further research and outcomes analysis is required in this regard.

The rate of intracranial infection in the VEM patients was low, likely due to the rapid brain growth that can quickly fill the retrofrontal dead space. Relapse in the very young can be an issue but it occurred mainly at the facial (not cranial/orbital)

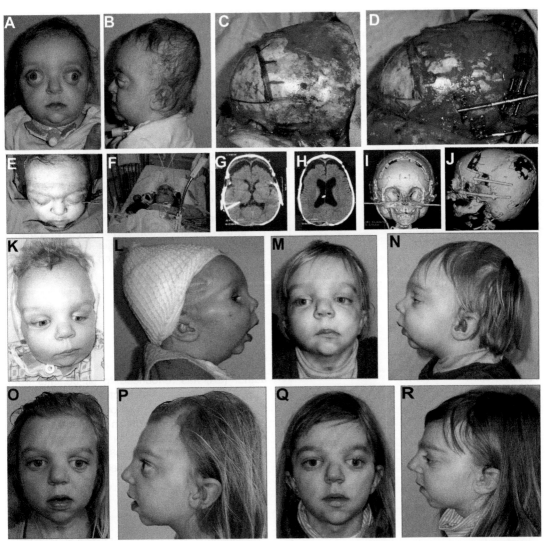

Fig. 2. A 11-month-old girl with Pfeiffer syndrome presenting with severe maxillary hypoplasia and exorbitism (*A, B*). Surgical history includes tracheostomy, posterior skull vault expansion, and ventriculoperitoneal shunt. Very early monobloc distraction osteogenesis (VEMDO) was performed at age 11 months using 4 internal distractors and a transfacial pin (*C–E*). External traction was applied to the transfacial pin for 4 days (*F*). Head CT scan 2 weeks postoperatively shows fast reattachment of the dura to the advanced frontal bone (*G, H*). Significant overcorrection was achieved through distraction (*I–L*). Respiratory function normalized postoperatively, and decannulation was performed at age 28 months (*M, N*). Five years postoperatively, the overcorrected maxillary advancement became milder (*O, P*). Eight years after VEMDO with transfacial pin and external traction: normal breathing, regular school, normal social interactions (*Q, R*).

level. We therefore use 4 distractors even in the youngest patients and remove the devices after 6 months to get sufficient bony consolidation at the tongue/groove level as well as the zygoma and the pterygomaxillary junction. Following this protocol, cranial and orbital relapse occurred in only one secondary case with bone grafts reconstruction of the bandeau during VEMDO procedure. Significant relapse did not occur at the orbital level, with only a 5% relapse rate in the months after removal of distractors.[40] Relapse at the occlusal level was observed during follow-up, often associated with a deterioration of the AHI. The immediate or secondarily deteriorated airways impairment may be addressed by a secondary Le Fort 3 with distraction.[63]

Reossification after major craniofacial osteotomies is not always complete, although the very

Table 2
Demographic characteristics of patients undergoing very early monobloc distraction osteogenesis with transfacial pin and external traction

	Frequency (%) (n = 6)	Mean ± SD
Sex		
Male	3 (50%)	
Female	3 (50%)	
Age (mo)		11.2 ± 4.9
Syndrome		
Crouzon	2 (33%)	
Pfeiffer	3 (50%)	
Crouzon with Acanthosis nigricans	1 (17%)	
Tracheostomy at presentation	5 (83.3%)	
Turbinectomy before VEMDO[a]	1 (17%)	
Posterior vault decompression before VEMDO[a]	4 (67%)	
Foramen magnum decompression (Chiari) before VEMDO[a]	2 (33%)	
Shunt or endoscopic third ventriculostomy before VEMDO[a]	4 (67%)	

[a] VEMDO, very early monobloc distraction osteogenesis.

early age in the VEMDO population is a prominent contributing factor. Pfeiffer syndrome tend to reossify less in the facial sites such as the zygomatic arches. Possible contributors to these findings are the small size of the craniofacial bones at this age, resulting in a limited bone stock for osteogenesis. Nevertheless, the presence of mineralization has been observed in some cases of relapse, which may indicate a poor mechanical quality of mineralized bone. Conversely, it has been also observed that in the presence of many areas lacking reossification, stability in the structures could still be obtained. This observation is possibly because ossification at the tenon (tongue/groove) and at the pterygomaxillary junction was sufficient to provide bony stability.

CLINICS CARE POINTS

- Frontofacial monobloc advancement improves obstructive sleep apnea in patient with syndromic craniosynostosis.
- Internal distraction decreases the morbidity associated with frontofacial monobloc advancement.
- Decannulation of tracheostomy was possible in up to 70% of the cases, with the adjunction of other ancillary procedures.
- Very early monobloc with internal distraction and external traction was an eye saving procedures in children younger that 12months and significantly was a step to deccannulation.

DISCLOSURES

The authors have nothing to disclose. The main author (EA) has renounced to all benefits from KLS Martin for the distractors that carry his name. A partial funding had been obtained for 20 patients in the early part of this prospective studies from PHRC (Projet Hospitalier de Recherche clinique - Ref CRANIORESP 2008), Assistance Publique-Hopitaux de Paris, 3 avenue Victoria, 75004 Paris.

REFERENCES

1. Oldridge M, Lunt PW, Zackai EH, et al. Genotype-phenotype correlation for nucleotide substitutions in the IgII-IgIII linker of FGFR2. Hum Mol Genet 1997;6(1):137–43.
2. Rutland P, Pulleyn LJ, Reardon W, et al. Identical mutations in the FGFR2 gene cause both Pfeiffer and Crouzon syndrome phenotypes. Nat Genet 1995;9(2):173–6.
3. Apert E. De l'acrocéphalosyndactylie. Bull Soc Med Paris 1906;23:1310–30.
4. Crouzon O. La dysostose cranio-faciale héréditaire. Bulletins et Mémoires de la Société d'Anthropologie de Paris 1935;6(4):41–5.
5. Pfeiffer RA. Dominant erbliche Akrocephalosyndaktylie. Z Kinder-heilk 1964;90(4):301–20.
6. Tessier P. The definitive plastic surgical treatment of the severe facial deformities of craniofacial dysostosis. Crouzon's and Apert's diseases. Plast Reconstr Surg 1971;48(5):419–42.
7. Tessier P. [Treatment of facial dysmorphisms in craniofacial dysostosis (DCF). Crouzon and Apert

diseases. Total osteotomy of the facial massif. Sagittal displacement of the facial massif]. Neurochirurgie 1971;17(4):295–322.

8. Tessier P. [The treatment of facial dysmorphy peculiary to cranio-facial dysostosis (C.F.D.). Crouzon and Apert diseases. Total osteotomy and sagittal displacement of the facial mass]. Chirurgie 1970; 96(10):667–74.

9. Renier D, Sainte-Rose C, Marchac D, et al. Intracranial pressure in craniostenosis. J Neurosurg 1982; 57(3):370–7.

10. Spruijt B, Mathijssen IMJ, Bredero-Boelhouwer HH, et al. Sleep Architecture Linked to airway obstruction and intracranial hypertension in children with syndromic craniosynostosis. Plast Reconstr Surg 2016;138(6):1019e–29e.

11. Tay T, Martin F, Rowe N, et al. Prevalence and causes of visual impairment in craniosynostotic syndromes. Clin Exp Ophthalmol 2006;34(5):434–40.

12. Gault DT, Renier D, Marchac D, et al. Intracranial pressure and intracranial volume in children with craniosynostosis. Plast Reconstr Surg 1992;90(3): 377–81.

13. Gault DT, Renier D, Marchac D, et al. Intracranial volume in children with craniosynostosis. J Craniofac Surg 1990;1(1):1–3.

14. Abu-Sittah GS, Jeelani O, Dunaway D, et al. Raised intracranial pressure in Crouzon syndrome: incidence, causes, and management. J Neurosurg Pediatr 2016;17(4):469–75.

15. Gosain AK, McCarthy JG, Wisoff JH. Morbidity associated with increased intracranial pressure in Apert and Pfeiffer syndromes: the need for long-term evaluation. Plast Reconstr Surg 1996;97(2):292–301.

16. Hayward R, Gonsalez S. How low can you go? Intracranial pressure, cerebral perfusion pressure, and respiratory obstruction in children with complex craniosynostosis. J Neurosurg 2005;102(1 Suppl): 16–22.

17. Yokota A, Matsuoka S, Ishikawa T, et al. Overnight recordings of intracranial pressure and electroencephalography in neurosurgical patients. Part II: changes in intracranial pressure during sleep. J UOEH 1989;11(4):383–91.

18. Dunaway DJ, Britto JA, Abela C, et al. Complications of frontofacial advancement. Child's Nervous Syst 2012;28(9):1571–6.

19. Arnaud E, Marchac D, Renier D. Reduction of morbidity of the frontofacial monobloc advancement in children by the use of internal distraction. Plast Reconstr Surg 2007;120(4):1009–26.

20. Arnaud E, Di Rocco F. Faciocraniosynostosis: monobloc frontofacial osteotomy replacing the two-stage strategy? Childs Nerv Syst 2012;28(9):1557–64.

21. Marchac D, Renier D. [The "floating forehead". Early treatment of craniofacial stenosis]. Ann Chir Plast 1979;24(2):121–6.

22. Marchac D, Renier D. Cranio-facial surgery for cranio-synostosis. Scand J Plast Reconstr Surg 1981; 15(3):235–43.

23. Marchac D, Renier D. Craniofacial surgery for craniosynostosis improves facial growth: a personal case review. Ann Plast Surg 1985;14(1):43–54.

24. Marchac D, Renier D, Jones BM. Experience with the "floating forehead. Br J Plast Surg 1988;41(1): 1–15.

25. Kushner J, Alexander E, Davis CH, et al. Crouzon's disease (craniofacial dysostosis). Modern diagnosis and treatment. J Neurosurg 1972;37(4):434–41.

26. Allam KA, Wan DC, Khwanngern K, et al. Treatment of apert syndrome: a long-term follow-up study. Plast Reconstr Surg 2011;127(4):1601–11.

27. Renier D, Lajeunie E, Arnaud E, et al. Management of craniosynostoses. Childs Nerv Syst 2000;16(10–11):645–58.

28. Arnaud E, Paternoster G, James S, et al. [Craniofacial strategy for syndromic craniosynostosis]. Ann Chir Plast Esthet 2016;61(5):408–19.

29. Kahnberg K-E, Hagberg C. Orthognathic surgery in patients with craniofacial syndrome. I. A 5-year overview of combined orthodontic and surgical correction. J Plast Surg Hand Surg 2010;44(6):282–8.

30. Stavropoulos D, Tarnow P, Mohlin B, et al. Comparing patients with Apert and Crouzon syndromes–clinical features and cranio-maxillofacial surgical reconstruction. Swed Dent J 2012;36(1): 25–34.

31. Sancar B, Tanisik BH. Treatment of the patient with Crouzon syndrome with Orthognathic surgery. J Craniofac Surg 2020;31(3):806–8.

32. Inverso G, Brustowicz KA, Katz E, et al. The prevalence of obstructive sleep apnea in symptomatic patients with syndromic craniosynostosis. Int J Oral Maxillofac Surg 2016;45(2):167–9.

33. Couloigner V, Ayari Khalfallah S. Craniosynostosis and ENT. Neurochirurgie 2019;65(5):318–21.

34. Lo LJ, Chen YR. Airway obstruction in severe syndromic craniosynostosis. Ann Plast Surg 1999; 43(3):258–64.

35. Alli A, Gupta S, Elloy MD, et al. Laryngotracheal anomalies in children with syndromic craniosynostosis undergoing tracheostomy. J Craniofac Surg 2013;24(4):1423–7.

36. Mathews F, Shaffer AD, Georg MW, et al. Airway anomalies in patients with craniosynostosis. Laryngoscope 2019;129(11):2594–602.

37. Maunsell R, Avelino M, Caixeta Alves J, et al. Revealing the needs of children with tracheostomies. Eur Ann Otorhinolaryngol Head Neck Dis 2018;135(5S):S93–7.

38. Cohen SR, Suzman K, Simms C, et al. Sleep apnea surgery versus tracheostomy in children: an exploratory study of the comparative effects on quality of life. Plast Reconstr Surg 1998;102(6):1855–64.

39. Arnaud E, Paternoster G, Khonsari H, et al. SYM9.9E Necker experience of frontofacial monobloc advancement with distraction (FFMBA): 145 cases in faciocraniosynostotic children. Plast Reconstr Surg – Glob Open 2019;7(8S-2):8–9.

40. Cruz AAV, Akaishi PMS, Arnaud E, et al. Exorbitism correction of faciocraniosynostoses by monobloc frontofacial advancement with distraction osteogenesis. J Craniofac Surg 2007;18(2):355–60.

41. Cruz AAV, Akaishi PMS, Arnaud E, et al. Palpebral fissure changes after monobloc frontofacial advancement in faciocraniosynostosis. J Craniofac Surg 2008;19(1):106–9.

42. Wolfe SA, Morrison G, Page LK, et al. The monobloc frontofacial advancement: do the pluses outweigh the minuses? Plast Reconstr Surg 1993;91(6):977–87 [discussion: 988–9].

43. Cohen SR, Boydston W, Hudgins R, et al. Monobloc and facial bipartition distraction with internal devices. J Craniofac Surg 1999;10(3):244–51.

44. Figueroa AA, Polley JW, Figueroa AD. Biomechanical considerations for distraction of the monobloc, Le Fort III, and Le Fort I segments. Plast Reconstr Surg 2010;126(3):1005–13.

45. Polley JW, Figueroa AA, Charbel FT, et al. Monobloc craniomaxillofacial distraction osteogenesis in a newborn with severe craniofacial synostosis: a preliminary report. J Craniofac Surg 1995;6(5):421–3.

46. Fearon JA, Whitaker LA. Complications with facial advancement: a comparison between the Le Fort III and monobloc advancements. Plast Reconstr Surg 1993;91(6):990–5.

47. S3-12 SESSION 3: FACIOCRANIOSYNOSTOSIS – part I COMPLICATION...: plastic and reconstructive surgery – Global open [Internet]. Available at: https://journals.lww.com/prsgo/Fulltext/2019/08002/S3_12_SESSION_3__FACIOCRANIOSYNOSTOSIS__PART_I.62.aspx. Accessed July 26, 2020.

48. Arnaud E, Marchac D, Renier D. Complications of maxillary distraction in children and modification by internal device with transfacial pin. In: Proceedings of the 2nd International Congress on cranial and facial bone distraction processes PA Diner, M-P Vazquez, Ed. France, June 17-19, 1999. p. 211–215.

49. Alonso N, Goldenberg D, Fonseca AS, et al. Blindness as a complication of monobloc frontofacial advancement with distraction. J Craniofac Surg 2008;19(4):1170–3.

50. Bradley JP, Gabbay JS, Taub PJ, et al. Monobloc advancement by distraction osteogenesis decreases morbidity and relapse. Plast Reconstr Surg 2006;118(7):1585–97.

51. Choi M, Flores RL, Havlik RJ. Volumetric analysis of anterior versus posterior cranial vault expansion in patients with syndromic craniosynostosis. J Craniofac Surg 2012;23(2):455–8.

52. Derderian CA, Wink JD, McGrath JL, et al. Volumetric changes in cranial vault expansion: comparison of fronto-orbital advancement and posterior cranial vault distraction osteogenesis. Plast Reconstr Surg 2015;135(6):1665–72.

53. Nowinski D, Di Rocco F, Renier D, et al. Posterior cranial vault expansion in the treatment of craniosynostosis. Comparison of current techniques. Childs Nerv Syst 2012;28(9):1537–44.

54. Swanson JW, Samra F, Bauder A, et al. An Algorithm for managing syndromic craniosynostosis using posterior vault distraction osteogenesis. Plast Reconstr Surg 2016;137(5):829e–41e.

55. Cinalli G, Chumas P, Arnaud E, et al. Occipital remodeling and suboccipital decompression in severe craniosynostosis associated with tonsillar herniation. Neurosurgery 1998;42(1):66–71 [discussion: 71–3].

56. Khonsari RH, Haber S, Paternoster G, et al. S3-17 SESSION 3: faciocraniosynostosis – part i frontofacial monobloc advancement with distraction reduces severe obstructive sleep apnea in faciocraniosynostoses: prospective assessment of 109 cases. Plast Reconstr Surg – Glob Open 2019;7(8S-2):40.

57. Khonsari RH, Haber S, Paternoster G, et al. The influence of fronto-facial monobloc advancement on obstructive sleep apnea: an assessment of 109 syndromic craniosynostoses cases. J Cranio-Maxillofacial Surg 2020;48(6):536–47.

58. Arnaud E, Antunez S, Khonsari H, et al. SYM9.9F transfacial external traction and internal distraction for young and severe faciocraniosynostoses: the very early monobloc. Plast Reconstr Surg – Glob Open 2019;7(8S-2):9.

59. Ortiz-Monasterio F, del Campo AF, Carrillo A. Advancement of the orbits and the midface in one piece, combined with frontal repositioning, for the correction of Crouzon's deformities. Plast Reconstr Surg 1978;61(4):507–16.

60. Britto JA, Greig A, Abela C, et al. Frontofacial surgery in children and Adolescents: techniques, indications, outcomes. Semin Plast Surg 2014;28(3):121–9.

61. Morice A, Paternoster G, Ostertag A, et al. Anterior skull base and pericranial flap ossification after frontofacial monobloc advancement. Plast Reconstr Surg 2018;141(2):437–45.

62. Khonsari RH, Hennocq Q, Nysjö J, et al. Defining critical ages for orbital shape changes after frontofacial advancement in Crouzon syndrome. Plast Reconstr Surg 2019;144(5):841e–52e.

63. Haber SE, Khonsari RH, Leikola J, et al. S3-18 SESSION 3: FACIOCRANIOSYNOSTOSIS – PART I Secondary facial advancement in syndromic craniosynostoses: a prospective assessment of 109 cases. Plast Reconstr Surg Glob Open 2019;7(8S-2):40–1.

Monobloc Distraction and Facial Bipartition Distraction with External Devices

David J. Dunaway, MBChB, FDSRCS, FRCS(plast)[a],*,
Curtis Budden, MD, MEd, FRCSC[b], Juling Ong, FRCS(plast)[a],
Greg James, PhD, FRCS (Eng), FRCS (NeuroSurg)[a],
Noor ul Owase Jeelani, MBA, MPhil (Medical Law), FRCS (NeuroSurg)[a]

KEYWORDS

- External distraction • Frontofacial advancement • Monobloc osteotomy • Facial bipartition

KEY POINTS

- Monobloc and bipartition advancement by external distraction plays a major role in the treatment of syndromic craniosynostosis. Bipartition distraction was developed to address the midfacial deformities of Apert syndrome.
- These techniques can reverse the deformity associated with syndromic craniosynostosis and mitigate complications associated with ocular exposure, intracranial hypertension, and upper airway obstruction.
- The procedure is associated with relatively high complication rates principally related to ascending infection and persistent cerebrospinal fluid (CSF) leaks. Distraction protocols should be used to mitigate risks of CSF leak, infection, and relapse.
- Distraction allows greater stable advancements than conventional osteotomies.
- External distractors allow fine tuning of distraction vectors and improve outcome but are less well tolerated that internal distractors.

INTRODUCTION

The monobloc osteotomy effectively cleaves the entire midfacial skeleton from the skull base and mobilizes the forehead, allowing these segments of bone to be advanced in relation to the rest of the skull. It is particularly useful in treating many types of syndromic craniosynostosis. The monobloc enlarges orbital and intracranial volume, increases the size of the nasopharynx, and corrects deformity thus producing functional and aesthetic benefits. Facial bipartition is a modification of the monobloc osteotomy that cleaves the face into 2 segments through a midline osteotomy. Its main indication is to treat hypertelorism, but the bipartition also enables a differentially greater advancement of the midface, which has greatly improved the treatment of Apert syndrome.

Monobloc advancement remains a major operation with a relatively high complication rate. A monobloc osteotomy includes both a transcranial and a transfacial procedure and thus creates a

[a] Great Ormond Street Hospital for Children, Great Ormond Street, London WC1N 7JH, UK; [b] Department of Surgery, Faculty of Medicine and Dentistry, University of Alberta, 8440 112 Street, Edmonton, AB T6G 2B7, Canada
* Corresponding author.
E-mail address: David.dunaway@gosh.nhs.uk

Clin Plastic Surg 48 (2021) 507–519
https://doi.org/10.1016/j.cps.2021.03.004
0094-1298/21/© 2021 Elsevier Inc. All rights reserved.

potential connection between the nasopharynx and intracranial cavity. Unless great care is taken to repair this connection, there is significant risk of ascending infection and cerebrospinal fluid (CSF) leak.

The advent of distraction has made frontofacial advancement both safer by reducing the risk of ascending infection and more predictable by allowing in treatment adjustments to the degree and vector of advancement. Both internal and external distractors are used, each with their pros and cons. Internal distractors are more convenient for the patient and allow prolonged fixation in the consolidation period but is difficult to adjust distraction vectors and distractor removal requires a second operation. External distractors are more cumbersome but allow fine tuning the distraction advancement.

HISTORY OF EXTERNAL DISTRACTION AND FRONTOFACIAL ADVANCEMENT

Distraction osteogenesis, the technique of bone lengthening by gradual tensile stress across a bone gap, was first described in the early 1900s.[1] Initially implemented in orthopedic surgery by Illizarov in lower extremity reconstruction, its application has since been broadened to include distraction of the craniofacial skeleton.

External craniofacial distraction was first reported by Synder (1973)[2] in a canine mandibular model. The technique entered general clinical use after McCarthy published his experience with mandibular distraction in 4 children.[3] In these early reports, distraction was performed using external distractors anchored into the bone using 4 screw half-pins. The external fixator remained in place for 8 to 10 weeks postdistraction without reported complications.[3]

Internal devices were soon developed in an attempt to provide greater stability, decreased facial scarring, and less cumbersome hardware leading to greater patient comfort.[4] Initially used in the mandible by Diner in 1996 these devices have been developed for use in the midface and other parts of the craniofacial skeleton.[5] Over the past 3 decades, however, numerous advances have refined skeletal advancement techniques.[6–8] Its utilization in the craniofacial skeleton has increased significantly, with most centers performing some form of craniofacial distraction.[9]

Frontofacial advancement has been enhanced significantly by the implementation of external distraction osteogenesis.[6,10–14] The initial description of monobloc advancement by Ortiz Monasterio in 1978 and the modification to include facial bipartition by van der Meulen resulted in midface correction but with a high complication rate.[7,15,16] These techniques were built on the early techniques of Gillies and Tessier.[15,17] Facial bipartition allows for the correction of the central concavity that is seen in Apert syndrome and represents an early attempt to both advance the midface and correct intrinsic bony deformities.[14,18] Because of the high morbidity and risk, this procedure was initially performed in only limited centers,[19] but with the advent of craniofacial distraction, these transcranial frontofacial advancements have been performed more widely with reduced morbidity.[20]

INDICATIONS

The precise indications for craniofacial distraction remain controversial.[21,22] Frontofacial advancement by distraction may be indicated in syndromic craniosynostosis to correct deformity or treat functional problems including the following:

- Intracranial hypertension by correcting craniocerebral disproportion
- Exorbitism by enlarging the orbits
- Airway, speech, and feeding difficulties by advancing the midface

Frontofacial advancement can be used to treat any of these functional problems, but there are often simpler less extensive alternatives. In view of the magnitude of the procedure, it is commonly used only where there is a combination of functional problems or where an individual problem is so severe that there is no other realistic alternative.

Frontofacial distraction may be performed at any age from early infancy to adulthood, and the indications vary with age with a focus on function in the young and deformity in older patients (**Fig. 1**). Monobloc advancement in infancy is challenging. The fragility and pliability of the infant skull make stable advancements problematic particularly in the central part of the midface. External distraction provides stable fixation with central pull, which differentially advances the midface producing a better correction of deformity and greater enlargement of the airway. Internal distractors by contrast push laterally to move the midface and thus bend the face unfavourably. Monobloc is favored over bipartition in the very young, as the midline osteotomy of the bipartition increases instability. Monobloc advancement in very young children is indicated where there is vision-threatening exorbitism characterized by globe subluxation and exposure keratopathy[23–25] and in cases of severe midface retrusion with airway compromise and raised intracranial pressure.[13]

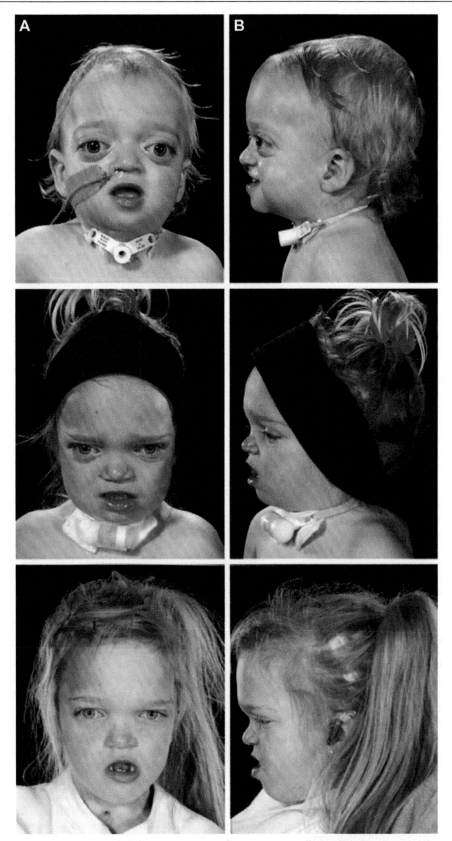

Fig. 1. Monobloc distraction and deformity improves function especially in the very young. (*A*) Preoperative photograph showing midfacial retrusion, ocular exposure. (*B*) Postoperative correction of deformity and

TIMING OF SURGERY

The timing for frontofacial advancement is determined by the functional and aesthetic goals of the procedure. For an infant with recurrent globe subluxation and severe midface hypoplasia, the frontofacial advancement can be performed at a young age (see **Fig. 1**).

Some surgeons feel that young children do not tolerate the consolidation period when wearing an external device. The experience at Great Ormond Street Hospital is that young children adapt and cope very well with the external, halo-type frame. An increasing number of units are performing frontofacial distraction at a younger age.[24,26]

Some centers do limit the use of frontofacial advancement to later childhood and teenage years.[27] The rationale is that there is an increased rate of relapse and requirement for secondary midface advancement when performed in children younger than 9 years.[24,27] Anterior midfacial growth is arrested after advancement, and with ongoing mandibular growth there is a risk for mandibulo-maxillary disproportion. Undertaking surgery toward the end of facial growth reduces this risk and overcorrection of midface advancement is recommended in the growing child. Disadvantages of later surgery include the fact that bone regeneration is more complete at a younger age and that complication rates increase with age. The authors' current philosophy on timing is as follows:

- Surgery for functional reasons when indicated at any age
- To correct severe deformity
- Surgery at 8 to 12 years when upper midfacial growth is almost complete
- Accept that Le Fort I or bimaxillary osteotomy may be needed at 18 years

SURGICAL PLANNING AND CHOICE OF PROCEDURE

Midfacial advancement may be achieved using transcranial procedures (monobloc, bipartition) or subcranial procedures (Le Fort II with zygomatic osteotomies, Le Fort III). Advancement may be obtained either conventionally, using bone grafts, or by distraction. The best form of correction will achieve the maximum functional anesthetic gains with the fewest complications and minimum inconvenience to the patient and family. To achieve these aims, static procedures (midface advancement with or without bone graft) are preferred to distraction and subcranial procedures to transcranial operations.

The limitations of static and subcranial procedures often make them unsuitable for the treatment of severe midfacial retrusion. It is difficult to achieve stable advancements greater than 1 cm with conventional advancement, and harmonious correction of the orbits and forehead often mandates transcranial corrections.

All children undergoing frontofacial advancement, whether subcranial or dura exposing, should undergo a computed tomography (CT) scan preoperatively. The predicted amount of advancement required at the orbital level determines whether advancement is performed in a static fashion using bone graft or using distraction osteogenesis. Any patient requiring more than 10 mm of advancement will undergo advancement via distraction. Distraction is also indicated in the very young where facial bones are too pliable to achieve stable fixation. It is also useful to allow fine tuning of the endpoint of advancement.

OPERATIVE TECHNIQUE

A summary of the authors' approach to frontofacial advancement by distraction is as follows:

Positioning

- Supine
- Head ring and a shoulder roll is placed to ensure mild neck extension to prevent compression of neck veins
- he head of bed facilitates venous drainage

Setup

- Circummandibular wire to secure the armoured endotracheal tube
- Temporary tarsorrhaphies to protect the corneas
- The nares and oral cavity washed with betadine
- Intraoperative cell salvage to reduce blood product donor exposure
- Tranexamic acid is given at the start of each case

correction of functional problems. (*From* Ahmad F, Cobb ARM, Mills C, Jones BM, Hayward RD, Dunaway DJ. Frontofacial monobloc distraction in the very young: a review of 12 consecutive cases. Plast Reconstr Surg. 2012 Mar;129(3):488e-497e; with permission.)

Exposure

- Bicoronal incision and upper buccal sulcus incision
- kin is incised using monopolar cautery and raised in a subgaleal plane
- An anteriorly based pericranial flap is preserved and used later in the anterior cranial fossa floor reconstruction
- The coronal flap is taken down to expose the nasal bones, entire orbit, and zygomatic arch. It is our preference to leave the medial canthi attached to prevent postoperative telecanthus. With the soft tissue protected, a reciprocating saw is used to complete the osteotomy cuts. A detailed technical summary of the techniques is presented elsewhere.[28]

An alternative to the coronal incision has been proposed by Maercks and colleagues.[29] They have described a minimal access technique of monobloc osteotomy. They used an ultrasonic scalpel and endoscope to perform the osteotomies while minimizing soft tissue dissection.

Midface Osteotomies and Disimpaction

- Monobloc osteotomies are undertaken in the following order:
  - Division of zygomatic arch
  - Circumorbital osteotomies
  - Completion of anterior skull base cut across the midline
  - Pterygomaxillary osteotomy
  - Separation of nasal septum from skull base
- Our preference is to perform the pterygomaxillary disjunction from an intraoral approach, which gives better control and reduces the risk of significant hemorrhage.[30]
- The monobloc osteotomy is then mobilized.
- A facial bipartition may now be completed if indicated by removing a midline wedge of bone superiorly and dividing the hard palate and maxillary alveolus in the midline. The bipartition fragments are then mobilized and fixed with a titanium plate placed in the glabella region.

Attachments for the distractor wire are now placed using a combination of drill holes and titanium plates. Our preference is generally to place 3 fixation points above the orbit positioned in the midline and just lateral to the supraorbital notch. Fixation at the lower maxillary level is through drill holes in the inferior lateral part of the piriform aperture (**Fig. 2**). Many clinicians prefer the use of a fixation to the upper dental arch using a splint, which is an effective method, but, in our experience, the pyriform aperture wires are more comfortable for the patient.

Reconstruction of the anterior cranial base with calvarial bone graft and a pericranial flap is an essential step to reduce the risk ascending infection and CSF leak into the nose (**Fig. 3**).

Closure

It is important to support the midfacial soft tissues before closure to prevent descent of the soft tissue envelope. Unfavorable soft tissue movements can be partially mitigated by limiting elevation of the soft tissue at the access stage. Soft tissue support should include suspending midfacial soft tissues to the temporal fascia and lateral canthopexies secured through drill holes in the lateral orbit. The scalp wounds are closed in a layered fashion. Topical antibiotic ointment is applied to the scalp incision. The intraoral incisions are closed, and no further dressings are applied.

Distractor Application

On a side table the RED frame is assembled. The frames can be adjusted to fit the patient, and it accommodates all patient sizes. Four to five cranial fixation pins on each side are used to secure the

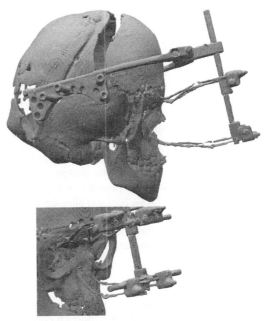

Fig. 2. Application of RED external distraction device. The frame is angled upward from the Frankfurt plane to compensate for the tendency for the midfacial segment to descend during distraction. The midfacial osteotomy segment is attached to the distractor via wires secured to the supraorbital region and pyriform fossae.

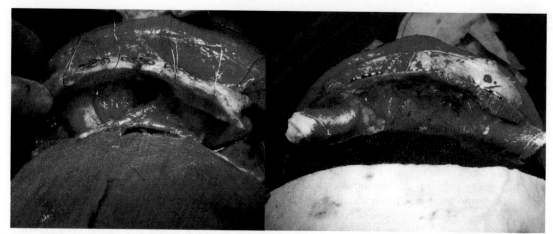

Fig. 3. The monobloc osteotomy creates a communication between the anterior cranial fossa and nasal cavity risking ascending infection. The communication is closed with a pericranial flap or graft and reinforced with bone graft.

frame. The frame is positioned in a slightly elevated plane (approximately 2.5 cm above the Frankfurt plane). There is a tendency for the construct to slip inferiorly, and this must be checked daily postprocedure. In the case of very young children, consideration is made to place a titanium mesh in the temporal region in order to prevent transcranial pin placement. Soft silicone tubing is placed over the wires to minimize soft tissue trauma from the wire at the level of the nares.

TYPES OF DISTRACTORS

There are now an increasing number of external device systems available for use. The appliance used in most publications is the Rigid External Distractor (RED II) frame (KLS Martin Group, Jacksonville, USA). This device was introduced by Figueroa and Polley for use in cleft maxillary advancement.[11] Several commercially available alternatives are now available. The device consists of a U-shaped partial halo to provide fixation to the cranium combined with vertical rod situated in the midline anteriorly, which holds distraction-actuating devices connected to the osteotomy segment by stainless steel wires (see **Fig. 2**).

DISTRACTION PROTOCOL

Distraction osteogenesis can be divided into 3 stages: (1) latency, (2) activation, and (3) consolidation.[31] Distraction protocols vary. Most published protocols include a 5- to 7-day latency period, an activation of 0.5 to 2 mm per day and a consolidation period of 6 to 12 weeks. Our preferred protocol is to distract at 1 mm per day after a 7-day latency. Marchac and Arnaud in Paris

have reported a consolidation period with internal distractors of 6 months. The latency period in transcranial procedures allows for a period of callus formation and healing of the nasal mucosa and any potential dural tear. CSF leak development is thought to be mitigated by the latency period. Commencing distraction at 1 day postop in very young children resulted in a 50% CSF leak rate.[32] Conversion to a 7-day latency in this group of patients reduced the risk of CSF leak.[24]

DISCUSSION
External Versus Internal Distractors

Each craniofacial center has developed an individualized familiarity with the various devices and approaches used for frontofacial advancement. The selection of internal and/or external devices largely depends on local familiarity and opinion. Published advantages and disadvantages of each device are reviewed here.[8,9,33–35]

In 2015, Goldstein and colleagues[36] published the complications of 54 frontofacial distraction cases and included an analysis based on type of distraction system used. They reported that major infections requiring surgical intervention were greater in the semiburied (internal) distraction group when compared with the halo group. Overall, the investigators advocate for external device selection for its "improved vector choice" and "beneficial force conveyance." Internal distractors apply a force to the lateral part of the facial skeleton, which in young patients can cause and adverse bending of the facial bones exacerbating the central midfacial retrusion seen as part of most craniofacial syndromes. External distractors provide central pull to the facial bones and so avoid this potential problem of overadvancement of the zygomatic area.

There are times when a combination of internal and external distractions is thought to offer an enhanced distraction ability. Marchac and Arnaud suggest a combination of internal and external distractions (an RED frame is used as well as internal distractors) for severe midface hypoplasia in select cases. The details of this protocol are described elsewhere in this issue of Clinics in Plastic Surgery. The external frame is removed after 8 weeks, and the internal distractors left in situ for 6 months in an effort to prevent relapse.

Meling and colleagues[33] reviewed clinical outcomes in midface advancement based on the type of distraction apparatus used. Surgical time was approximately 60 minutes shorter in the external distraction group. Other aspects of clinical outcomes including blood loss, length of hospitalization, and consolidation time were similar between groups. Fifty percent of the external distractor group required frame repositioning. The investigators advocate the use of both types of distractors.

The advantages and disadvantages of internal and external distractors are summarized as follows:

- Internal distractors
  - Patient convenience, long consolidation times possible. Low displacement risk
  - More prone to infection. Do not allow distractor vector adjustment. Second operation to remove distractors
- External distractors
  - Adjustable distraction vectors, favorable facial bending in infants. Shorter consolidation times
  - Prone to displacement. Patient inconvenience

Complications

Most investigators report a relatively high complication rate with frontofacial advancement by distraction. Complications may be attributed to the surgery or distraction.

Distraction problems include under- or overadvancement, relapse, loss of appropriate distraction vector, unintended bone fracture, wire breakage, need for repositioning of the external device, need for early frame removal, poor tolerance, intracranial pin migration, pin-site infection, and visible scarring. There are several reports of intracranial pin migration and one instance of temporal bone fracture with dural injury associated with RED frame use.[37–39] In these cases a full recovery was made without permanent neurologic sequelae. The investigators have suggested technical advice to avoid serious pin-related complications,[36,40] which includes (1) using 4 pins to better distribute the forces, (2) avoid the cranial fixation at the site of prior temporal bone osteotomies, (3) parent education of pin depth, (4) limit activity of patient with the external distractor, and (5) use a titanium mesh or subgaleal washer to prevent transcranial pin migration.[36,41]

Surgery-related risks include infection, bleeding, hematoma, seroma, abscess, CSF leak, meningitis, brain injury, blood loss, and tooth and/or tooth bud injury during pterygomaxillary disjunction. In addition, corneal abrasion, chemosis, need for tracheostomy, and rare complications including internal carotid area dissection and skull base fracture leading to blindness have been reported.[30,42] A major inherent weakness of the monobloc osteotomy is the creation of a potential communication between the anterior cranial fossa and the nasal cavity via the anterior skull base osteotomies. Failure to repair this communication leads to a significant risk of prolonged CSF leak or ascending infection. If these problems persist, there is a risk of frontal bone flap infection. The advent of distraction osteogenesis has reduced these risks by preventing postoperative anterior cranial fossa dead space seen in conventional osteotomies and promoting soft tissue healing in the latent phase of distraction.

Several deaths have been reported related to monobloc frontofacial distraction.[19,26] A recent publication from Los Angeles compared complication rates in subcranial and intracranial midface advancement surgery.[43] Although the intracranial group experienced more dural tears, the rates of CSF leak were not significantly different. The initial descriptions of craniofacial surgery in the late 1970s showed death rates ranging from 0.64% to 4.3%.[19,44,45] Today, deaths are rare but are still reported.

Clinical Outcomes Using External Distraction

Frontofacial advancement is undertaken both to correct deformity and treat functional problems, principally upper airway obstruction, ocular exposure, and intracranial hypertension. In the authors' own review of 142 cases of frontofacial distraction, 65% of cases had functional indications for surgery. Ninety-seven percent of affected patients achieved ocular protection. In a separate review of patients in this cohort Saxby and colleagues observed 71% of patients achieved an improvement in apnoea/hypopnea index. Multivariate analysis of functional outcome showed that younger patients achieved the greatest functional gains but that the type of procedure, underlying condition, gender, and complications were not associated with changes in functional score.

Distraction allows for a greater advancement than conventional advancement with bone grafting.[11] It does so by distracting the soft tissue along with the bony segment. The soft tissue is often the limiting factor when a static advancement is performed. One concern about distraction is the potential for relapse following such a long advancement. Marchac and Arnaud report that in their experience using internal distraction they observed that the forehead maintains its position over time whereas the midface relapses.[21] This observation of relapse is more likely a function of an arrest of subsequent anterior midface growth rather than posterior displacement of the midface in relation to the skull base. A long-term study by Gwanmesia and colleagues[13] in 20 patients with a mean follow-up of 10.2 years showed that advancements with external distraction were stable based on cephalometric measurements. Most of the functional gains achieved from the midface advancement were present long term; however, there was a functional decrease over time in patients of young age. Bradley and colleagues[20] compared relapse rates for static and distraction osteogenesis monobloc advancement and observed lower relapse rates in the distraction group.

Raposo-Amaral and colleagues reported that once the midface is advanced there is no further facial growth in the sagittal plane.[13,27] Rates of reoperation are not well documented in the literature.[46] In general, long-term stability is achieved when growth is almost complete making relapse at the orbital level unlikely if surgery is undertaken in late childhood, whereas apparent relapse in the lower face is common after surgery in adolescence because of continued mandibular growth. It is often better to accept that a bimaxillary osteotomy will be necessary at skeletal maturity rather than severely overcorrect a monobloc advancement to compensate for anticipated mandibular growth.

BIPARTITION WITH EXTERNAL DISTRACTION

For most patients with syndromic craniosynostosis, monobloc advancement is an excellent procedure for advancing the midface. It treats midfacial retrusion at all levels and is a rigid osteotomy segment that can be stably advanced even in infants.

Patients with Apert syndrome frequently achieve suboptimal corrections with monobloc osteotomy because of the intrinsic deformities of the face. These intrinsic deformities include hypertelorism, a negative canthal axis, and central midfacial hypoplasia, resulting in a biconcave face. In addition, midfacial height is abnormal, and the negative canthal axis is a reflection of the fact that the medial canthal attachment is elevated toward the skull base rather than the scent of the lateral canthi. The facial bipartition can correct all of these deformities to some degree (**Fig. 4**) and is

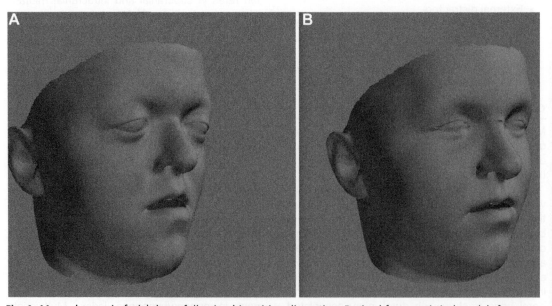

Fig. 4. Mean changes in facial shape following bipartition distraction. Derived from statistical models from preoperative and postoperative CT scans. (*A*) Preop. (*B*) Postop. Bipartition distraction corrects hypertelorism, negative canthal axis, biconcave facial form, and midfacial height disproportion.

therefore our procedure of choice when undertaking midfacial advancement in Apert syndrome (**Figs. 5 and 6**). A subcranial alternative to the bipartition is a Le Fort II osteotomy with zygomatic repositioning, and this procedure is separately described in this issue of Clinics in Plastic Surgery. Because external distraction "pulls" the face and the distraction points are centrally located, the process of distraction enhances the midfacial unbending effect of the facial bipartition.

THERAPEUTIC ADVANCES

Researchers continue to search for novel interventions that enhance the healing process during distraction osteogenesis. Recent trials using bone morphogenic protein, low-intensity pulsed ultrasound, plasma derivatives, and transcutaneous carbon dioxide have produced mixed results.[47–50] The stability of the bony construct relies on the process of osteogenesis and bone consolidation. Products that can enhance the development of rigid, new bone may improve the overall stability of the skeleton and help prevent bony relapse.

The use of virtual planning has also been applied to distraction of the craniofacial skeleton.[46,51,52] Cutting guides, splints, and/or implants can be 3-dimensionally printed preoperatively to increase precision intraoperatively.[51] These guides are made from high-quality plastic or titanium and are sterilized before use. This virtual computerized preparation can improve the speed and precision at which the procedure is performed. Although the advantages of this technology have been investigated in less complex craniofacial bony reconstructions, the benefits to midface advancement with or without distraction has yet to be realized.

CONCLUSION

Monobloc and bipartition advancement by external distraction play a major role in the treatment of syndromic craniosynostosis. They can reverse the deformity and play a role in the management of ocular exposure, intracranial hypertension, and upper airway obstruction. Both procedures are associated with relatively high complication rates principally related to ascending infection and persistent CSF leaks. Modern

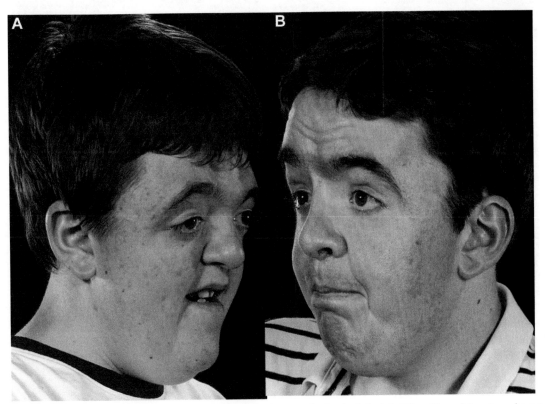

Fig. 5. Bipartition distraction advances the midface and treats the intrinsic facial deformities of Apert syndrome including hypertelorism central midfacial retrusion midfacial height disproportion. (*A*) Preop. (*B*) Postop.

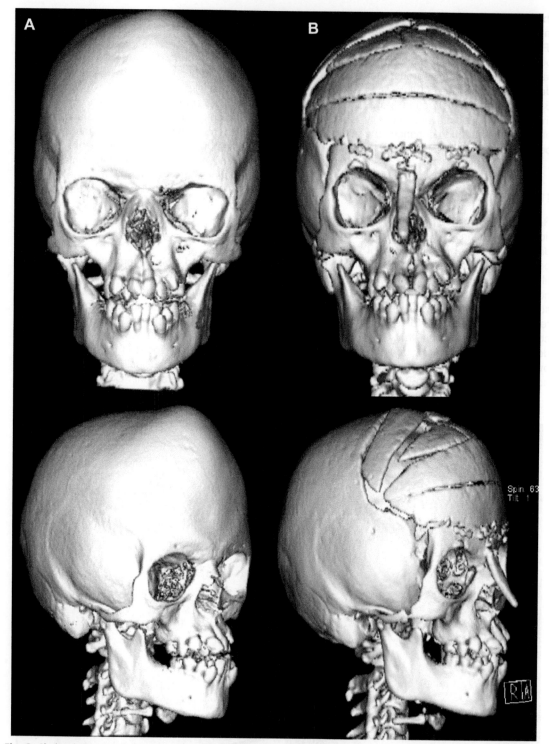

Fig. 6. Skeletal changes following bipartition distraction. (*A*) Preop. (*B*) Postop. Note the correction of hypertelorism and differential advancement of the central part of the midface. Segmentation of the frontal bone flap and a cantilevered nasal bone graft provide additional correction of the nasal deformity.

perioperative management has resulted in a significant decline in complications.

External distractors allow fine tuning of distraction vectors and improve outcome but are less well tolerated than internal distractors.

CLINICS CARE POINTS

- Distraction is indicated for monobloc and bipartition in syndromic craniosynostosis where advancements of greater than 1 cm are required. External distraction allows fine tuning of distraction vectors and outcome.

- Bipartition distraction is principally indicated in the management of Apert syndrome to treat hypertelorism and the biconcave facial deformity associated with the condition. Bipartition may not be suitable for the very young where the craniofacial skeleton is insufficiently rigid to secure the osteotomy.

- Prevention of infection and CSF leaks are key to the success of frontofacial distraction. Infection protection measures including individualized perioperative antibiotic regimes and antiseptic preparation of the nasal and oral mucosa are mandatory. Careful repair of the anterior cranial fossa with bone graft and pericranial graft, along with gradual distraction after a 1-week latency period, also reduces infections and CSF leakage.

- Intraoperative cell salvage and the use of tranexamic acid reduce blood transfusion volumes and donor exposure

- Great care must be taken to resuspend the soft tissues on wound closure to prevent soft tissue descent in the lateral orbital and midfacial region during distraction.

DISCLOSURE

The authors have nothing to disclose.

REFERENCES

1. Codivilla A. On the means of lengthening, in the lower limbs, the muscles and tissues which are shortened through deformity. 1904. Clin Orthop Relat Res 1994;(301):4–9.
2. Snyder CC, Levine GA, Swanson HM, et al. Mandibular lengthening by gradual distraction. Preliminary report. Plast Reconstr Surg 1973;51(5):506–8.
3. McCarthy JG, Schreiber J, Karp N, et al. Lengthening the human mandible by gradual distraction.

Plast Reconstr Surg 1992;89(1):1–8 [discussion 9-10].
4. Cohen SR, Rutrick RE, Burstein FD. Distraction osteogenesis of the human craniofacial skeleton: initial experience with new distraction system. J Craniofac Surg 1995;6(5):368–74.
5. Gosain AK, Santoro TD, Havlik RJ, et al. Midface distraction following Le Fort III and monobloc osteotomies: problems and solutions. Plast Reconstr Surg 2002;109(6):1797–808.
6. Hopper R, Ettinger R, Purnell C, et al. Thirty years later: what has craniofacial distraction osteogenesis surgery replaced? Plast Reconstr Surg 2020;145(6):1073e–88e.
7. Goel P, Munabi NCO, Nagengast ES, et al. The monobloc distraction with facial bipartition: outcomes of simultaneous multidimensional facial movement compared with monobloc distraction or facial bipartition alone. Ann Plast Surg 2020;84(5S Suppl 4):S288–94.
8. Al-Namnam NMN, Hariri F, Rahman ZA. Distraction osteogenesis in the surgical management of syndromic craniosynostosis: a comprehensive review of published papers. Br J Oral Maxillofac Surg 2018;56(5):353–66.
9. Mathijssen IMJ. Guideline for care of patients with the diagnoses of craniosynostosis: working group on craniosynostosis. J Craniofac Surg 2015;26(6):1735–807.
10. Sant'Anna EF, Cury-Saramago A, Lau GWT, et al. Treatment of midfacial hypoplasia in syndromic and cleft lip and palate patients by means of a rigid external distractor (RED). Dental Press J Orthod 2013;18(4):134–43.
11. Polley JW, Figueroa AA. Rigid external distraction: its application in cleft maxillary deformities. Plast Reconstr Surg 1998;102(5):1360–72 [discussion 1373-1374].
12. Hopper RA. New trends in cranio-orbital and midface distraction for craniofacial dysostosis. [Miscellaneous Article]. Curr Opin Otolaryngol Head Neck Surg 2012;20(4):298–303.
13. Gwanmesia I, Jeelani O, Hayward R, et al. Frontofacial advancement by distraction osteogenesis: a long-term review. Plast Reconstr Surg 2015;135(2):553–60.
14. Glass GE, Ruff CF, Crombag GAJC, et al. The role of bipartition distraction in the treatment of Apert syndrome. Plast Reconstr Surg 2018;141(3):747–50.
15. Ortiz-Monasterio F, del Campo AF, Carrillo A. Advancement of the orbits and the midface in one piece, combined with frontal repositioning, for the correction of Crouzon's deformities. Plast Reconstr Surg 1978;61(4):507–16.
16. van der Meulen JC. Medial faciotomy. Br J Plast Surg 1979;32(4):339–42.
17. Gillies H, Harrison SH. Operative correction by osteotomy of recessed malar maxillary compound in

a case of oxycephaly. Br J Plast Surg 1950;3(2):123–7.

18. Witherow H, Thiessen F, Evans R, et al. Relapse following frontofacial advancement using the rigid external distractor. J Craniofac Surg 2008;19(1):113–20.

19. Poole MD. Complications in craniofacial surgery. Br J Plast Surg 1988;41(6):608–13.

20. Bradley JP, Gabbay JS, Taub PJ, et al. Monobloc advancement by distraction osteogenesis decreases morbidity and relapse. Plast Reconstr Surg 2006;118(7):1585–97.

21. Marchac A, Arnaud E. Cranium and midface distraction osteogenesis: current practices, controversies, and future applications. J Craniofac Surg 2012;23(1):235–8.

22. Tahiri Y, Viezel-Mathieu A, Aldekhayel S, et al. The effectiveness of mandibular distraction in improving airway obstruction in the pediatric population. Plast Reconstr Surg 2014;133(3):352e–9e.

23. Hopper RA. Discussion: frontofacial monobloc distraction in the very young: a review of 12 consecutive cases. Plast Reconstr Surg 2012;129(3):498e–501e.

24. Ahmad F, Cobb ARM, Mills C, et al. Frontofacial monobloc distraction in the very young: a review of 12 consecutive cases. Plast Reconstr Surg 2012;129(3):488e–97e.

25. Arnaud E, Marchac D, Renier D. Reduction of morbidity of the frontofacial monobloc advancement in children by the use of internal distraction. Plast Reconstr Surg 2007;120(4):1009–26.

26. Arnaud E, Di Rocco F. Faciocraniosynostosis: monobloc frontofacial osteotomy replacing the two-stage strategy? Childs Nerv Syst 2012;28(9):1557–64.

27. Raposo-Amaral C, Denadai R, Zanco G, et al. Long-term follow-up on bone stability and complication rate after monobloc advancement in syndromic craniosynostosis. Plast Reconstr Surg 2020;145(4):1025–34.

28. Raposo-Amaral C, Denadai R, Ghizoni E, et al. Treating craniofacial dysostoses with hypertelorism by monobloc facial bipartition distraction: surgical and educational Videos. Plast Reconstr Surg 2019;144(2):433–8.

29. Maercks RA, Taylor JA, Gordon CB. Endoscopic monobloc advancement with ultrasonic osteotomy: a feasibility study. J Craniofac Surg 2010;21(2):479–82.

30. Matsumoto K, Nakanishi H, Seike T, et al. Intracranial hemorrhage resulting from skull base fracture as a complication of Le Fort III osteotomy. J Craniofac Surg 2003;14(4):545–8.

31. Ilizarov GA. The principles of the Ilizarov method. Bull Hosp Jt Dis Orthop Inst 1988;48(1):1–11.

32. Witherow H, Dunaway D, Evans R, et al. Functional outcomes in monobloc advancement by distraction using the rigid external distractor device. Plast Reconstr Surg 2008;121(4):1311–22.

33. Meling TR, Høgevold H-E, Due-Tønnessen BJ, et al. Midface distraction osteogenesis: internal vs. external devices. Int J Oral Maxillofac Surg 2011;40(2):139–45.

34. Kuroda S, Araki Y, Oya S, et al. Maxillary distraction osteogenesis to treat maxillary hypoplasia: comparison of an internal and an external system. Am J Orthod Dentofacial Orthop 2005;127(4):493–8.

35. Rachmiel A, Nseir S, Emodi O, et al. External versus internal distraction devices in treatment of obstructive sleep apnea in craniofacial anomalies. Plast Reconstr Surg Glob Open 2014;2(7):e188.

36. Goldstein JA, Paliga JT, Taylor JA, et al. Complications in 54 frontofacial distraction procedures in patients with syndromic craniosynostosis. J Craniofac Surg 2015;26(1):124–8.

37. Rieger J, Jackson IT, Topf JS, et al. Traumatic cranial injury sustained from a fall on the rigid external distraction device. J Craniofac Surg 2001;12(3):237–41.

38. Le BT, Eyre JM, Wehby MC, et al. Intracranial migration of halo fixation pins: a complication of using an extraoral distraction device. Cleft Palate Craniofac J 2001;38(4):401–4.

39. van der Meulen J, Wolvius E, van der Wal K, et al. Prevention of halo pin complications in post-cranioplasty patients. J Craniomaxillofac Surg 2005;33(3):145–9.

40. Aizenbud D, Rachmiel A, Emodi O. Minimizing pin complications when using the rigid external distraction (RED) system for midface distraction. Oral Surg Oral Med Oral Pathol Oral Radiol Endod 2008;105(2):149–54.

41. Witherow H, Dunaway D, Ponniah A, et al. Monobloc distraction in an infant, using the rigid external distractor: problems and solutions—a case report. J Cranio-Maxillofacial Surg 2008;36(1):15–20.

42. Britto JA, Greig A, Abela C, et al. Frontofacial surgery in children and adolescents: techniques, indications, outcomes. Semin Plast Surg 2014;28(3):121–9.

43. Munabi NCO, Williams M, Nagengast ES, et al. Outcomes of intracranial versus subcranial approaches to the frontofacial skeleton. J Oral Maxillofac Surg 2020;78(9):1609–16.

44. Matthews D. Craniofacial surgery–indications, assessment and complications. Br J Plast Surg 1979;32(2):96–105.

45. Munro IR, Sabatier RE. An analysis of 12 years of craniomaxillofacial surgery in Toronto. Plast Reconstr Surg 1985;76(1):29–35.

46. Adolphs N, Haberl E-J, Liu W, et al. Virtual planning for craniomaxillofacial surgery–7 years of experience. J Craniomaxillofac Surg 2014;42(5):e289–95.

47. Ramly EP, Alfonso AR, Kantar RS, et al. Safety and efficacy of recombinant human bone morphogenetic

protein-2 (rhBMP-2) in craniofacial surgery. Plast Reconstr Surg Glob Open 2019;7(8):e2347.

48. Sant'Anna EF, Leven RM, Virdi AS, et al. Effect of low intensity pulsed ultrasound and BMP-2 on rat bone marrow stromal cell gene expression. J Orthop Res 2005;23(3):646–52.

49. Kusnoto B, Figueroa AA, Polley JW, et al. Radiographic evaluation of bone formation in the pterygoid region after maxillary distraction with a rigid external distraction (RED) device. J Craniofac Surg 2001;12(2):109–17.

50. Kumabe Y, Fukui T, Takahara S, et al. Percutaneous CO_2 treatment accelerates bone Generation during distraction osteogenesis in rabbits. Clin Orthop Relat Res 2020;478(8):1922–35.

51. Steinbacher DM. Three-Dimensional analysis and surgical planning in craniomaxillofacial surgery. J Oral Maxillofac Surg 2015;73(12, Supplement):S40–56.

52. Ponniah AJT, Witherow H, Richards R, et al. Three-dimensional image analysis of facial skeletal changes after monobloc and bipartition distraction. Plast Reconstr Surg 2008;122(1):225–31.

Treating Syndromic Craniosynostosis with Monobloc Facial Bipartition and Internal Distractor Devices
Destigmatizing the Syndromic Face

Cassio Eduardo Raposo-Amaral, MD, PhD[a,b],*, Pedro Henrique Vieira, MD[a],
Rafael Denadai, MD[a], Enrico Ghizoni, MD, PhD[a,b],
Cesar Augusto Raposo-Amaral, MD[a]

KEYWORDS

- Syndromic craniosynostosis • Apert syndrome • Crouzon syndrome • Pfeiffer syndrome
- Craniofacial dysostosis • Monobloc advancement • Facial bipartition

KEY POINTS

- Monobloc Facial Bipartition Distraction Osteogenesis is a highly complex operation requiring a multidisciplinary team having both craniofacial and neurosurgical expertise.
- Syndromic patients operated on at 9 years of age or older present greater bony stability and therefore will most likely have lower relapse rates.
- The myriad of stigmatic facial features characteristic of Apert syndrome can be greatly improved with Monobloc Facial Bipartition Distraction Osteogenesis and internal devices.

INTRODUCTION

Monobloc facial bipartition (MFB) was predominantly used before the distraction osteogenesis (DO) era to simultaneously address midface retrusion accompanied by hypertelorism. MFB is a technique that combines 2 other landmark techniques based on specific principles originated by Tessier.[1–3] Facial bipartition was added to frontofacial monobloc advancement in order to treat certain syndromic clinical features that could not be resolved by monobloc advancement alone.

Because DO was applied to the skull[4] and other areas of the craniofacial skeleton, the increased bony stability and lower complication rates associated with monobloc DO compared with monobloc advancement became increasingly recognized.[5] In the late 1990s, DO was added to MFB to create a novel technique named monobloc and facial bipartition advancement with distraction osteogenesis (MFBDO).[6]

Patients whose syndromic craniosynostosis (SC), such as Apert, Crouzon, and Pfeiffer, with significant hypertelorism, are among those who benefit from medialization of hemi-halves of the face, in combination with midface advancement in a single bloc.[7–9] Moreover, this technique is particularly effective for those syndromic patients simultaneously presenting a combination of midface retrusion and

Funding: None.

Conflict of interest: The authors have no personal, financial, or institutional interest in any of the drugs, materials, or devices described in this article.

[a] Institute of Plastic and Craniofacial Surgery, SOBRAPAR Hospital, Av Adolpho Lutz, 100, Caixa Postal: 6028, Campinas, São Paulo 13084-880, Brazil; [b] Department of Neurology, University of Campinas (UNICAMP), São Paulo, Brazil

* Corresponding author. Institute of Plastic and Craniofacial Surgery, SOBRAPAR Hospital, Av Adolpho Lutz, 100, Caixa Postal: 6028, Campinas, São Paulo 13084-880, Brazil.

E-mail address: cassioraposo@hotmail.com

Clin Plastic Surg 48 (2021) 521–529
https://doi.org/10.1016/j.cps.2021.03.002

hypertelorism, vertical orbital dystopias, downslanting of the palpebral fissure, associated divergent strabismus, or a collapsed maxillary arch with an inverted "V" deformity.[10] Among the syndromes referenced above, patients with Apert syndrome most commonly present features that are characteristic of the syndromic face, and frequently benefit from the palatal expansion generated by hemifacial medialization.[10,11] Although MFBDO is a proven effective technique that corrects the aforementioned clinical features in SC patients, this technique is not currently used by most craniofacial centers worldwide.

The objective of this study is to describe the authors' experience using MFBDO in patients with SC and provide in detail the surgical planning used to achieve medialization of the orbits and destigmatize the syndromic face.

PATIENTS AND METHODS

A retrospective study was performed on consecutive patients with SC who underwent MFBDO between 2007 and 2019 performed by the same craniofacial plastic surgeon and neurosurgeon (C.E.R.-A. and E.G.) working in tandem. Patients who solely underwent monobloc advancement and patients with incomplete medical records were excluded from this study.

Demographic data (patient gender and age when the procedure was performed), diagnosis, surgical-related data, and outcome data (mean midface advancement and mean interorbital distance before and after facial medialization) were verified via medical records, clinical photographs, and frontal and lateral cephalograms. Intraoperative complications related to orbital medialization, an inability to bring the midface forward during the distraction activation period (described as a collapse of the face), and improvement of strabismus, were all recorded.

Indications for MFBDO included SC patients with mild to severe exorbitism and/or midface retrusion, patients with recessive brow position, with or without clinical signs of elevated intracranial pressure, and patients who presented at least one of the following clinical features: hypertelorism, vertical orbital dystopias, marked downslanting of the palpebral fissure whether or not associated with divergent strabismus, or a collapsed maxillary arch with an inverted "V" deformity.

Distraction Protocol

After surgery, there is a 5- to 7-day latency period to facilitate sealing of the anterior cranial base. The latency period is followed by an activation period during which the midface is advanced at a rate of 1 mm per day. After the activation period is concluded, there is an 8-week consolidation period. In this study, the average total distraction advancement during the activation period ranged from 9 to 17 mm, depending on clinical need and patient age.

Distraction End Points

The endpoint for distraction was the orbital level, which left those patients operated on at skeletal immaturity with mild enophthalmos, to be corrected later. Conversely, patients who underwent surgery at skeletal maturity did not need subsequent overcorrection. The technical details of the surgery have been described in other articles by the authors.[10,12]

All subjects enrolled in this study completed a consent form signed either by each adult patient or by the patient's parents for patients younger than 18 years of age, in accordance with the Helsinki Declaration of 1975, as amended in 1983. Local institutional research ethics board approval was obtained for this study.

Surgical Technique

The 5 main specific surgical steps that are necessary in order to successfully perform an MFBDO were recently described in detail and demonstrated in 5 educational videos. The key component of the combined MFBDO technique is separation of the cranial segment, which is then followed by medialization of the face. These 2 important steps consisting of facial bipartition and facial medialization are further discussed later and are specifically referred to as facial bipartition and medialization of the facial segments.

Facial bipartition

Before bipartition, the interdacryon distance is measured with a caliper, and a V-shaped osteotomy is marked and performed via reciprocating saw from the upper medial orbital border toward the nasal bone. An approximate average of between 5.5 and 9.5 mm of bone is maintained as a margin between each medial orbital wall, leaving between 11 and 19 mm of bone separating the medial canthi. The larger the degree of hypertelorism, the wider the angle of the midline "V" needs to be, in order to adequately medialize the hemifacial halves. Thus, it is essential to accurately determine the amount of residual bone that will be left in place, rather than the amount of bone that needs to be resected. If the patient also presents vertical orbital dystopia, this factor should be taken into account during the medialization maneuver in order to compensate for the vertical discrepancy between the orbits.

The hard palate is osteotomized at the midline, followed by an alveolar osteotomy between the frontal incisors, using a smaller osteotome. These midline palatal and alveolar osteotomies usually result in a frontal incisor diastema or in some cases a height discrepancy between the frontal teeth.

The pericranial flap is inserted into the midline region at the anterior cranial base in order to keep the oral and nasal cavities separate from the brain, and the flap is then sutured to the dura mater. Alternatively, a periosteum patch can be sutured to the dura mater at the anterior cranial base.

Medialization of Facial Segments

The facial segments are moved medially and vertically as needed to achieve facial convexity. There is also a small degree of rotation along the vertical axis (yaw) that also restored facial convexity. All bone in the midline, beginning at the frontal bone of the supraorbital rim, across the ethmoid bone, up to and including the nasal bone, needs to be removed in order to enable facial segment medialization. Facial segment stability is ensured by fixation with 2.0-mm titanium plates and screws at the midline region, and by wires at the maxillary region. Nasal bone grafts as needed can also be placed in the midline region. Interdacryon distance is remeasured. Medial canthopexy with wires is performed to enable the redundant midline tissue to shrink and provide better definition to the midline region. The authors' preference is to use Kawamoto midface internal distraction devices (KLS Martin, Jacksonville, FL, USA), which are placed anteriorly in the inferior region of the lateral orbital wall, posteriorly behind the zygomatic root, and above the auditory canal, as these areas of the craniofacial skeleton and cranial base are particularly thick. An external halo device can also be considered.

After placement of 2 drains below the scalp between the periosteum and galea tissue, the distractors are partially activated and then reversed to test for bony stability, and incisions are sutured. The frontal bone flap is carefully trimmed in order to closely correspond with the new orbital bar position, which usually has a V shape. The inferior border of the frontal bone must be trimmed into an inverted V shape to securely attach to the superior orbital bar (**Fig. 1**).

RESULTS

Among the 18 patients who underwent monobloc advancement during the study period, 9 patients underwent MFBDO. The average patient age at MFBDO surgery was 11.6 ± 6.6 years. The average length of hospital stay was 5 days. Mean distraction advancement was 14.3 ± 2.68 mm. The mean preoperative interorbital distance measured intraoperatively was 32.2 ± 1.85 mm, and the mean postoperative interorbital distance was 14.4 ± 2.45 mm.

Hypertelorism, vertical orbital dystopia, and downslanting of the palpebral fissure were corrected in all patients. Divergent strabismus, which was presented by 5 of the 9 patients who underwent MFBDO, was corrected without the need for separate ophthalmologic surgery.

During the medialization maneuver, an unexpected fracture line of the orbital bar occurred with 1 Apert patient, which extended to the medial, superior, and lateral orbits. The upper facial segment, where the fracture line occurred, was affixed laterally with a 2.0-titanium plate and medially to the contralateral side and maintained stability throughout activation process; there was no collapse or disruption of the bony segments. This particular patient did not present divergent strabismus preoperatively but developed convergent strabismus postoperatively (**Figs. 2–5, Table 1**).

DISCUSSION

MFB was first developed by Tessier in order to address clinical characteristics of the Apert face. Medialization of the hemi-halves of the face enables surgeons to remove significant syndromic facial features typical the Apert face, such as hypertelorism, vertically short central face, and facial convexity. One of the guiding principles developed by Tessier related to SC was to make all patients look as normal as possible. This goal could not be achieved without effectively addressing orbital rotation, deviation, altered horizontal and vertical distance among both orbits, and their associated functional issues. Once DO had been introduced as an effective technique to treat midface anomalies, MFBDO was eventually developed.[6]

The addition of a modified internal midface Kawamoto device by the UCLA group enabled the performance of the first series of patients who underwent MFBDO, demonstrating substantial stability during the distraction process.[9] The Kawamoto device is secured to lateral aspects of the facial skeleton. The central portion of the facial bipartition segments is affixed with rigid fixation techniques to avoid midline facial collapse during the distraction process. The Great Ormond Street Hospital (GOSH) described a similar technique using an external halo device and popularized the procedure with sequential studies demonstrating potential advantages of their external device over internal devices.[8,13–15] According to proponents

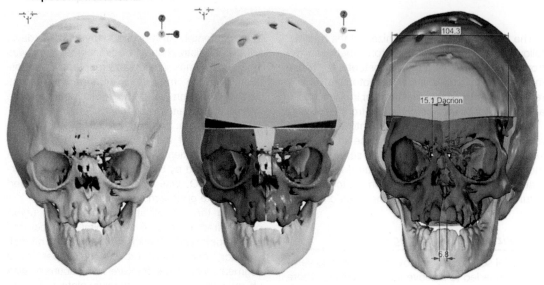

Fig. 1. Virtual planning of MFBDO. (*left*) Preoperative frontal view of the craniofacial skeleton of a 9-year-old Apert patient, showing hypertelorism and vertical orbital dystopia. The right orbit is lower than the left orbit, leading to an imbalance of extraocular muscle and divergent strabismus. (*center*) The frontal bone must be trimmed into an inverted V shape (*red*) in order to fit into the new orbital bar. The midline bone (*yellow*) should also be resected. (*right*) The authors planned to reduce the interorbital distance to 15.1 mm, which would result in a frontal incisor diastema of 6.8 mm.

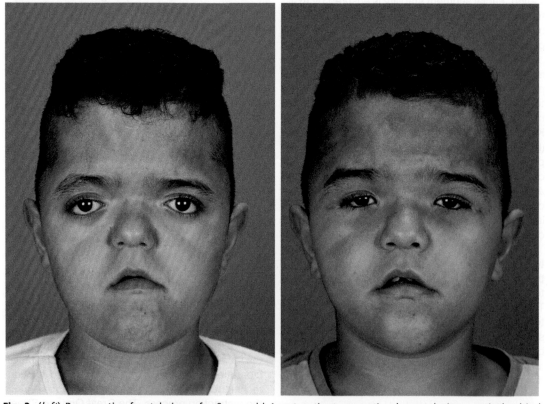

Fig. 2. (*left*) Preoperative frontal view of a 9-year-old Apert patient presenting hypertelorism, vertical orbital dystopia, divergent strabismus, downslanting of the palpebral fissure, and an inverted V-shaped maxillary arch, all clinical features for an optimal candidate to receive MFBDO. (*right*) Postoperative frontal view of the same patient showing correction of hypertelorism, correction of vertical orbital dystopia by elevation of the right orbit, correction of the divergent strabismus, and improvement of visual acuity, a change in position of the lateral canthi that became higher than the medial canthi, and finally expansion of the maxillary arch, which corrected the posterior crossbite at the expense of creating a frontal incisor diastema of 10 mm, which should be addressed postoperatively during orthodontia care.

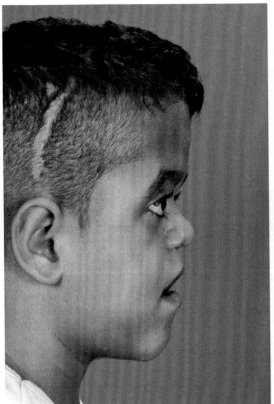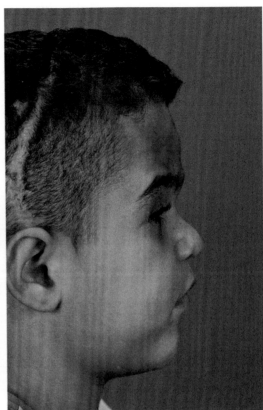

Fig. 3. (*left*) Preoperative lateral view of the same patient and (*right*) postoperative lateral view.

at GOSH, an external device maximizes the "unbending" of the face by pulling the face in different proportions with increased force at the central regions of the face, rather than at the lateral regions.[8] In addition, external halo devices facilitate final adjustments during the distraction process. As stressed by the GOSH group, an internal device, in contrast with the pulling force of an external halo device, pushes the zygomatic bone, which consequently tends to worsen facial collapse and augments facial concavity.[8]

Facial unbending begins with facial medialization. Reduction of the interorbital distance pushes the central part of the face forward, and the face tends to unbend. In order to achieve a stable medialization movement and maintain facial unbending during the distraction activation process, a surgeon needs to be meticulous during the lateral orbital wall osteotomies and work deep inside the inferior orbital fissure and the roof toward the anterior cranial base, in order to provide sufficient bone support for craniofacial disjunction and advancement. If there is sufficient bone support laterally and superiorly, the face can be safely medialized without jeopardizing bone stability. Inadequate bone support both laterally and superiorly could result in an unexpected bone fracture, because the force necessary to approximate the facial halves must be lesser than the force necessary to fracture the orbital buttresses. As described above, this type of unexpected fracture occurred with 1 Apert patient in the authors' study, as the lateral osteotomies provided bone support that was inadequate for successful orbital medialization.

The authors' preferred intraoperative interorbital distance (measured with a caliper during surgery before and after facial bipartition) varies between 11 and 19 mm and includes a titanium box plate that is affixed to the midline region superiorly between the 2 hemi-facial halves. Certainly, a degree of overcorrection is preferable. The authors use wire between the inferior osteotomies in the maxilla, right above the frontal incisor diastema. A semi-rigid fixation in this region enables precise postoperative movements by the orthodontia team during follow-up care, in order to close the midline frontal diastema. Using both upper face rigid fixation and lower face semi-rigid fixation prevents facial collapse during the internal device DO activation process and facilitates postoperative diastema correction. Patient age at surgery might

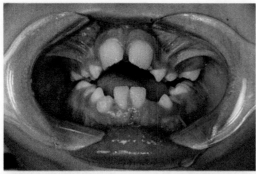

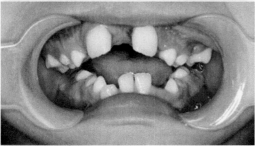

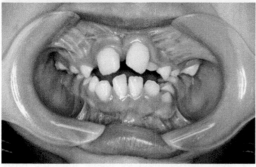

Fig. 4. (*top*) Preoperative frontal view of the same patient, showing the occlusion, and immediate postoperative frontal view showing the diastema of 10 mm (*center*). Orthodontia for this patient following surgery was indicated but could not be performed because of the COVID-19 outbreak. However, frontal incisor diastema decreased from 10 mm to 5 mm, alleviating any need for further intervention at 6-month postoperative follow-up. Interestingly, the posterior palate remained expanded without posterior crossbite relapse (*bottom*).

also be a critical factor in bone stability as performing this study closer to the time of facial maturity will result in less phenotypic relapse.

It is important to distinguish between cases where only monobloc advancement with DO is indicated, and those cases where the addition of facial bipartition is indicated. There are 4 major bony and soft tissue features that are important variables that must be considered before an appropriate surgical plan can be implemented. These variables are described as follows:

1. Whether the patient presents increased horizontal (hypertelorism) and vertical distances (vertical orbital dystopias) between the orbits. Vertical orbital dystopia is clinically characterized by a height discrepancy between both canthi, either medial or lateral. A computed tomographic image can show orbital cone mispositioning.
2. Whether the patient presents downslanting of the palpebral fissure, commonly characterized by rotation of the orbital axis, which brings the lateral canthi into a lower position than the medial canthi.
3. Whether the patient presents divergent strabismus.
4. Whether the patient presents a narrow or inverted V-shape maxilla with posterior crossbite and medially inclined frontal incisors, which are characteristic of an Apert face.

The presentation of a syndromic face may be characterized by one or more of these features. From a surgical standpoint, syndromic patients who present all these features are those who are most likely to have maximum beneficial aesthetic and functional outcomes from an MFBDO.[16] Conversely, a Crouzon patient who presents only one of these features (eg, mild hypertelorism) will not appreciably benefit postoperatively from an MFBDO surgical approach. Therefore, during preoperative planning, craniofacial surgeons must carefully consider the variables involved and determine whether the overall potential benefits of extending the operation to medialize the face via a facial bipartition maneuver outweigh the risks involved.

The bipartition maneuver necessitates additional steps during the surgery. Detailed trimming and adjustments must be made so that the frontal bone flap properly fits into the "new" V-shaped orbital bar. In addition to midline fixation, nasal bone grafting is often necessary to provide height to the midline.[17,18] It is also necessary to perform a medial canthopexy in order to adjust the new medial canthi position and remove any redundant midline soft tissue that might impede medial canthi definition. These 3 important steps often accompany facial medialization.[17]

When treating hypertelorism in patients with rare facial clefts and craniofrontonasal dysplasia, the authors have anecdotally observed that divergent hypertelorism tends to improve with orbital medialization, but convergent strabismus tends to worsen after facial bipartition. Improvement of divergent strabismus also results in improved visual acuity, which has a tremendous impact on a patient's quality of life.

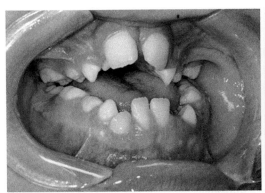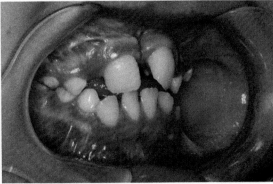

Fig. 5. (*left*) Preoperative oblique view of the occlusion and (*right*) postoperative oblique view.

For Apert patients, downslanting of the palpebral fissure is especially difficult to correct without performing facial bipartition. Lateral canthopexy can certainly improve the position of the lateral canthi but bringing the lateral canthi into a higher position than the medial canthi is nearly impossible by monobloc alone, if the orbital axis is severely rotated. The facial bipartition maneuver significantly contributes to lateral canthi elevation, as lateral canthopexy by itself is not sufficient to lift the lateral canthi to a higher position than the medial canthi.

The complication rate for MFBDO was not significantly higher than the complication rate for monobloc alone; however, as previously described by the authors' group and Children's Hospital of Philadelphia, the MFBDO complication rate was significantly higher than the subcranial Le Fort III complication rate.[19–21] Surgical strategies to prevent and treat complications were discussed at length in a recent article.[12]

Our study is not without limitations. Most of the patients in the authors' recent studies did not undergo surgery until 9 years of age or older, and this is especially true for those patients who also underwent MFBDO. It is likely that patients who undergo MFBDO before 9 years of age may present insufficient bone stability to support large bony medializations and sagittal movements during the activation forces from internal devices, which may result in fractures. Because of the mean age of the patients, and the focus on ensuring maximum bone support for the orbital buttress, facial collapse was not observed in the authors' series.

Table 1
Demographics of syndromic patients who underwent facial bipartition monobloc

Patient	Diagnosis	Age (y)	Advancement (mm)	Pre-IOD (mm)	Post-IOD (mm)	Previous Surgery (Y/N)	Divergent Strabismus (Y/N)
1	Apert	12	13	31	12	Yes	Yes
2	Apert	8	14.5	33	16	Yes	Yes
3	Crouzon	12	17	30	15	No	No
4	Apert	8	12	35	15	Yes	No
5	Apert	9	15	31	15	Yes	Yes
6	Apert	9	17	35	15	Yes	Yes
7	Pfeiffer	29	9	33	11	No	Yes
8	Crouzon	10	17	31	19	No	No
9	Apert	8	14.5	31	12	Yes	No
Mean	—	11.6	14.3	32.2	14.4	—	—

All patients underwent surgery with internal distractor devices.

Abbreviations: advancement (mm), millimeters of advancement with DO; age (y), age at surgery in years; post-IOD, postoperative interorbital distance; pre-IOD, preoperative interorbital distance; previous surgery (y/n), previous surgery yes or no.

Apert patients usually present a wide range of delayed development issues,[22] and the authors believe that patients and their families better tolerate internal devices, as internal devices enable patients to resume school and social activities during the consolidation period, showing satisfactory quality of life.[23] In addition, as seen in the authors' subcranial Le Fort III series, there is always a risk of halo pin migration into the brain, which could result in a fatal outcome. Internal devices can also support a longer consolidation period, although this issue has not been studied by the authors' group. Major complications, and a detailed description of the monobloc advancement procedure, were recently described by the authors' group[12] and are beyond the scope of this article.

Notwithstanding the limitations referenced above, this article provides detailed information and important technical details to prevent complications, accomplishes a successful medialization of the facial segment before advancing the face forward, and may guide craniofacial surgeons in selecting the best candidates for MFBDO.

SUMMARY

MFBDO with the aid of internal distractor devices is a technique that comprehensively addresses significant visible clinical features that characterize a syndromic face.

CLINICS CARE POINTS

Monobloc Facial Bipartition Distraction Osteogenesis:

- Significantly advances the midface forward.
- Reduces elevated intracranial pressure, exorbitism, and obstructive sleep apnea.
- Provides long-lasting maxillary changes and expansion resulting in correction of both hypertelorism and inverted "V" shaped maxilla.
- Reduces malocclusion and related maxillary-mandibular discrepancies.
- Improves positional relationship of medial and lateral canthi via bony medialization and orbital rotation, destigmatizing the Apert syndrome face.
- Can reduce degree of divergent strabismus.
- Despite these advantages, this particular intracranial procedure presents a higher complication rate than other subcranial procedures.

- Intraoperative and postoperative complications associated with this procedure include bone infection and subsequent frontal bone loss, dural tear and cerebrospinal fluid (CSF) leak resulting in meningitis, postoperative seizures possibly due to brain manipulation, as well as intraoperative massive bleeding, epidural hematoma, nerve palsy, orbital overcorrection resulting in long-lasting enophthalmos, undercorrection of the maxillary region, and unforeseen facial fracture following the craniofacial disjunction maneuver. This procedure also presents a risk of fatal outcome.

REFERENCES

1. Tessier P. Experiences in the treatment of orbital hypertelorism. Plast Reconstr Surg 1974;53:1–18.
2. Tessier P. Orbital hypertelorism. I. Successive surgical attempts. Material and methods. Causes and mechanisms. Scand J Plast Reconstr 1972;6:135–55.
3. Tessier P. [The cranio-facio-stenoses (CFS): Crouzon's disease and Apert's disease]. Ann Laringol Otol Rinol Faringol 1979;77:19–30.
4. Raposo do Amaral CM, Di Domizio G, Tiziani V, et al. Gradual bone distraction in craniosynostosis. Preliminary results in seven cases. Scand J Plast Reconstr Hand Surg 1997;31:25–37.
5. Bradley JP, Gabbay JS, Taub PJ, et al. Monobloc advancement by distraction osteogenesis decreases morbidity and relapse. Plast Reconstr Surg 2006;118:1585–97.
6. Cohen SR, Boydston W, Hudgins R, et al. Monobloc and facial bipartition distraction with internal devices. J Craniofac Surg 1999;10:244–51.
7. Raposo-Amaral CE, Raposo-Amaral CA, Garcia Neto JJ, et al. Apert syndrome: quality of life and challenges of a management protocol in Brazil. J Craniofac Surg 2012;23:1104–8.
8. Greig AV, Britto JA, Abela C, et al. Correcting the typical Apert face: combining bipartition with monobloc distraction. Plast Reconstr Surg 2013;131:219e–30e.
9. Bradley JP, Levitt A, Nguyen J, et al. Roman arch, keystone fixation for facial bipartition with monobloc distraction. Plast Reconstr Surg 2008;122:1514–23.
10. Raposo-Amaral CE, Denadai R, Ghizoni E, et al. Treating craniofacial dysostoses with hypertelorism by monobloc facial bipartition distraction: surgical and educational videos. Plast Reconstr Surg 2019; 144:433–8.
11. Raposo-Amaral CE, Denadai R, Oliveira YM, et al. Apert syndrome management: changing treatment algorithm. J Craniofac Surg 2020;31:648–52.
12. Raposo-Amaral CE, Denadai R, Zanco GL, et al. Long-term follow-up on bone stability and

complication rate after monobloc advancement in syndromic craniosynostosis. Plast Reconstr Surg 2020;145:1025–34.

13. Khonsari RH, Way B, Nysjo J, et al. Fronto-facial advancement and bipartition in Crouzon-Pfeiffer and Apert syndromes: impact of fronto-facial surgery upon orbital and airway parameters in FGFR2 syndromes. J Craniomaxillofac Surg 2016;44: 1567–75.

14. Cobb AR, Boavida P, Docherty R, et al. Monobloc and bipartition in craniofacial surgery. J Craniofac Surg 2013;24:242–6.

15. Glass GE, Ruff CF, Crombag G, et al. The role of bipartition distraction in the treatment of Apert syndrome. Plast Reconstr Surg 2018;141:747–50.

16. Raposo-Amaral CE, Denadai R, Ghizoni E, et al. Family of Crouzon syndrome represents the evolution of the frontofacial monobloc advancement technique: from immediate movement to monobloc distraction to monobloc bipartition distraction. J Craniofac Surg 2015;26:1940–3.

17. Raposo-Amaral CE, Denadai R, Ghizoni E, et al. Surgical strategies for soft tissue management in hypertelorbitism. Ann Plast Surg 2017;78:421–7.

18. Raposo-Amaral CE, Raposo-Amaral CM, Raposo-Amaral CA, et al. Age at surgery significantly impacts the amount of orbital relapse following hypertelorbitism correction: a 30-year longitudinal study. Plast Reconstr Surg 2011;127:1620–30.

19. Zhang RS, Lin LO, Hoppe IC, et al. Retrospective review of the complication profile associated with 71 subcranial and transcranial midface distraction procedures at a single institution. Plast Reconstr Surg 2019;143:521–30.

20. Zhang R, Taylor JA. Reply: retrospective review of the complication profile associated with 71 subcranial and transcranial midface distraction procedures at a single institution. Plast Reconstr Surg 2019;144: 1118e–9e.

21. Hopper RA. Discussion: retrospective review of the complication profile associated with 71 subcranial and transcranial midface distraction procedures at a single institution. Plast Reconstr Surg 2019;143: 531–2.

22. Fearon JA, Podner C. Apert syndrome: evaluation of a treatment algorithm. Plast Reconstr Surg 2013; 131:132–42.

23. Raposo-Amaral CE, Neto JG, Denadai R, et al. Patient-reported quality of life in highest-functioning Apert and Crouzon syndromes: a comparative study. Plast Reconstr Surg 2014;133:182e–91e.

Craniofacial Distraction
Orthodontic Considerations

Shayna Avinoam, DDS, MS, Pradip R. Shetye, DDS, BDS, MDS*

KEYWORDS

- Midface distraction • Mandibular distraction • Outcomes • Surgical planning
- Orthodontic considerations

KEY POINTS

- Dental occlusion is a valuable factor in stability of distraction.
- Reliable outcomes can be achieved with good teamwork between the surgeon and orthodontist.
- Orthodontic management is critical to the success of craniofacial distraction.

INTRODUCTION

Since its advent in 1989, distraction osteogenesis of the craniofacial bones has been a valuable intervention for treating patients requiring extension of the mandible, maxilla, zygomas, or cranial vault.[1] A distraction procedure that transports the maxilla and/or mandible changes the dental occlusion, which can affect patient function and long-term stability of the result. An orthodontist should be involved in distraction procedures from the start of the planning through to the follow-up stages, because dental occlusion is an important factor in the stability of the eventual result and acts as the cornerstone in achieving the final jaw position. Orthodontics can play an essential role during activation, consolidation, and follow-up phases of distraction.

MANDIBULAR DISTRACTION
Types of Mandibular Distraction

Tooth borne

Tooth-borne interdental distractors have been used in midface or mandibular procedures, both in the anteroposterior and transverse dimensions. They can be useful in closing large bony defects, both in clefts and after tumor resection.[2] The devices are fitted by cementing stainless steel crowns with an expansion screw between them to the teeth adjacent to the osteotomy site. This technique creates large spaces that are difficult to close orthodontically, and often results in open bites because of poor vertical control and molar extrusion.[3] These devices are useful for increasing alveolar length and volume, but exert forces through the dentition and can cause unwanted dental side effects. It should be noted that their morbidity is significantly less than full jaw distraction[4] (examples of this device can be seen in the Elçin Esenlik and Evellyn M. DeMitchell-Rodriguez's article, "Alveolar Distraction," in this issue).

Bone borne

Bone-borne devices for mandibular distraction exert forces directly through the osteotomized bone and are fixated on either side of the osteotomy site with the activation screw spanning the bony segments. These devices can be external or internal, and each has its own benefits and drawbacks. The choice of external or internal devices must be considered based on size, shape, and the needs of the patient. External distractors allow movement in 3 planes, are versatile, and are ideal for severely hypoplastic mandibles or for those requiring bone graft reconstruction. However, the device is visible, can cause additional scarring, and is prone to traumatic dislodgement. In contrast, internal or semiburied distractors apply forces directly to the bone, reduce scarring, and are more effective for the vertical vector of movement. They can only distract

Hansjörg Wyss Department of Plastic Surgery, NYU Langone Health, New York, NY 10017, USA
* Corresponding author. Hansjörg Wyss Department of Plastic Surgery, NYU Langone Health, 222 East 41st Street, 22nd Floor, New York, NY 10017.
E-mail address: pradip.shetye@nyulangone.org

Clin Plastic Surg 48 (2021) 531–541
https://doi.org/10.1016/j.cps.2021.02.009

unidirectionally. Internal devices are fixated by self-tapping screws or pins on either side of the osteotomy and have an arm with an activation screw that extends percutaneously for accessibility.[3] However, they have limited use in severely hypoplastic mandibles.[5]

Hybrid

Hybrid distraction devices are a subset of internal distractors that are anchored to both the teeth and the bone. They can be used in mandibular symphyseal distraction in the transverse plane as well as alveolar distraction in the anteroposterior dimension.

Timing of Distraction

Neonatal

Mandibular distraction can be used in at its earliest stage in neonates. In infants, a severely compromised airway associated with a micrognathia are the usual indications. Mandibular distraction has been used to avoid a tracheostomy or to decannulate patients diagnosed with Pierre Robin sequence.[6] Neonatal and infant mandibular distraction has been shown to be a safe and effective intervention in properly selected patients. However, the developing tooth buds can be damaged, displaced, or destroyed by use of the devices, negatively affecting occlusion in the future. Therefore, families should be appropriately informed when considering this intervention.

Primary/mixed dentition

Distraction of the mandible can be used in patients in primary and mixed dentition with no increase in side effects or complications compared with infants. Note that these patients will continue their current growth pattern, whether it be asymmetric or restricted, and overcorrection should be considered. Tooth buds are more easily visualized at this stage and proper planning of device placement can minimize trauma to the developing teeth.

Permanent dentition

Mandibular distraction of the adult dentition can be performed in response to airway obstruction at the tongue base, severe retrognathia, or trauma. It is planned much the same way, with consideration taken for amount of growth remaining, if any. It may also be planned in conjunction with orthognathic surgical procedures such a genioplasty or Le Fort I for occlusal cants and yaw correction.

Planning Distraction Vectors

The vector of placement is of the utmost importance to ensure movements are executed as expected. In mandibular distraction, the devices are placed in reference to the stable maxillary occlusal plane. The device placement must be stable to avoid deviation to the unstable side or rotation on activation.[6] The planning of these vectors is complex because they relate not only to the position of the mandible but to the occlusal plane as well. For example, planned vertical distraction of the ramus will result in an oblique vector on activation if the device is placed parallel to the posterior border of the ramus rather than exactly perpendicular to the occlusal plane. In contrast, planned horizontal distraction will result in an oblique vector if the device is placed parallel to the inferior border of the mandible rather than exactly parallel to the occlusal plane. In addition, neuromuscular forces alter these vectors on activation and consolidation, which is a reason why continued orthodontic intervention throughout the distraction process is critical to achieving a favorable result. In addition, care must be taken to place paired devices in identical (parallel) positions to avoid creating an asymmetry.[7]

Horizontal

A horizontal vector results in anteroposterior movement and, when a unilateral device is applied, mandibular midline shift to the contralateral side. There are minimal effects on the ramus height, and this is a favorable vector in patients with Pierre Robin sequence.

Vertical

A vertical vector is more useful for counterclockwise rotation of the mandible, causing an increase in ramus height without a marked midline shift. This approach benefits patients with craniofacial microsomia or Treacher Collins syndrome, who tend to have vertically deficient ramus height (**Figs. 1–4**).

Oblique

An oblique vector can be applied to mandibular distraction to establish a change in both the anteroposterior and vertical planes.[8–10]

Curvilinear

Curvilinear devices use multidirectional distraction to mimic a more anatomic growth pattern. The devices produce three-dimensional (3D), rotational, and translational movement in the vertical and sagittal planes.[11] Patients with Treacher Collins syndrome can benefit from curvilinear distraction of the mandible, as detailed elsewhere in this issue.

Pretreatment Orthodontics

Planning for the preoperative, intraoperative, and postoperative phases is critical from an

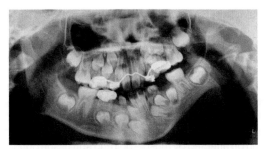

Fig. 1. Preoperative panoramic radiograph before initiation of mandibular distraction. Note the reduced ramus height and amorphic condyle of the left mandible.

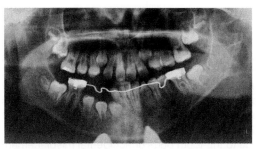

Fig. 3. One-year follow-up panoramic radiograph after mandibular distraction. Note the remodeling of the gonial angle, condyle, and mild relapse over the 1-year period.

orthodontic standpoint to ensure optimal results. Orthodontic evaluation is required preoperatively to assess the skeletal and dental relationships, preparation of the dentition and occlusion, and ideal vector of movement. The assessment is of hard and soft tissues, including position of the lips, corneal exposure, distance from lateral and inferior orbital rims to the globe, occlusal cant, interocclusal relationship, mandibular range of motion, interincisal path of opening, and temporomandibular joint (TMJ) function. Syndromic patients may require ophthalmologic and neurosurgical evaluation before the distraction devices are inserted.[12] All patients must be cleared by a dentist for carious decay and adequate oral hygiene.

Comprehensive records are required for good planning, including two-dimensional/3D photographs, medical-grade computed tomography (CT) or cone-beam CT (CBCT) scan, and dental study models. These records are used to evaluate the craniofacial morphology and idealize placement of the distraction devices. However, soft tissue response and muscle pull are unpredictable by 3D simulation and will have an effect on the final skeletal morphology.[12] CBCT scans can be used for design of cutting and placement guides. If

occlusal splints are necessary, these are fabricated using the preoperative records. Orthodontics plays a key role in both planning and execution of the distraction osteogenesis protocol. Orthodontists aim to modify the dentition in relation to the projected skeletal changes, and decompensate the occlusion to fit the final skeletal position.[7]

Maxillary expansion

Orthodontic appliances are often used in order to align the teeth, coordinate the maxillary and mandibular arches, and decompensate the dentition. The narrow maxillary dentition frequently requires expansion to develop sufficient transverse width, because failure to do so will result in an occlusal interference of the dentition during mandibular translation, otherwise known as a functional shift. It is important that the dental relationships aid in good distraction rather than hinder it.[7] Patients often require predistraction expansion of the maxilla to allow sufficient forward movement of the mandible without interference. This approach allows better stabilization of the occlusion through well-coordinated arch forms.

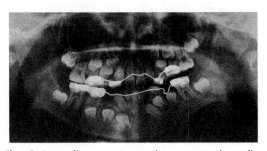

Fig. 2. Immediate postoperative panoramic radiograph following mandibular distraction. Note the increase in ramus height and improvement in mandibular morphologic symmetry.

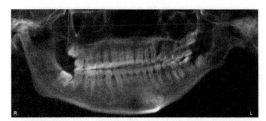

Fig. 4. Five-year follow-up panoramic radiograph after mandibular distraction. Note differential growth in the mandible between the less affected and more affected sides, resulting in the return of the asymmetry. Coronoid hypertrophy can be noted as well on the distracted side from increased action of the temporalis versus the masseter.

Developing tooth buds

Through 3D surgical planning, orthodontists can idealize device placement to mitigate the negative dental effects of distraction. 3D planning allows visualization of the tooth buds, roots of teeth, and inferior alveolar nerve for proper placement and vector of the distraction device. If extractions are indicated, they should be completed at least 6 months before device placement to avoid damage to the tooth buds or accidental misplacement and to allow sufficient time for bone healing to occur. The tooth buds are not spared in early distraction of the mandible if a mandibular body osteotomy is used. In this case it is usually prudent to extract the second molar tooth buds before treatment. The younger the patient, the more difficult it is to visualize these developing teeth and thus dental injury and future deleterious effects are more likely to occur.[13]

Orthodontics During the Active Phase

Serial radiographs and superimposition

During activation, the skeletal changes must be monitored to ensure the advancement is as planned. There is a latency period of 5 to 7 days that occurs immediately postoperatively, followed by the activation of the distractors. The protocol the authors follow involves a lateral cephalogram taken at the seventh day and every week following until the end of the activation period. Usual activation for mandibular distractors is 0.5 mm twice daily until target mandibular length is achieved.[14] The serial cephalograms are superimposed on one another to track direction and magnitude of movement and ensure fulfillment of the presurgical plan.

Elastics

During activation, orthodontic elastics can be useful to guide the occlusion or individual teeth into ideal position with the newly positioned mandible. They are often used through the consolidation phase to reestablish a stable occlusion and act as a counterbalance to neuromuscular forces.

End point of distraction/planning for growth and relapse

Clinical judgment is required along with analysis of the lateral cephalograms to determine the correct time to stop activation. In order to assess the activation success of a unilateral device mandibular distraction, the notable changes are lowering of the lip commissure, chin deviation to contralateral side, and leveling of occlusal plane. Patients with craniofacial microsomia should be overcorrected beyond the midline to a deviation to the contralateral side to account for the differential rate of growth as the patient ages. When accounting for planned overcorrection, it has been shown that up to 25% of distraction length is lost on average at 1-year follow-up. Therefore, at least 25% overcorrection is required as well as extra accounted for by the remaining growth on the unaffected side. Bilateral devices should be activated equally and monitored for the desired forward or counterclockwise movement of the mandible, depending on the vector of choice.[12] As mentioned, the vector of movement can be affected by muscle pull and soft tissue during activation. It is imperative to monitor for unanticipated vector changes and apply orthodontic elastics as needed to improve direction of distraction.[12]

Orthodontics During the Consolidation Phase

Management of transient malocclusion

There may be interferences unaccounted for or unpredicted movement during activation requiring intervention to mold the generate during the consolidation phase. The consolidation period usually spans 8 weeks after activation is deemed complete. During consolidation and postoperatively, the occlusion must be idealized and the patient should be closely followed by the orthodontist. Often there is significant occlusal adjustment required to establish a stable bite after activation is complete. Note that the actual vector observed often differs from the one planned presurgically, and can be affected by the biomechanics of the individual device, the differences in individual mandibular anatomy, neuromuscular effects, and external force.[7] Fixed braces can be used for patients with adult dentition, whereas bonded splints with hooks may be necessary in patients with short clinical crowns or multiple missing teeth. Temporary anchorage devices (TADs) or intermaxillary fixation screws are useful in all patients for the application of bone-borne forces (**Figs. 5** and **6**). The forces are ideally

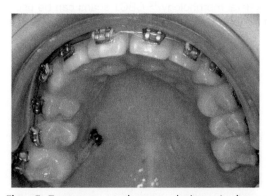

Fig. 5. Temporary anchorage device. A bone-anchored miniscrew that does not osseointegrate and provides transient anchorage for orthodontic movement without dispelling forces through teeth.

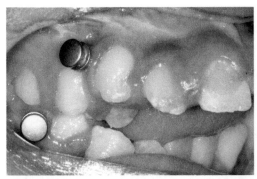

Fig. 6. Intermaxillary fixation screws. More commonly used intraoperatively for stable fixation of postoperative occlusal splints.

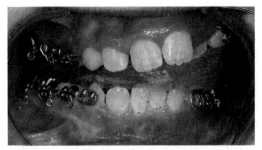

Fig. 7. Bite block for releveling of occlusal plane in mandibular distraction. This block is required secondary to lateral open bite development on the distracted side. Acrylic can be relieved from the occlusal surfaces to facilitate passive eruption of the maxillary teeth.

distributed over the basilar portion of the jaws to avoid extrusion of individual teeth, and TADs achieve this effectively.[12] Interdental orthodontic elastics used in conjunction with any of the appliances mentioned earlier can assist in molding the bony generate during both the activation and consolidation phases.[15–17] Heavy elastic forces should be applied immediately during the consolidation phase because they are deemed ineffective at idealizing the alveolus once the bone has consolidated. It is recommended that the distractors remain while elastic forces are being used during the full consolidation period; if removed too early, there can be bending of the bony generate and buckling from the weakness.[6] Interestingly, orthopedic and orthodontic forces are more efficient and effective during these healing phases, likely because of increased bone metabolism after surgical trauma. This finding results in a window of opportunity during which time orthodontic visits should be frequent in order to accomplish treatment goals.[7]

Bite blocks

In unilateral mandibular distraction, a common appliance is the acrylic bite block conformed to the occlusal surfaces of the mandibular dentition to ensure occlusal stability (**Fig. 7**). This block is fabricated either preoperatively or from the consolidation phase onward and is intended to level the preoperative occlusal plane to its new optimal position, and to prevent any lateral shift of the segment during activation while maintaining the planned transverse relationship.[7] This function is commonly needed in patients with craniofacial (hemifacial) microsomia. Most importantly, the position of distracted mandible must be maintained during the consolidation phase. If there is a resultant lateral open bite postactivation, it is necessary to allow for supraeruption of the maxillary molars to establish a new,

leveled occlusal plane. Closure of the lateral open bite is accomplished either passively by reducing the bite block acrylic under the dentition planned for eruption, or actively by applying orthodontic forces to fixed appliances using vertical elastics.[12] These mechanics can be executed after the consolidation period, and lateral open bite closure can take 6 to 12 months. The splint permits molding of the regenerate and disperses masticatory compressive forces that can cause resorption during the consolidation period.[18] When fabricating the occlusal bite block, a bite registration should be taken in order for the appliance to fit passively, ultimately maintaining a balanced occlusion and ensuring minimal interfering forces on the bony generate. The surface contacting the maxillary dentition can be gradually reduced to facilitate eruption of the opposing teeth until occlusal contact is made with the mandibular teeth.

Jaw-opening exercises

Mandibular range of motion should be assessed at the time of device removal. Any limitation in the opening should be combatted with aggressive physical therapy and jaw-opening exercises. These techniques may help to avoid ankylosis from prolonged lack of motion at the condyle–glenoid fossa junction.

Orthodontics Postdistraction

Patients usually tolerate intraoral distractors for longer, and in these cases the consolidation period can be lengthened, if required. A radiograph confirming appropriate jaw position should be obtained before device removal. The remodeling period occurs postconsolidation, once distractors are removed. During this time, the healed generate undergoes normal physiologic forces and allows the final reshaping of the functional bone.[19] After device removal, the remaining orthodontic treatment goals should be achieved by reassessing the treatment plan and using traditional mechanics.

Passive versus active eruption

During and after consolidation, the use of bite blocks aids in stabilization of occlusion. If primary or mixed dentition is to be stabilized, passive eruption of the teeth into the bite block should be sufficient. Permanent teeth are likely to require active force to erupt and reestablish the occlusal plane.

Monitoring growth

In skeletally immature patients, growth of the mandible should continue postdistraction and should be monitored for growth deficiency or relapse. Retention is best achieved with a functional appliance, either fixed or removable, to maintain the forward position of the mandible, and allows continued remodeling at the glenoid fossa as the patient grows. Twin blocks, Frankl II, or Herbst can be used and followed up by the orthodontist.[20]

MIDFACE DISTRACTION
Types of Midface Distraction

Midface distraction can involve a Le Fort I, II, or III osteotomy, or monobloc distraction including the frontal bone. Each of these surgical procedures is detailed elsewhere in this issue. Similar to mandibular distraction techniques, external and internal devices are also available for midface distraction. Maxillary distractors can be an external halo device, also called a rigid external distraction (RED) device, or paired internal distractors. The external halo is more stable and was designed for large advancements or for patients with a cleft who have significant palatal scarring.[3] It allows better controlled movements compared with the internal devices (**Figs. 8** and **9**). In general, tooth injury can be avoided with preoperative planning, as well as osteotomy and distractor pins placed far from the developing tooth buds.[21] Internal distraction devices are better tolerated, are less visible, and can be more easily kept in place if an extended period of consolidation is required.

Biomechanics

When considering midface distraction, the center of resistance of the Le Fort III segment is the halfway point between the tip of the upper incisor and nasion, or 55% of the distance between the maxillary occlusal plane and nasion.[22] When the planned vector is a directly forward anteroposterior movement, there should be no changes to the occlusal plane. If the force is directed below

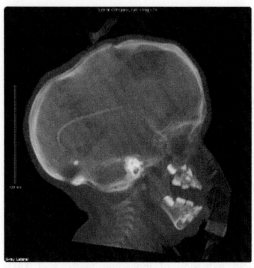

Fig. 8. Preoperative cephalometric radiograph before initiation of midface distraction. Note the retruded position of the maxilla and infraorbital rims.

the center of resistance, there is a resultant counterclockwise rotation of the maxilla causing open bite. In contrast, should the force be applied above the center of resistance, clockwise rotation occurs and causes the advancement of the infraorbital rims and zygomas. The center of resistance is slightly varied between patients and is affected by the individual's soft tissue and muscle pull.

Midface distraction requires precise control during the activation phase. Note that the procedure is not as accurate as traditional surgical advancement and repositioning with rigid fixation. The vertical plane is the most difficult to control, and its

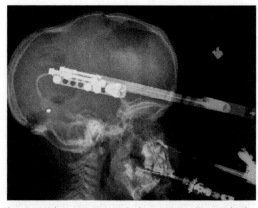

Fig. 9. Midtreatment cephalometric radiograph during activation phase of midface distraction. Note the significant advancement of the maxilla and infraorbital rims relative to the cranial base. This patient was distracted using a dental cemented rigid maxillary splint as well as suspensory wires for added stability.

final position depends on the vector of force relative to the maxillary occlusal plane. The success of the activation is assessed by clinical advancement of the orbitozygomatic contour, correction of exorbitism, as well as the dental occlusal relationship measured in the lateral cephalogram. The expected overcorrection in overjet is usually 5 to 6 mm excess in skeletally immature patients. It is important to halt activation when the infraorbital rim extends just beyond the cornea to prevent enophthalmos, although in very young patients, a greater degree of advancement has been advocated by some surgeons. The soft tissue changes during distraction include muscle lengthening, which affects the resulting function and resistance to relapse. Striated muscles parallel to the plane of distraction stretch with the forward movement, creating new sarcomeres. This procedure is best accomplished by multiple smaller staged activations to minimize muscle damage and allow DNA synthesis of the new muscle cells.[19]

Orthodontic Appliances

The range of orthodontic appliances used in midface distraction osteogenesis procedures is vast and their use should be customized to the needs of the individual patient. These appliances assist in distraction and can include occlusal splints, bite blocks, fixed appliances, bone plates, and TADs.[18] Splints are used in midface distraction procedures to transfer translational forces to the osteotomized zygomas and nasomaxillary complex during activation. There are 2 types of occlusal splints: traditional (nonrigid) and rigid. Nonrigid splints are fabricated by adapting a headgear inner bow to the maxillary dentition and the outer bow is bent into anterosuperiorly angulated hooks. The inner bow is then lined in acrylic to the contours of the maxillary occlusal teeth surfaces. Steel ligature wire ties connect the splint hooks to the vertical rod of the RED device (**Fig. 10**). In contrast, rigid splints have a rigid connection to the RED vertical rod instead of a wire connector. This design allows better control of the occlusal plane and improved stability of the midface during activation. The intraoral component is composed of a wire mesh framework adapted to the maxillary dental arch and lined in acrylic to conform to the dentition. The extraoral component is a horizontal metal extension attached to a vertical rod, which is then attached to the vertical rod of the RED by a screw[12] (**Fig. 11**).

Procedurally, the Le Fort III is osteotomized and mobilized, followed by suturing of the lateral orbital wall with an absorbable suture to set the vertical height of the Le Fort III segment. The occlusal splint is cemented to maxillary dentition and the RED

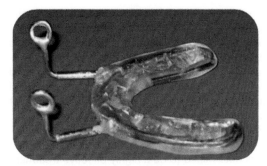

Fig. 10. Nonrigid maxillary distraction splint.

device is pinned to the cranium. The splint is then attached to the vertical bar of the RED device using 0.26-gauge stainless steel ligature wires.

Two-Jaw Distraction

Midface advancement has been considered in conjunction with mandibular distraction in cases where the underdevelopment of the lower jaw coincides with restricted maxillary growth and is combined with clockwise rotation of the upper and lower jaws. In these patients, distraction is either applied to both jaws concurrently in intermaxillary fixation or with heavy orthodontic elastics during activation to maintain the maxilla-mandibular relationship.[13] An article elsewhere in this issue describes counterclockwise craniofacial distraction to decannulate patients with severe airway obstruction caused by Treacher Collins syndrome. This technique involves simultaneous Le Fort II and mandibular osteotomies to rotate both segments forward and counterclockwise with the planned distraction vector.[23]

CLINICAL OUTCOMES
Mandibular Distraction Outcomes

Several studies have examined the longitudinal outcomes of distraction osteogenesis procedures,

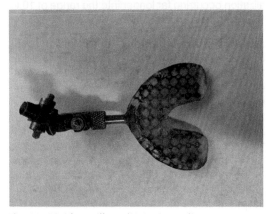

Fig. 11. Rigid maxillary distraction splint.

most of them with positive results. A systematic review of 1185 patients observed the treatment protocols for mandibular distraction for patients with syndromic craniofacial deformities and resultant airway obstruction. The patients included were approximately evenly split between unilateral and bilateral distraction treatment, and the most common diagnoses were craniofacial microsomia, Pierre Robin sequence, Treacher Collins syndrome, and sleep apnea. Mandibular distraction was determined to be a highly effective treatment of these patients by improving facial asymmetry and retrognathia, correcting slanted lip commissure, leveling the mandibular occlusal plane, preventing tracheostomies, and relieving symptoms of obstructive sleep apnea.[24]

Outcomes

In a 5-year to 10-year follow-up on a retrospective sample of 12 patients undergoing mandibular distraction for craniofacial microsomia, the patients' average age was 48 months.[20] The usual activation rate was 1 mm/d,[24] and the mean total activation length was 21.7 mm.[20] In mandibular distraction, the need for bone grafts is eliminated, which reduces the risk of infection and failure to integrate; the native bone is more stable.[25]

Ideal consolidation period

Overall there is a wide range in consolidation periods. When distraction is performed in neonates, the consolidation period can be foreshortened. When significant and complex movements are performed in adults, the consolidation period can be extended. The mean latency period in 1 report is 6.1 days with a subsequent mean consolidation of 60.6 days.[20] On evaluation of distraction protocol in another study, the latency period after device insertion ranged from 3 to 7 days, and the typical consolidation period was 6 to 8 weeks.[24] Although the common recommendation is 6 weeks of consolidation, scintigraphy scans detect mineralization occurring far longer into the range of 10 to 14 weeks before completion.[26]

Stability, relapse, and long-term growth

In patients with craniofacial microsomia, it has been reported that ramal length (condyle to gonion) increased by an average of 13.04 mm postdistraction. This length had decreased by 3.46 mm at the timepoint 1 year later, but subsequently increased by 3.83 mm at 5 years and 3.10 mm at 10 years. This finding averages to a growth rate of 0.77 mm/y compared with 1.3 mm/y on the patient's unaffected side. By this inference, it is evident that the asymmetry regresses over time despite a stable distraction result because of the difference in growth rate on the affected side. It

is therefore pertinent to plan for overcorrection during distraction. If the asymmetry returns, there is still significant reduction in the extent of the deformity, making secondary correction less severe in the future.[20]

Another literature review investigated the stability of mandibular distraction and ventured that relapse could be attributed to true relapse, return to the bone's original morphology, or phenotypic relapse, which is a reappearance of the bony deformity over time caused by defective growth patterns of the affected bone. True relapse was defined as resorption during the consolidation phase caused by masticatory muscle forces.[26]

The original morphology can relapse because of soft tissue resistance to distraction and it is known that these soft tissue changes are variable and unpredictable in presurgical planning.[26] Growth patterns remain disturbed despite distraction; growth on the affected side may proceed but at a slower rate, causing recurrence of the asymmetry and occlusal cant. It was determined that nonsyndromic patients had a more favorable response to distraction, but some forms of this relapse are not preventable in any patient.[26] However, long-term follow-ups showed more successful distraction outcomes if the patients had adequate mandibular bone volume, good vector of distraction, sufficient overcorrection, and comprehensive orthodontic treatment.[27]

Complications

The complications of distraction have been studied, specifically those involving the TMJ and developing tooth buds. In a review of 40 articles, the most common complications were tooth injury (22.5%), scarring (15.6%), nerve injury (11.4%), infection (9.5%), device failure (7.9%), premature consolidation or nonunion (2.4%), and TMJ injury (0.7%).[21] Regarding TMJ complications, a study of 28 patients with TMJ ankylosis showed that 27 patients had a syndrome, namely craniofacial microsomia, Goldenhar, Nager, Pierre Robin, Treacher Collins, Crouzon, or Hecht. Of the 16 patients who experienced iatrogenic ankylosis of the TMJ, 11 had undergone mandibular distraction. It is speculated that distraction can result in flattening of the posterior condylar head and a thinning of the cartilage. In addition, damage to the glenoid fossa and the articular disc can lead to ankylosis. The recurrence rate of ankylosis was 75% and was potentially predicted by younger age at first operation.[28] It is also suggested that ankylosis postdistraction could be caused by the condyles being displaced upward and backward with heavy force, causing resorption of the condyle. This stress could be avoided by unloading condyles during the distraction process, ensuring the appropriate vector, and performing the osteotomy below the sigmoid notch to prevent coronoid process impingement on the zygomatic arch.[29] It has also been noted that active physiotherapy is required postoperatively for all patients in order to manage the deleterious effects that muscle spasm or edema can have on mandibular hypomobility.[19]

Maxillary Distraction Outcomes

Evolution of midface advancement procedures

A long-term study at new York University evaluated the clinical and cephalometric outcomes of 60 patients with a mean age of 6.2 years undergoing Le Fort III advancements from 1973 to 2006. The first phase in the Le Fort III protocol, from 1977 to 1987, involved intraosseous wiring and intermaxillary fixation after traditional osteotomy and repositioning. The second phase, from 1987 to 1996, used rigid plate fixation instead of wiring. The most recent protocol, from 2000 to 2005, used the RED device for distraction osteogenesis of the midface. Although there was no difference in outcome noted from the first 2 phases of traditional Le Fort III advancement, there was a significant difference between the traditional and distraction treatments. The distraction protocol is less invasive and avoids the need for bone grafts, which significantly reduced operating room time, blood loss, and length of stay in hospital. All 3 techniques show minimal to no relapse at 1-year follow-up.[5]

Stability, relapse, and long-term growth

Several studies have reviewed the stability of midface distraction procedures with respect to growth of the maxilla. In one study, Le Fort III distraction was completed in 15 patients with syndromic craniosynostosis. Lateral cephalograms exposed preoperatively, postoperatively, and at 1-year, 5-year, and 10-year follow-ups were superimposed. The average advancement was 14.86 mm at point A and 10.54 mm at orbitale, and this measurement remained unchanged. This finding implies that there was no maxillary growth anteroposteriorly, which is consistent with the known deficiency in sutural or displacement growth of the midface. It was determined that relapse occurred to a phenotypic class III pattern by late mandibular growth rather than true relapse of the distracted midface.[30] In the same sample of patients, proptosis was measured as the distance from the anterior globe to orbitale and the lateral orbit. It was discovered that there was a decrease by 7.41 mm from orbitale and 6.6 mm from lateral orbit immediately postoperative, suggesting

adequate advancement to reduce proptosis. At the 10-year follow-up, this distance had increased by 4.18 mm, which signifies there was no midface growth anteroposteriorly but continued normal forward growth of the globe.[31]

Soft tissue changes

Soft tissue profile changes with RED devices were studied in 20 patients with a mean age 5.7 years. Lateral cephalograms were exposed preoperatively, postconsolidation, and at 1-year follow-up. The ratio of change of soft tissue to hard tissue was 0.73:1 for the nasal dorsum to orbitale, 0.86:1 for the tip of the nose to the anterior nasal spine (ANS), 0.88:1 at point A, 0.88:1 from the upper lip position to the labial surface of the upper incisor, and 0.27:1 vertically from the nasal tip elevation to the ANS. It was concluded that, in terms of horizontal change, there is a linear relationship of hard to soft tissue advancement. However, in the vertical dimension, this relationship is nonlinear.[32]

Airway

Upper respiratory tract obstruction has been shown to improve with advancement of the midface as well, which consequently lessens the symptoms of sleep apnea. Postdistraction, there was evidence of an increased angle between the velum and the cranial base, and the nasopharyngeal and velopharyngeal spaces were expanded. The ratio of advancement to airway expansion is 1:0.5 in the nasopharynx and 1:0.25 in the velopharynx. Therefore, substantial midface advancements would be required in order to significantly improve the airway volume. In addition, there is improvement in the constriction of the lateral airspace behind the velum.[33]

Complications

Traditional Le Fort III osteotomy, advancement, and rigid fixation often results in more soft tissue resistance, longer operative time, increased bleeding, and increased length of stay in hospital, and necessitates bone graft harvesting from a donor site. In contrast, the osteotomy and distraction does not require grafts or rigid fixation, allows for larger advancement, requires less blood transfusion, and results in shorter length of stay in hospital.[34] Therefore, the Le Fort distraction procedure has less overall morbidity and maintains a predictable and stable result.[35]

A retrospective analysis was completed of 30 patients who underwent early Le Fort III advancement with rigid fixation versus 30 patients who underwent early Le Fort III distraction. In the traditional advancement group, 93% of maxillary second molars and 28% of first molars experienced disturbed eruption, compared with 82% of second molars and 20% of first molars in the distraction group. Compared with late surgical advancement, only 26% of second molars and no first molars were affected. This finding is expected given the position of developing tooth buds high in the maxilla in young patients, and families should be educated regarding this potential associated morbidity of Le Fort III osteotomy.[36]

SUMMARY

Orthodontists and surgeons should work together in the planning and execution of craniofacial distraction to ensure a stable occlusion and proper vectors of activation.

CLINICS CARE POINTS

- Overcorrection is key to the planning of distraction
- An adequate consolidation period is necessary to minimize relapse
- The postactivation occlusal stability must be managed orthodontically
- Planned vectors of distraction should be planned jointly with the surgeon and orthodontist
- Close collaboration with a craniofacial orthodontist is critical to achieving optimal results

DISCLOSURE

The authors have no conflicts of interest or disclosures.

REFERENCES

1. McCarthy JG, Schreiber J, Karp N, et al. Lengthening the human mandible by gradual distraction. Plast Reconstr Surg 1992;89(1):1–10 [discussion: 9–10].
2. Bousdras VA, Liyanage C, Mars M, et al. Segmental maxillary distraction with a novel device for closure of a wide alveolar cleft. Ann Maxillofac Surg 2014; 4(1):60–3.
3. Maull DJ. Review of devices for distraction osteogenesis of the craniofacial complex. Semin Orthod 1999;5(1):64–73.
4. Sunitha C, Gunaseelan R, Anusha V, et al. Maxillary movement in cleft patients treated with internal tooth borne distractor. J Maxillofac Oral Surg 2013;12(3): 266–72.
5. Davidson EH, Brown D, Shetye PR, et al. The evolution of mandibular distraction: device selection. Plast Reconstr Surg 2010;126(6):2061–70.
6. Yen S, Gaal A, Smith KS. Orthodontic and surgical principles for distraction osteogenesis in children with pierre-robin sequence. Oral Maxillofac Surg Clin North Am 2020;32(2):283–95.
7. Hanson PR, Melugin MB. Orthodontic management of the patient undergoing mandibular distraction osteogenesis. Semin Orthod 1999;5(1):25–34.
8. Grayson BH, Santiago PE. Treatment planning and biomechanics of distraction osteogenesis from an orthodontic perspective. Semin Orthod 1999;5(1): 9–24.
9. Dec W, Peltomaki T, Warren SM, et al. The importance of vector selection in preoperative planning of unilateral mandibular distraction. Plast Reconstr Surg 2008;121(6):2084–92 [discussion: 2093–4].
10. Vendittelli BL, Dec W, Warren SM, et al. The importance of vector selection in preoperative planning of bilateral mandibular distraction. Plast Reconstr Surg 2008;122(4):1144–53.
11. Aizenbud D, Hazan-Molina H, Thimmappa B, et al. Curvilinear mandibular distraction results and long-term stability effects in a group of 40 patients. Plast Reconstr Surg 2010;125(6):1771–80.
12. McCarthy J, editor. Craniofacial distraction. New York: Springer International Publishing AG; 2017.
13. McCarthy JG, Stelnicki EJ, Grayson BH. Distraction osteogenesis of the mandible: a ten-year experience. Semin Orthod 1999;5(1):3–8.
14. Jensen JN, McCarthy JG, Grayson BH, et al. Bone deposition/generation with LeFort III (midface) distraction. Plast Reconstr Surg 2007;119(1): 298–307.
15. Vendittelli BL. Moldability of the callus after distraction osteogenesis. J Oral Maxillofac Surg 2000; 58(7):828.
16. McCarthy JG, Hopper RA, Hollier LH, et al. Molding of the regenerate in mandibular distraction: clinical experience. Plast Reconstr Surg 2003;112(5): 1239–46.
17. Peltomaki T, Grayson BH, Vendittelli BL, et al. Moulding of the generate to control open bite during mandibular distraction osteogenesis. Eur J Orthod 2002;24(6):639–45.
18. Santiago PE, Grayson BH. Role of the craniofacial orthodontist on the craniofacial and cleft lip and palate team. Semin Orthod 2009;15(4):225–43.
19. Guerrero CA, Rivera H, Mujica EV, et al. Principles of distraction osteogenesis. Current Therapy in Oral and Maxillofacial Surgery. Philadelphia: Elsevier Saunders; 2012. p. 101–11.
20. Shetye PR, Grayson BH, Mackool RJ, et al. Long-term stability and growth following unilateral mandibular distraction in growing children with

craniofacial microsomia. Plast Reconstr Surg 2006; 118(4):985–95.

21. Master DL, Hanson PR, Gosain AK. Complications of mandibular distraction osteogenesis. J Craniofac Surg 2010;21(5):1565–70.

22. Shetye PR, Giannoutsos E, Grayson BH, et al. Le Fort III distraction: Part I. Controlling position and vectors of the midface segment. Plast Reconstr Surg 2009;124(3):871–8.

23. Hopper RA, Kapadia H, Susarla S, et al. Counter-clockwise craniofacial distraction osteogenesis for tracheostomy-dependent children with Treacher Collins Syndrome. Plast Reconstr Surg 2018; 142(2):447–57.

24. Ow AT, Cheung LK. Meta-analysis of mandibular distraction osteogenesis: clinical applications and functional outcomes. Plast Reconstr Surg 2008; 121(3):54e–69e.

25. Hanson PR, Melugin MB. Surgical/orthodontic treatment of mandibular asymmetries. Semin Orthod 2009;15(4):268–78.

26. Peltomaki T. Stability, adaptation and growth following distraction osteogenesis in the craniofacial region. Orthod Craniofac Res 2009;12(3):187–94.

27. Weichman KE, Jacobs J, Patel P, et al. Early distraction for mild to moderate unilateral craniofacial microsomia: long-term follow-up, outcomes, and recommendations. Plast Reconstr Surg 2017; 139(4):941e–53e.

28. Ramly EP, Yu JW, Eisemann BS, et al. Temporomandibular joint ankylosis in pediatric patients with craniofacial differences: causes, recurrence and clinical outcomes. J Craniofac Surg 2020;31(5): 1343–7.

29. Wu CC, Sakahara D, Imai K. Ankylosis of temporomandibular joints after mandibular distraction osteogenesis in patients with Nager syndrome: report of two cases and literature review. J Plast Reconstr Aesthet Surg 2017;70(10):1449–56.

30. Gibson TL, Grayson BH, McCarthy JG, et al. Maxillomandibular and occlusal relationships in preadolescent patients with syndromic craniosynostosis treated by LeFort III distraction osteogenesis: 10-year surgical and phenotypic stability. Am J Orthod Dentofacial Orthop 2019;156(6):779–90.

31. Gibson TL, Grayson BH, McCarthy JG, et al. Proptosis correction in pre-adolescent patients with syndromic craniosynostosis by Le Fort III distraction osteogenesis. J Craniofac Surg 2018;29(6): 1535–41.

32. Shetye PR, Caterson EJ, Grayson BH, et al. Soft-tissue profile changes following early Le Fort III distraction in growing children with syndromic craniosynostosis. Plast Reconstr Surg 2013;132(4): 945–54.

33. Flores RL, Shetye PR, Zeitler D, et al. Airway Changes following Le Fort III distraction osteogenesis for syndromic craniosynostosis: a clinical and cephalometric study. Plast Reconstr Surg 2009; 124(2):590–601.

34. Shetye PR, Davidson EH, Sorkin M, et al. Evaluation of three surgical techniques for advancement of the midface in growing children with syndromic craniosynostosis. Plast Reconstr Surg 2010;126(3): 982–94.

35. Figueroa AA, Polley JW. Management of severe cleft and syndromic midface hypoplasia. Semin Orthod 2009;15(4):244–56.

36. Gonchar MN, Bekisz JM, Grayson BH, et al. Eruption of maxillary posterior permanent molars following early conventional Le Fort III advancement and early Le Fort III distraction procedures compared to late surgical intervention. Plast Reconstr Surg 2019; 143(3):565e–71e.

Moving?

Make sure your subscription moves with you!

To notify us of your new address, find your **Clinics Account Number** (located on your mailing label above your name), and contact customer service at:

Email: journalscustomerservice-usa@elsevier.com

800-654-2452 (subscribers in the U.S. & Canada)
314-447-8871 (subscribers outside of the U.S. & Canada)

Fax number: 314-447-8029

Elsevier Health Sciences Division
Subscription Customer Service
3251 Riverport Lane
Maryland Heights, MO 63043

*To ensure uninterrupted delivery of your subscription, please notify us at least 4 weeks in advance of move.

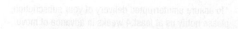

Printed and bound by CPI Group (UK) Ltd, Croydon, CR0 4YY

08/05/2025

01864697-0019